Communication & Ethics
for Bodywork Practitioners

Patricia M. Holland, LMT, MC
Dean of Students
Cortiva Institute—Tucson
Tucson, Arizona

Sandra K. Anderson, BA, LMT, ABT, NCTMB
Tucson, Arizona

 F.A. Davis Company • Philadelphia

F. A. Davis Company
1915 Arch Street
Philadelphia, PA 19103
www.fadavis.com

Printed in the United States of America

Last digit indicates print number: 10 9 8 7 6 5 4 3 2 1

Senior Acquisitions Editor: Christa Fratantoro
Manager of Content Development: George W. Lang
Developmental Editor: David Payne
Manager of Art and Design: Carolyn O'Brien

As new scientific information becomes available through basic and clinical research, recommended treatments and drug therapies undergo changes. The author(s) and publisher have done everything possible to make this book accurate, up to date, and in accord with accepted standards at the time of publication. The author(s), editors, and publisher are not responsible for errors or omissions or for consequences from application of the book, and make no warranty, expressed or implied, in regard to the contents of the book. Any practice described in this book should be applied by the reader in accordance with professional standards of care used in regard to the unique circumstances that may apply in each situation. The reader is advised always to check product information (package inserts) for changes and new information regarding dose and contraindications before administering any drug. Caution is especially urged when using new or infrequently ordered drugs.

Library of Congress Cataloging-in-Publication Data

Communication & ethics for bodywork practitioners / Patricia M. Holland, Sandra K. Anderson.
p. ; cm.
Includes bibliographical references and index.
ISBN 978-0-8036-2404-7 (pbk. : alk. paper)
 1. Massage therapy—Moral and ethical aspects. 2. Interpersonal communication.
3. Medical personnel and patient. I. Holland, Patricia M. II. Anderson, Sandra K. III. Title: Communication and ethics for bodywork practitioners.
 [DNLM: 1. Massage—ethics. 2. Communication. 3. Professional-Patient Relations—ethics. WB 537]
 RM722.C66 2012
 615.8'22—dc23

2011022319

This book is dedicated to Dianne Pecoraro (1952–2009), friend, mentor, and teacher. Her patience, kindness, resilience, and truth are legendary. Dianne may not have even truly known how many people she affected over the years, and what a tremendous joy she was to so many of us.

Preface

Introduction

Although a career in bodywork can be tremendously rewarding, there are also many problems and issues students and professional practitioners may face. These include, for example, the consequences of being unprofessional in dress and manner, misunderstandings surrounding the treatment plan, boundaries being crossed, and issues around payment for services, the navigation of dual role relationships, and how and when to refer clients to other practitioners. The root of most of these problems is usually a lack of effective communication skills.

Most people believe they communicate perfectly well and that if there is a problem it lies with the "other person." This can be true of bodywork students and professionals. However, effective communication skills and professional behavior do not just "happen." They need to be cultivated and nurtured. Continual self-evaluation and willingness to adjust methods and ways of thinking are essential to the cultivation process.

This text is a practical guide to assist bodywork students and professionals in the development of effective, ethical, and professional relationships. The chapters are designed to encourage practitioners to be honest and clear in their communication and to take responsibility for their actions and words. Old, inadequate communication styles can be discarded, and new communication tools can be acquired. Boundaries and ethics are discussed in detail. They are put in contexts that are understandable and relevant to bodywork practitioners, fostering the ability to discern and address ethical situations that may arise in their professional and personal lives. Complex concerns and topics, such as power differences, dual relationships, self-care, and financial aspects of the bodywork profession, are tackled head on. Real-life examples of issues and dilemmas that students and professionals have faced are used to illustrate points. There is an emphasis on creative problem solving. This is done through activities that encourage readers to discover personal biases and beliefs and to challenge them to reframe views that are limiting. Other activities stimulate self-reflection and group discussion of ethical dilemmas, and there is guidance for journaling to track one's own professional growth and emotional connection with clients and the profession.

Bodywork practitioners are not always accorded dignity and respect. Likewise, clients can suffer from less than expert practitioner-client interactions. The more communication skills practitioners have, the more clients and practitioners themselves will benefit. Having a clear sense of oneself as a bodywork professional will be translated through strong, clear boundaries and skillful, appropriate communication. In turn, this will lead to greater client satisfaction, and a more successful bodywork practice.

Communication & Ethics for Bodywork Practitioners is easy to read and offers numerous pedagogical features that support learning and information retention and increase interest in the subject matter. Readers are encouraged to make the information their own through various activities designed to integrate the subject matter into their own experience.

Contents and Organization

This text is divided into two parts. Part I, Chapters 1 to 4, focuses on aspects of communication; Part II, Chapters 6 to 10, focuses on aspects of ethics. The contents are described in greater detail as follows.

Part I: Communication

Chapter 1, "Communication: The Basics," emphasizes the importance of communication in bodywork, including the connection between communication and ethics. The components of communication are explored as well as what defines effective communication. Because being genuine is essential to establishing rapport with clients and, therefore, ensuring career longevity, a section on how to practice authentic communication is included. Communication styles round out the chapter.

Chapter 2, "Professional Presentation of Self," clarifies the messages sent by bodywork practitioners' personal appearance and defines professional dress. Methods to develop personal and professional verbal and nonverbal language are included. The impact of technology on communication is covered, including the use of telephones, e-mail, and Web sites. Just as important, written communication, such as business cards, brochures, business letters, and résumés, is discussed, along with how writing a mission statement can be a guiding framework for professional presentation.

Chapter 3, "Communication Skills for Successful Client Retention," defines the factors necessary for client retention, such as trust, rapport, education, and credibility. The chapter discusses when it is appropriate to use bodywork "lingo" with clients and methods for encouraging authentic feedback from clients. How to give feedback to clients and other practitioners rounds out the chapter.

Chapter 4, "Communication Gaps and Conflict Resolution," assists readers in bridging communication gaps due to, for example, generational, regional, and cultural differences. Also included is a section on managing difficult interactions using conflict resolution strategies and the intervention model.

Part II: Ethics

Chapter 5, "Ethics: The Basics," discusses the connection between professional work ethics and career longevity. Codes of ethics and codes of conduct are defined. How to transform the abstract concepts of ethics to specific behaviors is included, covering the topics of self-accountability and ethical congruency. Being able to recognize and resolve ethical dilemmas is crucial to the bodywork profession, and strategies for doing so are presented.

Chapter 6, "Power Differences," starts with the definition of and methods for recognizing power differences. Strategies for working within the power differences of client-practitioner relationships and workplace settings are included, along with managing difficult client behaviors. The chapter concludes with challenges each of the genders faces in the bodywork profession.

Chapter 7, "Ethical and Legal Parameters of Practice," includes the definition of scope of practice and the role it plays in client retention, as well as how to develop parameters for scope of practice. Confidentiality, especially legal factors related to it, including the Health Insurance Portability and Accountability Act (HIPAA), are covered as well as other legal parameters of practice, including informed consent, disclosure, documentation, licensure, accounting, and taxes.

Chapter 8, "Boundaries, Transference, Countertransference, and Dual Relationships," discusses the importance of boundaries in the bodywork profession. Included is how to develop and maintain personal and professional boundaries, including those involving self-care. Transference and countertransference are defined, and strategies to manage situations in which these occur are outlined. The risks and benefits of dual relationships are examined. Strategies for managing dual relationships among family, friends, coworkers, associates, acquaintances, and strangers are covered.

Chapter 9, "Touch Integrity," explores the different types of touch, and how one's personal history of touch influences present perceptions. Desexualized and safe touch are discussed, including healing mechanisms of bodywork in the context of safe touch. The continuum of sexual manipulation in the bodywork profession, from flirting all the way to sexual acts, is covered, including how to develop appropriate, nonsexualized interactions between practitioners and clients and between practitioners. Ways to educate clients about the purpose of bodywork, including an intervention model to use when a client exhibits inappropriate behavior, are discussed.

Chapter 10, "Support for Ethical Practice," discusses how bodywork practitioners can receive supervision and mentoring from more experienced professionals and how they can become mentors themselves. This chapter also identifies the roles peer support plays for bodyworkers, as well as how to build networks of peer support. Communicating effectively within the networks and using them effectively as resources is included.

Features

Each chapter has a number of pedagogical features designed to help readers generate interest in the material, retain information, and integrate the knowledge into their own experience. What follows is a list of the features and how to use them.

Chapter Learning Objectives

Each chapter opening page contains measurable objectives for readers. These objectives help them identify key goals and what information should be studied thoroughly. Readers can use these as a checklist for recall of important information. Those readers who are students can use the objectives in preparation for exams.

Key Terms

When key terms are initially introduced and defined within the text, they are boldfaced to highlight their importance. Readers can watch for these bolded key terms, knowing that these point to useful pieces of information.

Food for Thought

Food for Thought boxes are found throughout each chapter. These valuable self-reflection areas help readers identify personal emotions, biases, communication patterns, and ethics and to understand how these affect their bodywork careers.

Words of Wisdom

Words of Wisdom boxes contain field interviews with experienced bodyworkers on communication and ethical challenges they faced, how they dealt with them, and what they learned throughout their careers.

Case Profiles

A case profile, drawn from real-life experiences of professional bodywork practitioners, is in each chapter. These case profiles are designed to be situations readers are likely to encounter. Critical thinking skills are enhanced as readers answer the questions posed in the case profiles.

Guidance for Journaling

A section on journaling provides readers with guidance for tracking their individual professional growth and emotional connection with clients and the profession by writing their thoughts and feelings about the topics presented in the chapter.

Chapter Summary

Summaries at the end of each chapter provide an overview of major topics and information discussed. Readers can use these as quick references and for quick searches of the material presented in the chapter.

Activities

These activities are designed specifically for instructors and classes to assist students in developing critical thinking skills regarding communication challenges and ethical dilemmas. All activities are presented in ways that work with Gardner's multiple intelligences as well as for kinesthetic, visual, and auditory learners.

Review Questions

The review questions are in multiple-choice, fill-in-the-blank, and short-answer formats. Readers can use these as a method to retain the information presented in the chapter. Students can use these to prepare for exams.

Reviewers

Linda Delker, BA, MS, LMT, RMTI
Owner & Director
Crystal Mountain School of Therapeutic
  Massage
Albuquerque, New Mexico

Wendy G. Marsh, BA, LMBT
Licensed Massage & Bodywork Therapist
Fayetteville, North Carolina

Judith McDaniel, PhD, JD
Independent Consultant & Trainer
Tucson, Arizona

Lisa Mertz, PhD, LMT
Program Coordinator, Associate Professor
Health, Physical Education & Dance
Queensborough Community College/City
  University of New York
New York, New York

Jean E. Middleswarth, MSW, LMBT, NCTMB
Clinical Coordinator
Therapeutic Massage
Forsyth Technical Community College
Winston-Salem, North Carolina

Dawn M. Schmidt, BS, LMP
Director & Instructor
Education
Cortiva Institute–Brenneke School of Massage
Seattle, Washington

Judy Smith, NCTMB
Department Chair
Massage for Wellness Program
Dover Business College
Clifton, New Jersey

Tamela S. Voorhees, LMT, NCTMB
Program Director
Massage Therapy/Education
High Tech Institute
Las Vegas, Nevada

Acknowledgments

This book represents the contribution of the many clients, colleagues, and students Patricia and Sandra have worked with through the years. They have educated and inspired us with their words, ideas, open minds, open hearts, and kindness. We are grateful for their trust and willingness to share this journey with us. We would specifically like to thank the following:

Christa Fratantoro, for sharing our vision for this book and for her dedication to making this book a reality.

David Payne, for his commitment to an inclusive vision for this book and his ability to guide us toward that vision with his experience and expertise.

The staff of F.A. Davis, who guided our manuscript through the many stages of production.

Cortiva Institute–Tucson, formerly the Desert Institute of the Healing Arts, for providing us with the opportunity to teach and inspire students as they discover their professional and ethical voice.

Kathy Lee, Bonnie Fredenberg, David Anderson, Annie Gordon, Tee Wills, Barbara Grandstaff, Kathleen Smith, Julie Goodwin, Janna Harvey, and Sue Kauffman, for their invaluable "words of wisdom."

Kathy Lee and Joann Rockwell MacMaster, for their invaluable expertise about business operations and business communications.

Ashley Earnest and Dave Nelson, for their willingness to be photographed.

Jason Torres, for his excellent photography skills and great sense of humor.

Laurie Anne Calland, for enduring Patricia's process of creative writing, for walking with her every step of the way even when it meant Laurie lost sleep, for her insightful contributions, and for keeping the home fires burning so that Trio of Tabbies—Fannie, Cal, and Willie—and Patricia feel loved and cared for.

Sandy Anderson, friend, co-author, and Wizard of Calm Reassurance. Patricia is grateful for her patience and her mantra, "This is fixable," at times when Patricia was stuck and unable to reassure herself.

Patricia's family in Illinois and Ohio. It is with them that Patricia first experienced the process of identifying her values, feelings, and style of communication. Although all of them don't always get it right, Patricia is grateful that everyone keeps trying.

With deep gratitude and love, Patricia acknowledges her parents, Rosemary and Jerry Holland, for their profound influence on her life and for reminding her that she could do whatever she wanted as long as she worked hard with integrity and grace.

David Kent Anderson, a wonderful husband and business partner. He has taught Sandy the most about effective and healthy communication. His love, support, unending patience with Sandy's writing process, and meals brought to her while she spent yet another long night at the computer, have made this book possible.

Sue Kauffman, the best sister Sandy could ever want. Her sense of humor, wittiness, priceless common sense, and playfulness help make life wonderful.

Patricia Holland, friend, co-author and playmate. Sandy deeply respects her knowledge and wisdom, without which this book would not have been possible. Patricia's fresh and joyful approach make knowing her fun.

The staff and practitioners of Tucson Touch Therapies and the Arizona Chapter of the American Massage Therapy Association, for their knowledge, expertise, and willingness to give of themselves, share what they know, and help any way they can.

Contents

chapter 2   **Professional Presentation of Self**   **45**

chapter 3   **Communication Skills for Successful Client Retention**   *91*

chapter 4   **Communication Gaps and Conflict Resolution**   *125*

PART II   Ethics

PART I

Communications

Communication
The Basics

LEARNING OBJECTIVES

After studying this chapter, you will be able to:

1. Explain the importance of communication in bodywork.
2. Define *therapeutic relationships* and discuss how to create a therapeutic relationship.
3. Delineate the six components of communication, and define the different types of language.
4. Discuss the reasons communication fails.
5. Explain what good communication is and the roles intention, appropriate communication, and self-disclosure play in good communication.
6. Define *authentic communication* and the role it plays in the bodywork profession.
7. Discuss communication styles based on the senses and communication styles based on behavior.

CHAPTER OUTLINE

KEY TERMS

Auditory: a component of communication that involves hearing

Auditory processors: people who process information most effectively when they hear it spoken. They are very attentive to the tone and rhythm of speech and will often hum, talk to themselves, or listen with their eyes closed or gazing off.

Authentic communication: communication characterized by an honest presentation of oneself and a lack of pretension

Conscious communication: communication in which a person thoughtfully considers how what he or she says will affect the other people involved, both in the short term and the long term

Disclosure: revealing information

Intimacy: something of a personal or private nature; the quality or state of being familiar; acts of a sexual nature; the degree of closeness in a relationship

Kinesthetic processors: people who communicate most effectively when using touch and body language. When speaking, they tend to use "feel" words (such as "that hit me really hard" and "the story was really touching").

Language: a system of communicating ideas, thoughts, and feelings by the use of words, their pronunciations, and the methods of combining them as has been agreed upon by a community; communication using sounds, gestures, or symbols

Nonverbal communication: communication without using words, such as facial expressions or body gestures

Oral language: communication in which the lips and tongue form words

Self-disclosure: the process of deliberately revealing information about oneself that is significant and that would not normally be known by others

Therapeutic relationship: the bond formed between the practitioner and the client that is necessary for a positive treatment outcome for both the practitioner and the client

Verbal communication: communication using words, either written or spoken

Visual processors: people who communicate most effectively when creating pictures in their minds and using many descriptive words as they "paint" word pictures during conversation. They tend to use "see" words (such as, "Let's take a look at this," and "If we view it from this angle") and want to make eye contact when conversing.

One of the hallmarks of a professional bodywork practitioner is the ability to communicate clearly and effectively with clients and other health-care professionals. From arranging appointments and discussing a client's health conditions to explaining fees and establishing appropriate boundaries around relationships and touch, your communication skills can make or break your professional connection with the client. Fortunately, communication is a learned skill and can be improved with education, practice, and the willingness to work at it. Therefore, the purpose of this chapter is to introduce you to some basic concepts that can help you develop effective communication skills. Having these skills can lead to a long and productive bodywork career.

First, we consider how to establish therapeutic relationships using conscious communication. We explore the components of communication, discuss why communication can break down, and look at language in the context of communities. Because good communication depends on clarity of intent, appropriate disclosure, and authentic communication, we also cover these concepts in detail. Communication styles, based on the senses (visual, auditory, and kinesthetic processors) and behavior (analytical, driven, amicable, and peacemaker), are presented. All of these styles are defined and discussed and examples given so that you can determine for yourself what your style is and how you can communicate better with people who have styles different from your own.

Establishing Therapeutic Relationships

Communication plays a critical role in establishing a successful professional relationship with the client. Given the nature of bodywork, there is a unique set of challenges to establishing a successful professional relationship with a client. For example, how many other legitimate professions require the employee to be alone in a private room with a customer who is disrobed to his level of comfort, perhaps only 15 minutes after meeting that customer for the first time, and then to touch him for the next 30, 50, 60, or 90 minutes? Indeed, the bodywork profession requires almost instant intimacy. It is how this intimacy, and the communication around the intimacy, is handled by the practitioner that determines whether a therapeutic relationship is formed. A **therapeutic relationship** is the bond formed between the practitioner and the client that is necessary for a positive treatment outcome for both. Before examining what factors determine a therapeutic relationship, it is helpful to understand what intimacy is.

Intimacy

Intimacy has several different meanings, such as "something of a personal or private nature," "the quality or state of being familiar," and "acts of a sexual nature." Perhaps the best definition of intimacy is the degree of closeness in a relationship.[1] From these definitions, it is easy to see that there can be many different levels of intimacy and that people have different levels of intimacy with different people in their lives. For example, being in a family with members who know each other quite well is one level of intimacy. Having a friendship in which both people confide their deepest secrets and fears is another level of intimacy. A romantic relationship between two people who are in love is yet another level of intimacy.

Intimacy is communicated many different ways. It is expressed through words, written and spoken. Sometimes it involves a look passed between people. Facial expressions and body language also convey the levels of intimacy between people. One of the most common means of showing intimacy is through touch. Depending on cultural backgrounds (some cultures are more touch-oriented than others), close friends will touch each other on the back or the arm or even hold hands. Sometimes men give each other a playful punch. An arm around the shoulders of someone who is upset can be comforting and reassuring. Lovers who are physically intimate enjoy sexual touch. In Western culture, a standard greeting of respect is a handshake.

Food for Thought

Think back to a time when you did not receive clear communication about something. What was it? What resulted from the lack of clear communication? How did you feel about it? What specifically would have made the communication clearer for you?

It is through touch that bodywork has its effect. Even modalities in which practitioners are working exclusively in the client's energy field and not physically touching the client, such as Healing Touch, are energetically touching the client. It is important to keep in mind that, in bodywork, touch is much more than just applying techniques to the client's body. A great deal of communication in bodywork occurs through the practitioner's touch, and it is an important aspect of the therapeutic relationship. Chapter 9 discusses this in more detail.

Bodywork is an intimate act that requires professionalism to ensure that both the client and the practitioner have a shared understanding of the therapeutic relationship. One way this is accomplished is through informed consent. Obtaining informed consent, discussed in more detail in Chapter 7, is a standard procedure that a practitioner uses to establish safety for the client. It defines the structure of the bodywork session and clearly explains what the treatment will entail.

When the client is fully informed about what will happen during the treatment, the intimate nature of bodywork can unfold more easily. The practitioner respects the client by being clear and direct about the techniques used, benefits of the treatments, and possible side effects the client may experience. The client is also given the option of refusing the treatment or choosing to stop the treatment at any time. Because the client has been made aware of what to expect, he or she is more likely to have confidence in the practitioner's skills, and can relax and be present for the treatment. All of these factors encourage the formation of a healthy therapeutic relationship, and the likelihood of a positive treatment outcome.

Creating a Therapeutic Relationship

Sometimes bodywork students and new professionals have a difficult time creating therapeutic relationships with clients. They may be proficient at techniques but may feel they never quite "connect" with the client. Perhaps they are puzzled about why they do not have many repeat clients. Sometimes practitioners perform a treatment using the correct technique, but are surprised to learn that the client is not satisfied. Unfortunately, some practitioners blame clients for not being happy with the treatments they receive and are unwilling to evaluate themselves to see what they could have done better. Often, such failures to establish a therapeutic relationship are the result of poor communication with the client. Some examples include not providing the client with an opportunity to express specific treatment needs or to ask questions, or not listening to the client's feedback. Failures can also occur because of misunderstandings concerning the roles each party plays within the therapeutic relationship.

Consider the following:

Martin has asked Gisele, a friend, if he can practice Thai massage on her. Gisele is a massage therapist, so Martin assumes that she knows something about Thai massage. Martin performs a traditional 2-hour session, which involves many paired stretches and yoga-like poses in which the practitioner's body and the client's body are often touching. At the end of the session, Martin notices that his friend is not saying much. When he asks her what she thought of the treatment, she says quietly, while avoiding eye contact,

🥗 Food for Thought

Think of all the people with whom you consider you are intimate. What defines the intimacy? How would you characterize the level of intimacy? How do you demonstrate intimacy with each of the people? Do you think these levels of intimacy are appropriate with each person? Why or why not?

"I didn't know you would be so close to me all the time. It was really uncomfortable. If I had known it was going to be such a long treatment, I would have said something but I kept thinking it would end soon."

If Martin had taken the time to explain to Gisele what she should expect during a Thai massage, Gisele would have been more prepared for the intimate nature of the techniques, and for the length of the treatment. She may have then chosen to decline, and saved experiencing an uncomfortable 2-hour treatment. On the other hand, Gisele may have decided to proceed with the treatment. She might have been much more open to receiving the techniques because she would have known the practitioner-client body contact in Thai massage is normal. Even if she had decided to proceed with the treatment, but then started to feel uncomfortable, she might have said something to Martin rather than waiting for the treatment to end.

Overwhelming the client with too much information is another barrier to developing a sound therapeutic relationship. Often, this occurs during the pretreatment interview. For example, in an effort to find out where the client is experiencing pain, practitioners may use anatomical terms unfamiliar to the client. Some practitioners' interviewing styles involve firing questions at the client, barely giving him or her a chance to answer, let alone ask questions of the practitioners. Then there are those practitioners who enjoy practicing bodywork to such an extent that they feel the need to explain all the training they have received as well as all the details of the techniques they will be performing on the client. Unless the client is also a bodywork practitioner, much of this may go over the client's head, leaving him or her confused and no better informed than if the practitioner had said nothing.

Because they have been speaking to the client, these practitioners may assume or expect the client to feel at ease about receiving the treatment, which may not necessarily be the case. If the interview feels rushed or the client does not have his questions answered adequately, chances are the client is not feeling comfortable about receiving the treatment, will not benefit from it, and will most likely not return.

To avoid practitioner behaviors that can get in the way of developing a healthy therapeutic relationship, follow these guidelines:

- Do not interrupt and talk over your client.
- Do not dismiss the concerns of your client.
- Answer your client's questions adequately.
- Admit you do not know an answer to a question rather than pretend you do and potentially give out false information.
- Talk about only appropriate personal issues with your client.
- Be on time for every appointment.
- Make sure you are not taking long-term clients for granted.
- Do your best work with each and every session.
- Accommodate reasonable requests made during the session.
- Address difficult issues with clients, such as with those who do not follow your office policies.
- Find something new to do in each treatment instead of performing the same treatment over and over again.
- Represent your level of education and skills accurately.

Throughout the rest of the book, these and other methods of strengthening the therapeutic relationship are discussed in more detail.

Like any relationship, a therapeutic relationship requires the participation of everyone involved. The client participates by being willing to receive bodywork from the practitioner and by compensating the practitioner for the treatment. Being willing to receive bodywork puts the client in a vulnerable position because he or she is entrusting the care and safety of his or her body to the practitioner. The practitioner is the one with the knowledge and expertise. Therefore, practitioners have the responsibility of communicating and behaving professionally and ethically in therapeutic relationships. This is no small task; communication skills and professional, ethical behavior do not arise spontaneously. They must be cultivated and nurtured. The definition and components of communication are a good place to start.

Definition and Components of Communication

At its very simplest, communication is the exchange of information: intentions, emotions, and expectations. It is a process by which people assign and convey meaning in an attempt to create shared understanding and collaboration. Communication can occur one on one, with a few people, with large groups, and even worldwide.

Communication is a learned skill. Most babies are born with ability to make sounds but must learn to speak and communicate effectively. This process requires many abilities, including processing information internally as well as externally (with other people), speaking, questioning, analyzing, and evaluating. These abilities are all used in a split second during the actual act of communicating, which itself can be broken down into six parts (Fig. 1.1):

1. The *type* of information being communicated. For example, is it a thought, an emotion, or a fact?
2. The *source* of information. For example, where is it coming from or from whom?

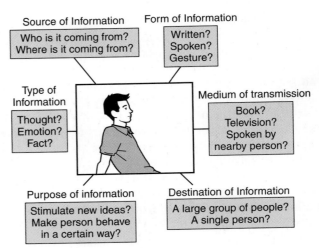

Figure 1.1 The six parts of communication.

3. What *form* the information is in. For example, is it written, spoken, or a gesture?

4. What *medium* the information is being transmitted through. For example, is it printed in book form, broadcast on television, or spoken by a person close by?

5. The *destination* of the information. For example, is it meant for a large group of people or a single person?

6. The *purpose* of the information. For example, is it to stimulate new ideas or to make a person behave in a certain way?

Put more simply, communication transmits messages in various forms toward a destination, such as oneself, another person, or another group of people, such as a corporation, church members, a political party, group of students, and so forth.

Next, we consider two key components of communication: language and communities.

Language

One critical component of communication is language. **Language** can be defined two ways. One way that language can be defined is as a system of communicating ideas, thoughts, and feelings by the use of words, their pronunciations, and the methods of combining them as has been agreed upon by a community. Language can also mean communication using sounds (grunting or snorts of contempt, for example), gestures (sign language and body language), or symbols, such as those used by ancient civilizations. Figure 1.2 shows an example of Hawaiian petroglyphs. Petroglyphs are rock engravings that are often (but not always) associated with prehistoric peoples. A symbol commonly understood today is shown in Figure 1.3. Even without words, the symbol on a yield sign is understood by most people.

Spoken language has both oral and auditory components. The **oral language** component is the part of communication in which the lips and tongue form the words. **Auditory** is the component of communication that involves hearing, such as the loudness and tone of the voice. Spoken language does not need to have both oral and auditory components for it to be understood. Hearing-impaired individuals who can read lips are able to interpret oral language, even though the auditory component is missing. Most hearing people can interpret a loud, angry tone even if no words are formed.

Nonverbal communication includes body language, sign language, touch, and eye contact. According to one study,[2] 55% of the impact of communication is determined by body language (postures, gestures, and eye contact), 38% by the tone of voice, and 7% by the actual words used in the communication process (although the exact percentage of influence may differ from person to person, depending on such things as family upbringing and cultural background). Taken together, this means that 93% of communication is nonverbal and only 7% has to do with the words used.

Language has a great deal of power; it is the foundation of all relationships. To interact successfully with one another, people need ways to express themselves so that they are understood. It may seem that communicating should be the easiest thing in the world. After all, it starts with a baby's first cry. But in

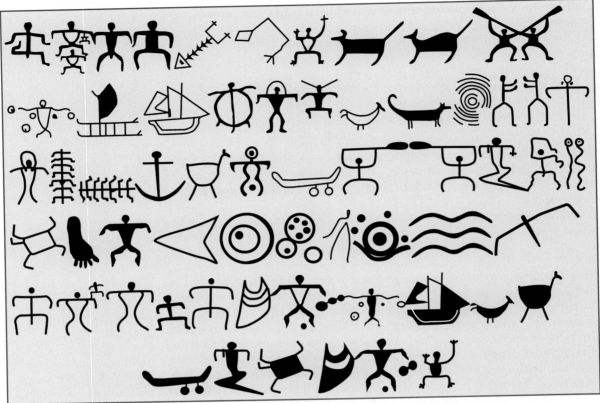

Figure 1.2 Symbols used in ancient Hawaiian petroglyphs. Images such as these have been found carved in lava. *Copyright Judith Sutcliffe. Available at http://www.identifont.com/show?4AQ. Accessed August 30, 2010.*

Figure 1.3 Even though there are no words on this symbol, it is understood by most people to be a yield sign.

reality, communication is made up of many different factors, such as personal perceptions, emotions, topic sensitivity, culture, and family dynamics, to name a few. Even though people may think they are being absolutely clear in what they are saying, writing, or demonstrating through body language, everything is subject to misinterpretation. Many issues that arise among people stem from a lack of clear communication.

Communities

The second component of communication is community, which is the context within which language is used. Interestingly, the root of the word *communicate* is the same as that for the word *community: communis,* Latin for "to participate." The members of a society need to be able to interact with others in the society to get their own needs met and for the society as a whole to function. This interaction takes the form of communication, and it is the communities into which people are born, in which they grow up, and in which they choose to live the rest of their lives that mold their communication styles.

Human beings have long chosen to live in communities. Although there are always exceptions to this, by and large we have congregated. Benefits of living together include safety, a sense of connection and belonging to one another, and the ability to find others for procreation. There are also many different communities within the larger societies. For example, there are work communities, religious communities, school communities, sports communities, professional association communities, and volunteer communities. Unless people decide to isolate themselves completely, they live at least some of their lives in group settings.

What, then, defines a community? Communities generally have laws and regulations stating what is acceptable behavior for its members and consequences if unacceptable behavior occurs. The members of communities tend to have similar values and similar overarching goals. Those within communities agree to cooperate with each other, with varying degrees of success, and have worked out methods to resolve conflicts. They have a common history or common social, economic, and political interests, meaning they have a generally agreed-upon form of government (although not necessarily the same political beliefs). Communities have also developed a commonly understood language and methods of communication. Certain communities may also require their members to act, dress, speak, and appear in specific ways. This is shown by, for example, sports teams, junior high school cliques, society clubs, cowboy culture, and religious affiliations.

In addition to the benefits of belonging to societies, there are, of course, challenges. Members may not wish to follow all the laws and regulations of a society; some may think such laws infringe on personal rights. Some members may think their personal needs override those of other members.

The bodywork profession is a community, both on national as well as regional levels. Members of this community may join national organizations (by choice or requirement), network within their own cities and towns, or choose to work in isolation. However, there are acceptable and unacceptable behaviors, ways to dress, and language for the members of the massage and bodywork community. Consequences for not following acceptable methods can range anywhere from losing clients to being ostracized.

For example, consider the following:

Lisa worked as a massage therapist for Central Bodyworks for 6 months. During her first 3-month evaluation, Lisa's supervisor talked with her about

Food for Thought

What are all the communities you belong to? Why are you in these communities? What is it you like about being in each of these communities, and what is it you don't like? Think about communities you have been in throughout your life. As you got older, were there communities that you outgrew?

her habit of arriving either just before or even late for her first appointment, how she smelled of cigarette smoke every time she came back from a break, and that she needed to wear tops with a higher neckline because her cleavage showed every time she bent over. The supervisor said that not only had he observed these behaviors and dress himself, he had also received complaints from the other practitioners and even from some clients. Lisa agreed to improve in these areas to continue employment at Central Bodyworks. For the first month after the evaluation, Lisa was a star employee. Gradually, however, she started to slide back into her previous habits and dressing less than professionally. At her 6-month evaluation, Lisa was told that she would be let go and would need to find another place to work.

Lisa's bodywork community—the clients, other practitioners, and the supervisor at Central Bodyworks—found her behavior and dress unacceptable. She was given the opportunity to change, which she did for a while, but then chose to return to her old ways. Because of her choices, she lost this bodywork community and had to find another.

Sometimes the consequences for unacceptable behavior as a bodywork practitioner can even include being arrested. For example, practitioners who overstep the boundaries for bodywork by touching their clients inappropriately or providing sexual services may find themselves behind bars.

Food for Thought
What would acceptable and unacceptable behaviors, ways to dress, and language be for the massage and bodywork community? In what ways could unacceptable behaviors result in losing clients, being ostracized, or being incarcerated?

Why Communication Fails

As discussed earlier, effective communication does not just happen. It takes a conscious effort on the part of both the sender and the receiver to get the right message across. Because everyone has different attitudes, experiences, filters, and perceptions affecting their communication, it is not guaranteed that the sender and the receiver will be in 100% agreement during any interaction. Therefore, Tubbs and Moss suggest that "we can't judge effectiveness if our intentions are not clear; we must know what we are trying to do . . . the goal of communicating is to bring about one or more of several possible outcomes as a way to determine when a person gets his or her point across."[3]

Possible outcomes of communicating with others include the following:

- Understanding—accurate reception of the content of the intended message
- Enjoyment—a sense of mutual well-being
- Attitude influence—changing and reformulating attitudes
- Improved relationships—seeking to understand motivation and social choices; developing trust and group cohesiveness
- Action—eliciting action on the part of another person

These potential outcomes suggest that it is the *process* of communication that matters more so than either the speaker or the receiver getting what he wants. Not all conversations will fit so nicely into a particular model or follow a specific theory of communication. However, it is possible for all people involved to be willing to have the conversation, to be open, to stay present in the process of the conversation no matter where it may lead, and to allow for an outcome to unfold. When there is a connection among the people, as well as appropriate behavior, a positive outcome of the conversation is likely. A positive outcome does not necessarily mean that everyone gets what he or she wants but that the effort was made. All parties felt heard and have an investment in the relationship.

Of course, the outcome of a conversation is not always positive. Often, there are gaps in communication and, sometimes, outright failures. These can sometimes be humorous, but can also lead to frustration, annoyance, anger, and conflict. There are as many different reasons communication fails as there are people. Although communication gaps and conflict resolution are discussed in more detail in Chapter 4, it is helpful to look at the five main reasons communication fails: language differences, cultural differences, personal differences, making assumptions, and lost information.

Language Differences

There is a myriad of languages around the world, and a myriad of differences within individual languages. The English spoken in England, for example, is not exactly the same as the English spoken in the United States, Australia, or Canada. Communication also, of course, has the potential to fail if the people involved do not even speak the same language. This is becoming more and more common as communities become more diverse.

In the bodywork profession, it is common for a non-English-speaking person to arrive at a treatment office that has only English-speaking practitioners. If the client does not bring an interpreter with him or her, it may seem that communication will definitely fail. However, with a little ingenuity and willingness on the part of everyone involved, most people can make themselves at least partially understood. For example, devise some nonverbal gestures that the client can use to indicate more or less pressure. Point to body charts to help the client communicate pain levels and areas of complaint. Learn a few common phrases in the client's language to address a client's potential discomforts. Remain confident, and do not be intimidated by the language barrier, because it projects a sense of calm and a willingness to communicate. Be sure to use nonverbal language (body language) as well.

The use of slang and lingo can also prove challenging. Not everyone understands current lingo, and these terms may not be appropriate for use in the bodywork profession. Each generation and each profession has its own particular terms that can be amusing, baffling, or frustrating to those who do not know the meaning. For example, the term "OMG" ("oh my god" or "oh my goodness") is well understood by those who text message often. However, those who do not text message are likely to have no idea what the term means. If a client should use that term when speaking to a practitioner who is not familiar with it, or vice versa, confusion can result, and communication can fail. A practitioner may use bodywork slang with a client who does not understand it. If a massage therapist should say, for example, "Your upper traps and levators are tight. I'm going to do stripping and t.p. work," then, unless the client is also a massage therapist, chances are that the client will not understand what the treatment will involve. The use of slang and lingo is discussed in more detail in Chapter 2.

Cultural Differences

Each culture has its own way of communicating and attaches meanings to words according to the norms of the culture. Sometimes cultural differences are very apparent; other times they may not be so easily discernible. For instance,

Muslim culture is quite different from Christian culture. However, among Christians, there are many different denominations and subcultures. Lutherans may have different religion-related language than, say, Catholics. Western culture is vastly different from Eastern culture. Within Western culture, traditions and communication among French citizens are different from those among Spanish citizens. There can be cultural differences even within regions or neighborhoods.

Cultural differences can have an impact on how bodywork is received. Feedback is a very important tool for bodywork practitioners to know how their work is affecting the client. However, some cultures feel it is disrespectful to tell another person directly how he or she should do something in a different manner. Other cultures value direct communications and honesty, sometimes to the point of rudeness in the eyes of those who are not members of that culture.

For example, a massage therapy student is having difficulty learning how to do proper draping procedures without inadvertently exposing his class partner. When his partner gives him feedback, he tells her that she is too heavy, and that the sheets are not large enough to cover her completely as she turns over. Although this may be perfectly acceptable to say to someone within his culture, his partner takes great offense and avoids him from that point on. He does not understand why until both students meet with the student adviser who has them discuss the issue openly.

It is important that practitioners be aware that cultural differences exist and be willing to respect them. It can be a fine line to walk, and practitioners should keep in mind that anything said should not be taken personally. Sometimes, the best way is simply to ask what the person's preferences are.

Personal Differences

Each piece of information received during communication will be colored by the recipient's personal opinions, tastes, thoughts, desires, and perceptions. This is natural and normal. What can be a barrier to good communication, though, is assuming that the other person has these same opinions, tastes, thoughts, desires, and perceptions. Personal differences can also be a huge barrier to successful communication if the people involved become invested in their way as the only way, and conversation stops. An important aspect of effective communication is to be willing to understand and not judge the other person's point of view. There is a time and place to share personal opinions but it is important to recognize when that is.

For example, Andre is very committed to working to stop global warming by doing what he can on a local level. He has made his entire practice "green" by following the guidelines of the local environmental group. He has even given up his vehicle and uses a bicycle to get around. Some of Andre's clients drive large SUVs that do not get great gas mileage. Each time one of these clients comes in for a treatment, Andre lectures the client on the carbon footprint his or her vehicle is leaving behind. He often gives out informative flyers and invites his clients to attend lectures on global warming and reducing carbon emissions at the local university. Over time, some of the clients feel free to engage him in conversation about his opinions, but many others have quietly left his practice, and have never come back.

✳ Making Assumptions

Making assumptions about what the other person is thinking or feeling about what the speaker is saying can lead to anticipating a specific response when a question is posed or a statement is made. In bodywork, this may occur if practitioners think their clients know more than they actually do about the treatment they are to receive. For example, in massage therapy, the client may be told to "disrobe to your level of comfort and slide under the top sheet." It may be perfectly clear to the practitioner what is expected, but the client may not understand. As has happened to many massage therapists, the practitioner comes into the room to find that the client has done any of the following:

- Left all clothes on and is lying on top of the top sheet with nothing covering him or her
- Left all clothes on and is lying under just the top sheet
- Left all clothes on and is lying under both the top and bottom sheet
- Taken the outer clothing off, left on underwear and socks, and is lying under the top sheet
- Taken the outer clothing off, left on underwear and socks, and is lying under both the top and bottom sheet
- Taken all clothes off and is lying on top of the top sheet with nothing covering him or her

It is, of course possible to give an effective treatment in each of these situations (although the client who has taken off all clothes and is lying on top of both sheets does need to be draped). However, with only one phrase from the practitioner, six different actions may be taken by the client. More than one practitioner has been surprised to discover that when they thought they could not have been clearer, the client had a vastly different interpretation about what was said.

✳ Lost Information

Information can be lost for several reasons: lack of clarity on the part of the speaker, more information given by the speaker than the receiver can take in, or lack of attention on the part of the receiver.

Lack of clarity can occur if the speaker is not exactly sure what he or she wants to say but hopes the message will eventually make sense if he or she talks long enough. Many times the receiver simply stops listening after a while. In bodywork treatments this can happen, for example, if the practitioner does not have a firm handle on anatomical terminology and tries to hide this fact by mixing in a lot of jargon. Or a practitioner does not understand a finding from an assessment, but believes he should offer some explanation so he makes up something that he hopes the client will not question. Another example is shown in Box 1.1.

As discussed in the section "Creating a Therapeutic Relationship," too much information given at once can result in lost information. Bodywork practitioners who are very passionate about their work can overwhelm a client with their enthusiasm. For instance, the practitioner may get so excited trying to explain what she has found in the client's soft tissue that it is causing the client to "check out," or feel so overwhelmed that he does not know

---

Box 1.1 | **LOST INFORMATION**

What the massage therapist says: "For your session today, I would like to do some myofascial work."

What the client hears: "For your session today, I would like to do some of my fast work."

What the client thinks: "Fast work?! I am paying $60 an hour and he is going to work fast? That's not right. I want a full hour."

What the client says: "No, I don't care for that. Why don't you just work slowly like you always do. I don't like it fast."

What the therapist thinks: "What on earth is he talking about?"

What the therapist says: "Okay. No myofascial work today."

In both of these examples, crucial pieces of information were lost or misunderstood. As a result, the massage therapist honors what the client requests, but does not understand the reason the client objects to his suggestion of myofascial work. The client is satisfied because he is assured he will receive a full hour, but does not receive the treatment that would be most beneficial to him. Communication has failed.

---

what to say. He may even be worried that the practitioner will injure him as she energetically addresses his soft tissues. It is important that practitioners balance the amount of information they know with the amount of information that the client needs at the time. Later, as the therapeutic relationship develops, there could be time to discuss the practitioner's findings and recommendations in depth.

Another barrier to communication is a lack of attention to what is being communicated. At a critical moment, a person may miss something crucial, and may not know it. He may even decide to fill in lost data with information of his own that is not necessarily correct. If, for example, a bodywork practitioner does not pay close attention to what the client says or has written on the intake form, then the client may view the practitioner as insensitive or too distracted to offer a safe treatment. This does not build trust. Further, it also means that the practitioner can perform a treatment that is harmful to the client. Lost information can completely change the dynamic as well as the intention of a treatment, prevent the therapeutic relationship from forming, and endanger the client.

Consider the following:

Priscilla has a busy day. Her last client, Sara, is coming to see Priscilla for the first time. When she arrives for her appointment she fills out the intake form, and then she waits. Priscilla greets Sara and invites her to follow her to the treatment room while she reads Sara's intake form. In the course of the interview, Priscilla asks Sara about the quality of her abdominal and low back pain, and how long she has been experiencing it. Sara looks at Priscilla with a very pained expression and says, "I wrote on the intake form that I had a miscarriage last week. It's been hurting since then." At this point, Sara starts to cry and excuses herself from the room to get a drink of water. She does not come back in for her treatment. After a few minutes, Priscilla comes out to the waiting area to find that Sara has left. Priscilla calls her later that evening to ask if she is okay. Sara tells her that she is offended that Priscilla had not noticed the miscarriage information on her form. She has been having a hard time accepting what had happened. She thought having a massage would be a way to escape for a while, but now says she does not think she will ever come back.

What Defines Effective Communication?

Now that we have established the basic components of and barriers to communication, we can explore what makes for effective communication and how we can communicate proficiently as bodywork practitioners. Many times people think they communicate just fine and that, if there is a problem, it lies with the other person. However, the root of good communication is self-responsibility for actions and words. Through continual, honest self-evaluation and willingness to adjust methods and ways of thinking, it is possible to discard old, inadequate communication styles and acquire new communication tools.

Some examples of old, inadequate communication styles include the following:

- Always having to have the last word. This involves valuing being right over understanding what the other person is thinking and feeling about the particular issue at hand. You can ask yourself, "Do I want or need to be right all the time, or do I want to have a successful conversation in which information is shared and understanding is increased?"
- Withdrawing from the conversation when not being understood or when not being agreed with. It may be out of fear that people choose to withdraw. However, each time a person does not stand up for her thoughts and ideas, she is communicating to others that her thoughts and ideas do not matter. A person may withdraw in an effort to get one's own way, which is a form of manipulation. The behavior of withdrawing can be subtle or dramatic. It is not professional or helpful to pout or sulk if the practitioner is in disagreement about how an issue should be dealt with. You can ask yourself, "Do I tend to withdraw from others? If so, why am I withdrawing? Am I afraid to speak up? Do I really think my thoughts and ideas have no worth? Am I trying to get my way in the same manner small children do?"
- Having a negative outlook in general can also hurt communication. Negative people tend to find fault in others and are not supportive. These feelings might arise out of jealousy, or perhaps out of low self-esteem. Some people think it is easier or better to point out all that is wrong in a given situation ("Hey! I'm just being realistic!"). Generally, though, negativity isolates the person, as others would rather not associate with them. Dealing with someone who is negative all the time can be frustrating and emotionally draining. You can ask yourself, "Do I always look at the dark side of things? Can I not be happy for someone else? If not, why not? What would happen if I looked at the bright side of things now and then?"

When defining the parameters of good communication, the place to start is with intention.

 Food for Thought
What are examples of how you have experienced miscommunication through each of the following: language differences, cultural differences, personal differences, making assumptions, and lost information? What successes in communication have you had despite these barriers?

Intention

A critical aspect of good communication is having appropriate intention. A therapeutic relationship can grow only through conscious, intentional communication. **Conscious communication** means being willing to think about how the communication will affect the other people involved, both in the short term and the long term, and choosing what is best for everyone involved, not just what is best for the practitioner. Conscious communication is an integral part of intention. For example, instead of saying to a client, "Wow, what a scar! No wonder your shoulders are so tight!" a more conscious way of communicating would be to say, "I notice you have a scar here along your right shoulder blade. I wonder if this is causing restrictions in your shoulder movement. What do you think?"

Practitioners are only responsible for their part of the conversation with a client. If a client forgets or chooses not to say something that seems important once the treatment has started, practitioners can ask what they need to know in a tactful manner. For people who are impulsive by nature and tend to express whatever is on their minds without censoring it or putting it through a filter, it would be wise to explore why they choose to communicate in this fashion and what impact it has on their relationships.

As can be seen, intention can be defined as a determination to act in a certain way. In the case of good communication, the way to act is with clarity of purpose. That is to say, the words, tone of voice, and body language used by the communicator need to match the goals of the communication. In the case of bodywork, the goals of the communication should be a positive experience in which both the practitioner and the client have their needs met appropriately.

Because body language is such a major part of communication, most humans, whether they know it or not, are experts at reading body language. Therefore, they instinctively know when they are being lied to or when there may be a hidden agenda, and many people feel this physically in some way. This is where the term "gut instinct" comes from. This is discussed in more detail in Chapter 2.

Clear communication as the foundation of successful professional relationships means that a minimum of misunderstanding and a maximum of creative interaction occur. There is an accurate transfer of information about what is thought and felt; all parties involved are clear about their intentions and maintain that clarity through all interactions. Another way to characterize this is having transparency of motives and intention.

Some questions you can ask yourself to make sure you are clear about your intentions include the following:

- What is my desired outcome?
- Why do I want this?
- Does getting this line up with my values?
- How do I benefit?
- What are the drawbacks to me?
- Would the other person(s) be harmed by this outcome?
- What am I willing to do to get this?
- Am I willing to do the work necessary to get this?

- Am I being truly honest and transparent about my intentions?
- Will my behavior be in alignment with my intentions?

Continuum of Appropriate Communication

Unconsciously, the depth and intimacy of relationships are measured by how much communication occurs. Intimacy and rapport with others, from strangers to friends to family members to clients to loved ones, exist on a continuum (Fig. 1.4). At one end of the continuum are low intimacy and rapport. Communication on this end usually remains polite, safe, and about superficial topics, such as a conversation about the weather one would have with a stranger in line at the bank. At the other end of the continuum is a great deal of intimacy, such as can occur between lifelong friends, life partners, and tight-knit family members. If the people involved trust one another and are willing to be vulnerable to each other, there can be a great deal of rapport and emotional connection. The communication can, in turns, be empathetic, intense, personal, emotional, and sometimes even angry.

Intimacy will increase along the continuum with the following factors in place:

- Being willing to connect on a deeper level with another person. Am I willing to be more vulnerable with this person so that he or she can see me more clearly? Am I willing to make myself more vulnerable even when there is no guarantee that it will be reciprocated?
- Being willing to devote time toward deepening the level of connection. Can I invest a significant amount of time out of my life to deepening this relationship? Am I willing to make this relationship such a priority that I will find the time? Is the other person willing to invest time toward getting to know me? If not, am I still willing?
- Making an effort. Am I willing to exert mental or physical energy, or both, to achieve a deeper connection with this person?

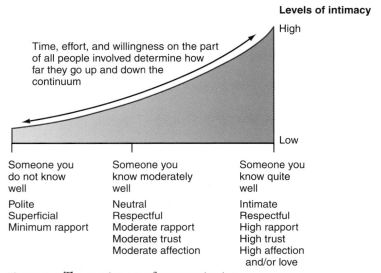

Figure 1.4 The continuum of communication.

Food for Thought
Think about a time when you felt that a person's body language did not match up with the words being said. How did you feel? How would you characterize that person's intention?

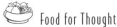

Food for Thought

Think about someone you are in love with or have been in love with. Also think about relationships you have had with a boss, coworkers, children, other family members, and friends. What type of language did you use to establish and maintain these relationships?

Movement along this continuum is dynamic. It is always changing, depending on the variables of who is involved and the purpose of increasing the level of intimacy. Expectations will also have an impact on how people move up or down the continuum of intimacy. If expectations are not met, people are likely to not feel the desire to deepen the connection. However, if expectations are met on a consistent basis it usually feels safe to continue moving closer to the person.

In the massage and bodywork profession, trust between the practitioner and client is necessary for a positive, therapeutic treatment to occur. Everyone has different levels of trust, different ways they trust, and different lengths of time it takes for them to trust someone else. However, the massage and bodywork profession is unique in that practitioners are basically asking clients to trust them immediately with their bodies and emotions. On the continuum of communication, this relationship is on the high end of intimacy almost at the outset of the practitioner and the client meeting.

It is sometimes a very fine line that practitioners walk between appropriate and inappropriate communication. The skill needed to know how deeply to communicate with a client is developed only with experience, and every practitioner makes mistakes along the way. Everyone has his or her own styles of communication, and they are different for different settings. For example, a practitioner can be more personal when talking with family, friends, and close colleagues. For less familiar and less casual environments, more formal communication may be called for. In the treatment setting, professional communication is necessary. Practitioners need to discern when personal, formal, and professional communication should be used; many times, miscommunication occurs if practitioners are not able to do this. Practitioners may inadvertently send out the wrong message, get a surprising (to say the least) response, offend clients, or degrade themselves or the profession.

Practitioners have many tools that can give them information on how to communicate with clients. The client's age, whether she has received massage previously, occupation, cultural background, medical history, and even permission from the client are all indicators of how far along the continuum the practitioner's communication may be. For example, if a client is an elderly gentleman, the practitioner may want to call him Mr. and use his last name (Mr. Smith), instead of calling him by his first name (Jim). If a client is one whom the practitioner has seen many times and is on a first name basis with, then asking about the client's family may be appropriate. Many times, however, either through inexperience or misconception, practitioners assume a great rapport when in fact it has not been established yet and clients can be offended.

Consider the following:

Marquez has been a shiatsu practitioner for 2 years. Recently, he started to work with Michiko. She is an elderly Japanese woman who had been a successful shiatsu practitioner in Japan for many years but is now retired. Marquez is so excited to be working with a master shiatsu practitioner that he finds himself asking Michiko all sorts of questions about shiatsu before, during, and after each treatment. Michiko is always very gracious and answers the questions politely but does not ask any questions of Marquez. After about 6 weeks of weekly sessions, Marquez asks Michiko if she would like to do a trade because he would love to experience her touch. Michiko becomes very annoyed. She states that she does not do trades with other practitioners, as her time is valuable. Besides, if she wanted to keep giving treatments she would not have retired. She then tells Marquez that she will no longer be receiving treatments from him because she is tired of all his questions and that he talks too much.

In this example, there is a combination of cues that Marquez should have picked up on to avoid the uneasy situation that culminated in losing a client. The cultural issue is foremost. In Japanese culture, there is deep regard and respect for masters of shiatsu. They are not to be quizzed and made to feel like a tutor. It was also not appropriate for Marquez to ask questions about shiatsu during Michiko's treatment. That Michiko did not ask Marquez any questions about himself should have been a clue that Michiko was not invested in a personal relationship with Marquez. Had Marquez not been so keen on getting as much information as he could immediately, he may have had a long and enriching therapeutic relationship with this client.

Disclosure

A final quality of effective communication is an appropriate level of disclosure. **Disclosure** means "revealing information." **Self-disclosure** is the process of deliberately revealing information about oneself that is significant and that would not normally be known by others. According to Adler and Rodman,[4] the reasons for self-disclosure include the following:

- Catharsis (release of issues by expressing them emotionally)
- Self-clarification
- Self-validation
- Reciprocity
- Impression management (trying to control how others view you)
- Relationship maintenance and enhancement
- Control

There are different amounts of self-disclosure in every different relationship a person has. In that sense, disclosure can form the framework of a relationship, whether it is casual, formal, has a lot of give and take among the people involved, or is somewhere in between. It can be used to build trust or, at the other end of the spectrum, to manipulate others and destroy relationships.

The following are examples of self-disclosure that bodywork practitioners may implement in various types of relationships:

Casual relationship: "I'm returning to school next quarter to finish my degree in Health Science. I'm planning on incorporating the degree into my bodywork practice."

Formal relationship: "Because you are my supervisor, I want you to know that I have been emotional at work because my relationship of seven years ended. My clients and coworkers have expressed a concern that I haven't been myself lately. I wanted to tell you this in confidence, and assure you that this has not nor will not affect my work performance."

A close friendship: "I'm feeling very attracted to one of my clients. I haven't acted on this but I want to talk with you about what I am feeling and thinking. I need to decide if this is real or if it's just a silly crush. If it's a crush, then please help support me in remaining professional when I work on the client. If it's real, then I'll need to refer my client to someone else."

Practitioner-client relationship: "I hear that you're feeling overwhelmed by the stress in your life, and that you're afraid you will have an emotional breakdown if you let yourself feel all you're up against. I'd like to share with you that there have been times in my life when I've felt overwhelmed and was also afraid to show my feelings. But I opened up to a friend I trust and I felt a lot better afterward. I encourage you to reach out to one of your friends and not carry this burden all alone."

A certain amount of disclosure is essential in the practitioner-client relationship. Clients disclose personal information to the practitioner as it relates to the presenting problem. For instance, to receive a client-centered treatment, the client needs to disclose where she is feeling pain and what may be the cause of the pain. The practitioner may need to disclose his training and credentials if a client requests them. During the treatment or series of treatments, the client may choose to disclose more about herself, and the practitioner may choose to disclose more about himself. This can occur as the client relaxes, feels more comfortable with the practitioner, and places more trust in the practitioner. If there is mutual trust, and if professional boundaries are maintained, then the relationship may develop into one of more rapport, and along the higher end of the continuum of communication.

Sometimes, however, the client's level of self-disclosure may be excessive and inappropriate. The client may start discussing, for example, more personal aspects of her relationship with her partner, money troubles, or mental health issues. In such cases, the practitioner may say, "I can be a good listener, but what you appear to be asking me about is out of my field of expertise. It would be unethical for me to give you any type of advice. I would be happy to give you a good referral source [counselor, chiropractor, accountant, etc.] regarding this matter."

Sometimes the practitioner's self-disclosure can be a very powerful therapeutic tool. For example, if the client is worried about certain money issues, the practitioner may say, "I was worried about money too until I saw an accountant. She really helped me straighten out my finances." Before sharing, however, the practitioner needs to ask himself, "Why am I revealing this information? Is it to benefit the client, is it in the hopes of gaining more information from the client, or is it to just talk about myself?" The answer should always be to benefit the client.

In the massage and bodywork profession, people sometimes think they need to disclose much about themselves to show that they are open and receptive to the massage experience. They may also think it is the shortest and best route to establishing rapport with clients. This "rush to intimacy" may, in fact, have the opposite effect. Instead of creating a conduit of communication flow, a wall of words (Fig. 1.5) blocking communication is built.

Consider the following:

Peggy had been Cheryl's massage therapist for a little over a month when Cheryl disclosed that she had just finished a 2-month stay at a rehabilitation center for drug addiction. Peggy gets very excited and tells Cheryl how proud she is of her for getting clean and sober. Peggy goes on to share her own

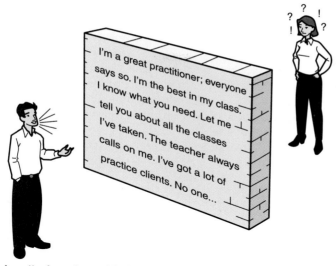

Figure 1.5 A wall of words can block communication.

experience as a drug addict and says she was lucky that she did not have to go a rehab center. She was able to kick the habit all on her own, but she is happy that Cheryl is turning around her life. After the session Peggy tells Cheryl that she is welcome to call her anytime she wants to talk about recovery. Cheryl thanks her and leaves the clinic. The following week Peggy notices that Cheryl has booked an appointment with another practitioner on staff. When she sees Cheryl in the lobby and says hello, Cheryl is distant and avoids eye contact.

■ **CASE PROFILE**

Benjamin was a school counselor for a middle school. Imani provided chair massage treatments each month to the teachers and staff at his school. Over the course of working at the school, Imani and Benjamin became very comfortable with each other by discussing the issues of stress reduction and mental health issues among the youth.

After two years of receiving Imani's chair treatments at the middle school, Benjamin left his job for another one and, because of the chair massage treatments he had received, began to see Imani for full body sessions to work on a chronic low-back condition. Benjamin felt tremendous relief in his back from the massages but also enjoyed the conversations before and after each session, and told Imani so. Over time, the massage appointments began with a checking in and some chatting about events from the last time they had seen each other, followed by a brief interview for the day's treatment. The massage would take place either in silence or with the conversation continuing throughout the treatment and posttreatment. Both think the talking has never interfered with the treatments. In fact, there were times it seemed to enhance it.

 Food for Thought

Have you ever had "disclosure remorse," or disclosed something about yourself to someone else and been sorry later? What did that feel like? What would you have done differently?

Case Study Continued to page 24

Case Study Continued from page 23

Benjamin has now been Imani's client for more than 10 years. He has paid promptly for his sessions and kept his appointments. If circumstances prevented him from doing so, he always called in advance to reschedule. Benjamin has frequently told Imani how much he appreciates her work and her professionalism. Consequently, Imani feels a great fondness for Benjamin and recognizes that they both have a shared goal of making sure Benjamin's treatments are effective.

What are three things that make this a successful therapeutic relationship?

What qualities does Imani have that have contributed to this success?

What qualities does Benjamin have that have contributed to this success?

Authentic Communication

Now I become myself.
It's taken time, many years and places:
I have been dissolved and shaken,
Worn other people's faces . . .

—MAY SARTON, from "Now I Become Myself" in *Collected Poems, 1930–1973*

Communication must not only be intentional, appropriate in level of intimacy, and appropriate in level of disclosure, it also must be authentic. Next we examine the definition of authentic communication, its role for massage therapists, and how to practice it. We also look at how to avoid using authenticity as an excuse for rudeness or self-centered communication.

Definition

✳ **Authentic communication** is being truly oneself in the conversation or interaction. There is no hiding behind masks, job titles, or perceived power; there is congruency between words and actions. This congruency, along with consistency, establishes credibility as a professional. An authentic person is comfortable in her own skin; she truly knows who she is. She can tolerate the fact that not everyone will like or agree with what she has to say, and she will express herself anyway because it would be untruthful to do otherwise.

When talking with such an authentic person there is an ease to the conversation. He is not trying to show off his expertise nor will he speak ill of others. This lack of pretension makes it easy to connect with others because there is no power play for position or need to be anyone other than who he is. He willingly shares credit for accomplishments with others, and does not need to draw attention to himself. He is genuine, dependable, and trustworthy.

The authentic person does not resort to bold ("in your face") tactics or put others down to ensure being heard. The speaker is able to let the power of his words speak for themselves. Communication is shared with respect for others and with respect for self. When this mutual respect exists between speakers, it increases the chance for successful and meaningful dialogues. Even though the outcome of conversations may not always be what is wanted, the ability to stay present and engaged is an accomplishment in and of itself.

This type of interaction feels good and is often described as warm and welcoming. It is easy to participate in these interactions because everyone involved feels respected and heard. The interaction can be as simple as a 2-minute conversation with the person behind the return desk at a department store or as lasting as an ongoing, lifetime friendship.

Consider the following examples of inauthentic and authentic conversations between two massage therapy students:

Inauthentic

Jose: It sounds like you're worried about passing your final.

Sue: Yeah, I just don't know if I can remember all the strokes and put them together in an integrated treatment.

Jose: I'm sure you'll do fine. You've been in class every day. You look good when you're working.

Sue: Easy for you to say. But I just don't feel ready!

Jose: You worry too much. You'll do fine.

Authentic

Jose: It sounds like you are worried about passing your final.

Sue: Yeah, I just don't know if I can remember all the strokes and put them together in an integrated treatment.

Jose: Tell me what you remember about putting together a complete and integrated treatment.

Sue: I know all the basic Swedish strokes. I can use either my hands or my forearms to apply them. I need to remember to use good body mechanics. I need to plan where I start the treatment on the client's body and where I finish it. And I should keep breathing and be present with my client.

Jose: Wow, it sounds like you remember a lot!

Sue: I guess I do. Maybe I'm just afraid because I haven't practiced as much as I've wanted to.

Jose: Ah, now that is something you can work on. Do you have time between now and the exam to give a couple of practice treatments?

Sue: Yes, I do. Thanks for the idea. Now I feel more like I'll be ready to take the exam.

The difference between these two conversations is that in the authentic dialogue Jose was genuinely interested in what Sue was saying, and asked her questions to help her figure out what is really bothering her. It was not that Sue did not know how to give a massage, it was that she felt that she had not had enough time to practice it. Once Jose heard that concern and followed up with an idea of practicing some more, Sue had a plan to manage her anxiety.

Being authentic in our connections with others does not have to be time consuming. Listening for content as well as the emotions in conversations will help you tune into what the client needs, as well as give you information on how to respond appropriately.

Role of Authentic Communication

The successful practitioner is one who is able to present a genuine and honest self to clients. Because the intimate nature of the bodywork profession requires immediate trust, it is essential that practitioners be able to communicate both verbally and nonverbally to clients that they will be respected and honored at all times. This can be done only if practitioners communicate authentically.

Practicing Authentic Communication

Just how is the authentic self accessed? How is this type of self-knowledge developed? What does it mean for someone to be comfortable in her skin?

People cannot communicate authentically unless they know themselves. It takes much effort and energy to maintain "masks," often to the point of exhaustion. Putting down the masks, being willing to take risks, being vulnerable, and allowing one's true self to be shown instead can be enormously freeing. It takes considerably less effort to be genuine, leaving more energy to connect with people on a real level. Most people can tell when someone is being genuine, and many, although not everyone, will respond in kind.

Being vulnerable means that one is willing to let down contrived protective devices constructed to feel safe and allow the true self to be seen. Being vulnerable means being willing and able to be honest with others about feelings, thoughts, desires, fear, likes and dislikes, values, and so forth. Allowing yourself to be seen in one or more of these areas is where the risk taking comes into play. There are the possibilities of being rejected, ridiculed, and hurt by those who do not agree with you, or by those who cannot or do not want to understand. Being vulnerable in relationships means taking the risk of losing them by not pretending to be something you are not or not choosing to adapt or accommodate to meet someone else's image of whom you should be.

It must be noted that being vulnerable in the appropriate way means that you are clear about your boundaries and your intentions. Vulnerability should not be confused with the behavior of someone who does not care what others think or is unaware of the fact that he is disclosing parts of himself without having done the necessary work of laying the foundation for a safe and trusting environment.

One way to get in touch with the authentic self is through answering the following questions. Answering them honestly will help practitioners define who they really are. Because it is sometimes difficult to look at certain parts of yourself, and even more difficult to share certain things with others, to be totally honest, you can answer the questions with the intent that only you will be reading the answers.

- How do you identify yourself? In other words, if you were to write out labels for yourself, what would they include? Be honest.
- Sometimes people start off with what may be considered simple labels, such as "I am female," "I am white [or Asian or African American, and so forth]," and "I am a student."
- From there, see if you can go deeper into yourself. For example, someone may come from a racist family, but does not share those views. Or

Food for Thought

What is the easiest thing for you to do when you connect with another person (i.e., shake hands, look him in the eye)? What made it possible for you to feel you could do this? Be specific.

someone may have experienced racism and carries anger about it around with him. Another example is a physically fit practitioner who harbors judgment and dislike for people who are overweight.

- What labels do you think friends, colleagues, and strangers would put on you? Are they all the same, or would different people use different labels? How would these labels differ?
- How have these labels formed the way you communicate? For example, someone who has experienced racism may hesitate to have a conversation with someone who seems to be a racist. The physically fit practitioner may use a dismissive or condescending tone when interviewing a client with a larger body size.
- In what ways have the labels enhanced your communication experiences? For example, at a party does it seem as if the other guests immediately feel comfortable talking with you when you say that you are a bodywork practitioner because they respect the knowledge and experience you have about alternative health-care ideas? Or if you are bilingual, can you facilitate an interview with a client whose first language is not English so that the bodywork session is successful for both you and the client?
- In what ways have the labels contributed to less-than-optimal communication experiences? For example, if you have a learning disability, have you had a teacher who talked to you in a patronizing tone when answering a question of yours? If you are quite muscular, have you had clients who were unsure of receiving a treatment from you because they thought that you might hurt them, and nothing you said seemed to put them at ease?

With the self-awareness that comes with answering these questions honestly, practitioners can begin or continue to practice authentic communication. The only way to do it is to just do it. If you are new at it, be patient with yourself. Like all skills, it requires practice and mistakes will be made along the way. After recognizing the mistakes and evaluating what could have been done differently, the experience needs to be let go.

Keep in mind the following while working at authentic communication:

- Do the best you can. Best gets better with practice. When you speak to clients from the heart, it paves the way to more powerful encounters in the future. Also, making an effort will feel better than avoidance. Avoiding difficult issues with clients tends to make them loom larger. When discussing such issues, assure yourself first, and then your client, that you are doing so to create a safe space for the therapy to happen.
- Know your strengths and weaknesses (i.e., do you become short with people when you're tired or overstressed? Are you able to engage strangers in conversation easily?) Do your weaknesses stem from lack of experience or do you need to acknowledge that you may still have reservations about being authentic because you fear people won't like the real you?
- Assess yourself. Authentic communication should feel good to the person practicing it. If an interchange does not feel good, identify your

role in it and be honest about your words and actions. Sometimes people do not respond in kind when authentic communication is used, so remember that there may have been simply nothing you could have done or said to change the outcome.

- Acknowledge what you are comfortable disclosing about yourself rather than thinking you must tell everything about yourself all the time. Recognize that every encounter you have with another person requires different levels of intimacy when communicating.
- Everyone makes mistakes, even those with lots of experience. Acknowledge the mistake and make amends if appropriate, then move on.

There will be times that we misjudge a situation or a person and we put our true selves out there, only to be rejected. This does not mean that we should never do it again, but simply that we must stay conscious about the reality of our therapeutic relationship with our clients. For example, a practitioner with 10 years of experience in the bodywork profession made the assumption that her client was asking her out on a date because he was telling her about an art opening he was hosting and told her he would really like for her to go. When she declined, stating that she did not date clients, he looked at her oddly and told her that he was in a committed relationship, and was, in fact, telling all the practitioners at the clinic about the opening. She was deeply embarrassed and had a hard time working with this client for a few months. Finally, she told him how awkward she felt and said she hoped he did not think less of her. His response was that he was just surprised but liked the fact that she had standards for how she socialized with clients. She was much more comfortable working with him after that.

This Is Just Who I Am; Deal With It

When recognizing certain truths about themselves, such as offending attitudes and behavior in particular, sometimes people respond with, "This is just who I am. Deal with it." For the person who says this, it is important that he evaluate the benefits and drawbacks of having this attitude. Does he behave this way to feel in control? Does he view any comment about how his attitude and behavior affects others as a threat? Has he never been made aware of other options in his behavior and attitudes?

Consider the following:

Joshua is a massage therapy student who is having a hard time getting along with his classmates. He is not well liked because his fellow students think he is too blunt in his assessment of their massage skills. In fact, he told one student that her feedback to him had nothing to teach him because he knew he gave a better massage than she did. A complaint is filed against Joshua stating that his behavior was interfering with the learning environment of the classroom. Joshua meets with the instructor to discuss the complaint. He says, "That's just how I am. If people don't like it, that's their problem, not mine. I know I'm right about what I should be doing in the classroom." The instructor points out to Joshua that although he has a right to his opinion it would be helpful for his professional development if he would look at the impact this behavior is having on his education as well as his ability to communicate with others. For example, his education is being

Words of Wisdom

The importance of developing the art of communication in the bodywork industry is too often under emphasized. This profession requires a significant amount of focus on professional and skillful interpersonal skills. The slightest misrepresentation of the facts or intention on the part of either party can compromise the integrity of the client–practitioner relationship.

From marketing a business in a brochure to setting personal boundaries during an intake interview, knowing how to communicate your intent when providing therapeutic treatment is crucial to your success. It can take years to build a successful practice but it takes only one bad experience to destroy it.

—KATHY LEE, BA,
  Licensed Massage Therapist
  since 1997, Bodywork
  Educator since 2001, and
  currently Director of Career
  Services at Cortiva
  Institute—Tucson, in
  Tucson, Arizona

limited because very few students are willing to work with him. He is missing out on a variety of experiences in which he could gain knowledge from other students, knowledge he could apply to clients when he graduates. In addition, his lack of concern about how others view him will likely be an attitude he carries into his professional practice. This could drive clients away if he insists on always being in charge and not caring about what his clients are experiencing. In short, the instructor informs Joshua that he could continue to act this way, but his behavior will isolate him in the profession and likely prevent him from making solid therapeutic relationships and connections. The instructor ended by saying that Joshua has a choice to make. "Do you want to be right all the time, or do you want to expand your knowledge and expertise in areas you are not aware of?"

To help someone grow in genuine awareness, a friend or colleague should honestly, kindly, and objectively mention to him specific examples of offending behavior and of how others felt and reacted. The next step is to ask him, without judgment, how he feels about hearing this sort of information about himself and how it feels to know that others are negatively affected. If the person is able to recognize and acknowledge the negative effects of his behavior, he may have an epiphany of sorts and ask for more information and even assistance to help unlearn the behavior.

If, however, this person is unwilling to do any self-examination and insists that the problem is not himself, but other people, then an impasse has been reached. At some point he may be held accountable for his actions and face consequences for the offending behavior. These can range from mildly uncomfortable interchanges all the way to incarceration, if the behavior is criminal. Ultimately, it is up to the communities in which the person lives to hold the person responsible for his words and actions.

As much as we strive to communicate effectively with our clients, there are times when it just does not happen. Sometimes practitioners forget what is said in the pretreatment interview, and work on an area that the client requested not be worked. Appointment times can become mixed up. A client's emotional outburst may not be handled well. However, if the practitioner has practiced effective communication in which the client is encouraged to speak up at any time during the treatment, the chances that a client will experience a satisfying treatment increase.

Communicator Styles

Personal processing styles affect the way information is both delivered and received. Some people prefer facts and order, whereas others may prefer concepts and ideas. Some people make decisions based primarily on processes of cause and effect and others in terms of people and social structure. How people prefer to communicate is determined by both genetic predisposition and experience. No one way to process information is better than another, only different.

There are several ways to categorize communicator styles, two of which are presented here. One method involves a person's tendency to rely on a particular physical sense in communication, such as vision, hearing, or touch. Another way is through behavior, or how the person responds to situations.

Communicator Styles Based on the Senses

People tend to rely on one particular physical sense more than the other senses in processing information, and this characteristic can significantly affect their communication with others. Our five senses are constantly informing us about the world around us. Some process information most effectively through what they see (visual processors), others through what they hear (auditory processors), and still others through what they touch (kinesthetic processors).

Visual Processors

Visual processors create pictures in their minds and use many descriptive words as they "paint" word pictures during conversation. They tend to use "see" words (such as, "Let's take a look at this," and "If we view it from this angle") and want to make eye contact when conversing.

Many visual processors do not do well when told how to do something. They need to see it and read it. In the classroom, bodywork instructors often have written information in some form (such as handouts) that go along with a hands-on demonstration of a particular technique. This can be problematic when the instructor organically adds some steps that are not included in the handouts. The visually astute students will notice the difference and may feel uneasy that they do not have all the information. However, there are a few ways to cope in such a situation. The instructor can be as careful as possible not to add new techniques while demonstrating techniques that the students have not yet mastered. The instructor may also add a disclaimer to the handouts, advising students that they will see the basics of the techniques but to be aware that, as a long-term practitioner, it is possible that some additional techniques will be performed, but the students are not required to replicate them at that time.

In a treatment office setting, practitioners who process visually find it helpful that important information be posted in memos where they can easily see them. These practitioners are also quite likely to want to see their schedules in a written format, such as a calendar. Being able to see the treatments they have for an entire week may help them plan better.

For clients who are visual processors, one method that is beneficial for communicating during the interview process is to have intake forms containing a diagram of the human body. The client can then mark where he or she is feeling stress or tension in his or her body. The diagram can then be used for further discussion about the treatment plan. If the practitioner is to give the client some stretches to do between sessions, the client will want to have them written down or in a handout format with drawings accompanying the instructions. When setting appointments with these clients it would be helpful to have a monthly calendar available. If a client has a mobile telephone/e-mail device, such as a smart phone, then he or she probably does this already.

Auditory Processors

Auditory processors are very attentive to the tone and rhythm of speech during a conversation. They will often hum, talk to themselves, and listen with their eyes closed or when gazing off into the distance.

Many auditory processors prefer to be told how to do something. They need to have information explained orally. If the information is in written form, they prefer to discuss it with someone else rather than to read it off the page. In the classroom, these students will want the bodywork instructors to explain each step as the instructor is doing it. If there are handouts, the auditory students may not read them or they may even discard them.

In a treatment office setting, practitioners who process auditorily find it helpful that important information be told to them directly. They are unlikely to read posted memos. These practitioners are also quite likely to want to hear their schedules rather than look at them.

Clients who are auditory processors will appreciate having the practitioner fully explain the goals and benefits of the session to make sure the client is aware of all aspects. This could cause a time management issue, however, if there is so much talking done before the treatment that it takes away actual treatment time. It will be important for practitioners to be mindful of this and develop strategies to wind down the interview and move on to the treatment. A simple way to do this is to say, "I have enough information to get started. If necessary, let's continue this conversation while you're on the table. Remember, you are always welcome to give me information throughout the treatment." This statement will give the client a chance to proceed with the treatment knowing that he or she can speak up at any time if necessary.

Kinesthetic Processors

Kinesthetic means "related to touch." Thus, **kinesthetic processors** learn and communicate through touch. When speaking, they use a lot of body language and "feel" words (such as "That hit me really hard" and "The story was really touching"). Often, they find that they have to physically touch something or someone while conversing to understand what is being said. Many bodywork practitioners are kinesthetic learners and communicators and so instinctively want to touch the people they are talking to. This is not necessarily always accepted in Western culture and can perhaps be off-putting to certain people. Kinesthetic processors may also find talking and listening for long periods of time fatiguing.

In the classroom, the student with kinesthetic strengths may tune out the lecture and miss key points before it is time to practice techniques. These students do not want to be told or to read how to do something; they want to try it for themselves. They, in fact, tend to learn best when performing techniques while the instructor is performing them. Instructors need to make sure there is a balance between lecture and hands-on demonstration and practice in the classroom.

In a treatment office setting, practitioners who process kinesthetically are unlikely to read posted information memos. The best way for them to retain information is if they are being touched or are touching someone or something while the information is being imparted. For example, if the office manager touches the kinesthetic practitioner on the shoulder while explaining changes in the schedule, the practitioner is more likely to remember it. If the kinesthetic practitioner has something to play with, such as a hand-strengthening tool, during staff meetings, he or she is more likely to be able to focus on the information being presented.

During the interview process the practitioner with kinesthetic preferences will likely ask the client if the practitioner may touch him or her to get a feeling for the location of the client's pain or discomfort. Also, if a client is having an emotional release during a session, the highly kinesthetic practitioner will naturally stay in physical contact with the client, seeking to comfort him or her. However, it would be wise for the practitioner, while keeping that physical connection, to ask the client what it is that he or she needs at this time. This is essential because it could be that the practitioner's touch somehow triggered the emotional release.

Clients who are kinesthetic processors tend to need to touch the practitioner to explain where their tension or pain is. If the practitioner suggests stretches or other exercises the client can do between treatment sessions, the practitioner must demonstrate them and the client must do them at the same time so that the client understands and remembers how to do them properly. When scheduling these clients in person, the practitioner may find it helpful to touch the client on the shoulder or the arm as the appointment is being made. This way, the kinesthetic processor client is more likely to remember the appointment.

Everyone processes information using all these methods, but certain ones dominate in each person. For example, almost everyone processes visual and auditory messages through the kinesthetic mode. The most common pattern is visual/kinesthetic, which means these people tend to see and feel to understand and transmit information. The second most common is auditory/kinesthetic, which means these people tend to hear and feel to understand and transmit information.

Communicator Styles Based on Behavior

There are four basic behavioral styles that describe how the majority of people communicate: analytical, driver, amicable, and peacemaker. Each style is a reflection of how a person interprets the world in which she lives and how successful she has been at getting her needs met. These styles are based on information found in *People Styles at Work . . . and Beyond: Making Bad Relationships Good and Good Relationships Better* by Bolton and Bolton.[5] One way to describe these styles is to compare each to a certain animal. Having an understanding of these different communication styles can increase a practitioner's awareness of how to work and interact with different clients, employers, and peers.

Analytical (Owl)

An analytical communicator is one who prefers to see the big picture (the "30,000-foot view"), like the owls, a high-soaring bird with keen vision. Owls are also perceived as wise and judicious in folklore. Analytical communicators like to have as many of the facts as possible before making a decision and speaking. They like to know all the details and tend to be reserved in their judgment. Owl communicators tend to observe a situation before taking action. People who are not focused on details may find it difficult to relate to Owl communicators. Therefore, one challenge an Owl faces is to avoid appearing as a know-it-all, which can create a communication barrier.

Owls appreciate quality and excellence. With such a huge focus on excellence, Owls may tend toward perfectionism and demand too much of themselves and others. Because Owls have such high standards, people with other communicator styles may feel that it is impossible to please an Owl. Owls want to be right. Owls can miss deadlines because they are focusing so intently on details and getting things absolutely right. At times, they may even miss the big picture. When Owls withdraw to process the situation, others may feel that they are disengaging, emotionally and otherwise.

To balance these tendencies, Owls can do the following:

- Watch that the tendency to be prudent does not turn into indecisiveness.
- Lessen concern over perfectionism. There is a fine line between painstaking attention to detail and being nitpicky.
- Shift from being purely task oriented to being more personable.
- Reassure others that they are still involved, even when needing time and space away to process things.

Owl practitioners are successful at visually assessing a client's physical posture and making connections concerning what would be the best treatment plan to address the needs of the client. They are also good at making detailed plans, such as for successive client treatments or a marketing plan for a business.

However, one challenge an Owl may face is working within a session's time frame. Owls may tend to work longer than necessary because the treatment did not feel complete to them. This may create problems for clients with time constraints and for other practitioners who may be scheduled to use the treatment room at a set time. Another challenge for Owl practitioners is to avoid being perceived as aloof. They can have, for example, quite a bit of knowledge about anatomy and techniques but fail to connect with the client on a personal level.

Driver (Lion)

People who are not afraid to state their needs, opinions, or ideas and who take pride in what they believe are Lions and exhibit the driver communicator style. Lions are known for their roar and for being "King of the Jungle." Lions like to be in charge. In fact, Lions are so comfortable speaking up that they could be perceived as controlling and intimidating when trying to get their point across. Lions also have strong leadership skills and are highly motivated in meeting their goals. As a communicator, Lions tend to be blunt and to the point; there is no beating around the bush. They are very aware of what is important to get across to others, sometimes at the risk of offending those with whom they are speaking. A challenge of communicating with a Lion is not to let her take over a conversation or a project.

Lions appreciate a direct approach. They are quick with a plan and comfortable in assuming a leadership position. They like to make things happen—now. A Lion's direct approach may intimidate or alienate others. Her conversational style may seem sterile and directed. The bluntness associated with Lions can be perceived as abrasive.

To balance these tendencies, a Lion can do the following:

- Slow down and allow others to contribute ideas and opinions.
- Take care to listen carefully and speak only as needed.
- Structure comments or ideas in ways that are less directive.
- Allow room for personal interaction.
- Focus on working collaboratively with others.

Lion practitioners can be successful in motivating clients to be invested in their bodywork process. They can also help move bodywork businesses forward by, for example, being the driving force behind expansion and trying new marketing methods. They also are committed to learning as much as they can about the bodywork profession. If they choose to volunteer for bodywork associations, they are happiest being chairs of committees or sitting on governing boards.

A challenge for Lions is to avoid being too directive in the development of the client's treatment plan, sometimes to the point of excluding the client's participation. Lion practitioners are sometimes so ready to start the treatment that they appear brusque during the pretreatment interview. They may also be too aggressive with the client when discussing lifestyle changes they think the client should make.

Amicable (Puppy)

The amicable communicator is one who expresses himself by being warm, friendly, and likeable, just like a puppy. Puppies are loyal and eager companions who constantly want to please their owners. Likewise, the amicable communicator, the Puppy, strives to please and say all the right things in an effort to fit in or to be accepted by others. He tends to be very willing to listen to the needs and ideas of others, but turns very little attention to his own ideas. He is often the communicator who will have lots of praise to give others while minimizing his own contributions. As a puppy is loyal, so is the amicable communicator. He has an investment in making sure that everyone gets along. He will tend to be the one in the group telling jokes or being silly as a means of diffusing tension or coping with anxiety. Puppies must be careful that they are not too agreeable or they will not be taken seriously. Puppies appreciate spontaneity. They may overcommit and therefore not get things done in a timely and thorough manner. This may lead to distrust by others.

Puppies tend to digress in conversations and avoid task completion, which may be perceived as a lack of commitment. Although Puppies are people oriented, they may tend to exclude others from organizational tasks. Sometimes they think participation takes too long. Puppies' fun-loving dispositions may cause others to question whether they can approach something in a serious manner.

To balance these tendencies, Puppies can do the following:

- Speak less and listen more; accept input and support from others.
- Slow down and make a game plan. Plan the work and work the plan.
- Break projects down into realistic action steps.
- Learn to manage time more effectively.

Puppy practitioners are successful at creating therapeutic relationships. It is easy for them because they are comfortable connecting with clients. They genuinely want to know what the client is experiencing, and most people respond positively to this authenticity. Puppies like ingenuity. They are always looking for ways to make their treatments more creative, and for techniques, information, and products that they think will be helpful to their clients.

A challenge for Puppies is to practice setting good boundaries so that they do not subsequently find themselves in uncomfortable situations. The practitioner wants to be liked by clients, but often does not know when to step back and not get personally involved in their issues. Puppies may also have problems with time management. For example, they so enjoy talking with their clients they may lose track of time.

Peacemaker (Turtle)

The hallmarks of the peacemaker communicator style are patience and thoroughness, making sure that all sides of an issue are discussed and considered. Turtles are slow and seemingly steady animals. They tend to take their time getting places but never stray from their course. The Turtle is the one who invites others to share, listens more than she speaks, and takes her time processing information before making a decision to speak up. By taking on the role of a peacemaker, the Turtle ensures that everyone's ideas and feelings are taken into consideration. In addition, the Turtle strives to be inclusive and collaborative. Like a turtle, this communicator can also be quick to "snap" if she does not believe that she has had enough time to process information. Therefore, others may view Turtles as temperamental.

Turtles appreciate harmony. They prefer to avoid conflict. They may try to maintain relationships with others by sweeping things under the rug or by not making waves. Turtles may in fact stifle their own opinions to achieve this.

Turtles usually see many sides to an issue and are diplomatic. They are sensitive to others and do not want to offend anyone with their words or actions. Turtles respond slowly and are more reactive than proactive.

To balance these tendencies, Turtles can do the following:

- Be prepared for interactions.
- Gather information ahead of time, think of their own position, and consider their own needs.
- Figure out a constructive way to be assertive.
- Expand options. Instead of choosing between being nice or assertive, they can be both. Turtles can be dependable and supportive without being stepped on.
- Take care to balance attention to others with attention to self and the task at hand.

Successful Turtle practitioners are interested in making sure they understand the client's physical, mental, and emotional concerns. They bring a balanced approach to their work, and are adept at creating therapeutic relationships because they honor clients' experiences. They also strive for harmony in their work settings.

A challenge Turtles face is to avoid allowing the client to be in complete charge of the session. Turtles do not want to assert their knowledge, and may be reluctant to suggest alternatives to the client. Turtles may not be able to set strong boundaries when needed, and can possibly be dominated by clients and coworkers.

Practitioners should remember that everyone exhibits elements of all these traits, but each prefers the one that is the most effective in meeting personal needs, as well as what each situation may require. For example, if there is a deadline to meet, driven Lion characteristics would be helpful to make sure things are done on time, whereas the analytical Owl will make sure all the details are taken care of. When a situation is less driven, a more amicable Puppy or peacemaker Turtle approach can be implemented.

Figure 1.6 shows a summary of how the different animal types communicate.

Box 1.2 has helpful reminders for interacting with those who have different communicator styles than yours.

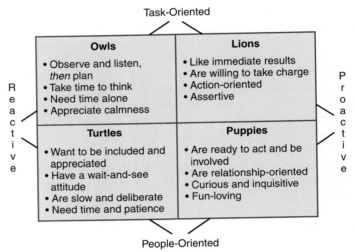

Figure 1.6 Summary of how the different animal types communicate.

Box 1.2	**REMINDERS WHEN INTERACTING WITH THOSE WHO HAVE DIFFERENT COMMUNICATOR STYLES**

- No communication style is better, worse, smarter, or dumber than the others.
- No one uses the same communication style all the time; everyone uses each of the different styles to a certain extent. However, one style is usually dominant.
- When people of two different communication styles do not get along, the issue is not always incompatibility. It is usually a lack of understanding of the other person's communication style.
- The bottom line for all styles includes respect, fairness, and honesty.
- Think about adapting personal communication styles to be more in sync with people who have different communication styles. It may help to improve the results of an interaction. Examples of adapting communication styles include the following:
  - Prepare ahead of time to communicate with someone of a different communication style by letting others know your communication style before communicating

| Box 1.2 | **REMINDERS WHEN INTERACTING WITH THOSE WHO HAVE DIFFERENT COMMUNICATOR STYLES—cont'd** |

with them. They may not be familiar with the concept of the four animals; if, for example, you are a Lion, you could explain that you prefer factual information, and that you process it quickly. Ask the other person ahead of time what his or her communication style is. If the person is unfamiliar with the specific behavioral types of communication, you can ask questions such as, "Do you prefer to know facts first and details later?" and "Do you prefer if we get to know each other a little before we start on the project?" The answers to these questions can indicate how the person prefers to communicate.

• Slow down or speed up speech.
• Talk less and listen more.
• Be more succinct or precise.
• Expand your comments.
• Expect a long story.
• Consider the time and place for your communication.
• Tone down.
• Focus more or less on facts.
• Be aware of nonverbal cues.

Chapter Summary

In this chapter, we have covered the basics for effective communication with clients and colleagues. Such effective communication requires understanding how to properly establish a therapeutic relationship and the definition and components of communication. You must also understand the primary reasons communication fails and the qualities of effective and authentic communication. Finally, you must recognize that people have different communication styles, which can greatly affect how we communicate with one another. In the coming chapters, we consider some of the finer points of communication in greater detail.

Review Questions

Multiple Choice

1. Being willing to think about how communication affects other people involved and what is the best choice for everyone involved, not just what is best for the practitioner, is the definition for:

   a. Conscious communication
   b. Disclosure
   c. Auditory processor
   d. Intimacy

2. Establishing and maintaining safe and respectful boundaries with clients, peers, coworkers, employers, and family members are components of:

   a. Communities
   b. Appropriate disclosure
   c. Therapeutic relationships
   d. Behavior

3. Which of the following is an example of inappropriate communication that a practitioner may use with a first-time client?

a. Discussing the weather

b. Asking about political views

c. Questioning about health history

d. Asking permission to massage the abdominal area

4. The communication style characterized by being willing to state needs, opinions, and ideas is which of the following?

a. Analytical

b. Amicable

c. Peacemaker

d. Driven

5. When choosing to disclose to a client, which of the following questions should the practitioner ask herself regarding revealing the information?

a. Why am I doing this?

b. How will I benefit?

c. Will the client like me more?

d. What will the client reveal to me?

6. Which of the following strategies can a Puppy use when interacting with an Owl?

a. Pick up the pace

b. Talk more

c. Emphasize feelings

d. Be systematic

7. Language that does not use words is considered:

a. Verbal

b. Auditory

c. Nonverbal

d. Oral

Fill in the Blank

1. The bond formed between the practitioner and the client that is necessary for a positive treatment outcome for both the practitioner and the client is called the ____therapeutic relationship____.

2. Clear communication as the foundation of successful professional relationships means that a minimum of ____misunderstanding____ and a maximum of _____ occur.

3. During communication, the strongest messages are delivered through _____.

4. Being truly oneself in a conversation or interaction describes _____.

5. Being patient and being sure that all sides of an issue are discussed and considered describes a ____turtle____ communicator.

6. Language that uses words is considered ____verbal____.

7. The root of good communication is self-responsibility for _____ and ____actions, words____.

Short Answer

1. Describe the participation required of both practitioners and clients in the therapeutic relationship.

2. Explain each of the three communication styles based on the senses.

3. List and explain the six parts of communication.

☀**4.** Discuss at least four main reasons communication fails. (pg 12)

5. Describe at least four ways to ensure authentic communication.

6. List the four behavioral communication styles and the animal associated with each. List two or three traits associated with each style.

7. Explain at least five ways the practitioner can develop a healthy therapeutic relationship.

Activities

1. Self-Disclosure Activity
This exercise is designed to make you aware of your comfort levels for what you are willing to share with others. If you would be more comfortable, you may write your answers on a separate sheet of paper or even just keep them in your thoughts. The results of this exercise are not intended to be shared with anyone.

Fill in the following:

Write down something you think is very safe to disclose about yourself (e.g., I went to the movies last night).

_____

_____

With whom are you willing to share this and why? _____

_____

_____

Write down something you are selective about disclosing (e.g., My boyfriend and I are fighting and may separate).

_____

_____

With whom are you willing to share this and why? _____

_____

_____

Write down something you tell very few people (e.g., I am a sexual assault survivor).

_____

_____

With whom are you willing to share this and why? _____

_____

_____

_____

Write down something no one else knows about you. _____

_____

_____

Why are you not willing to share this with anyone? _____

_____

2. Self-Assessment Activity

People cannot communicate authentically unless they know who they themselves are. This activity is designed to encourage you to discover personal biases and beliefs, as well as to discern blaming, shaming, and judgmental language and behavior. It involves a series of questions regarding assumptions you may have about various races, religions, heritages, age groups, sexual orientations, and socioeconomic classes.

For each of the following, write what immediately comes to mind. Answer right away; do not stop and think about each one. Answering right away will show what you really think about each one.

Fat people   _____

Thin people   _____

Old people   _____

Young people (in their twenties) _____

Middle-aged people   _____

Teenagers   _____

Children   _____

Babies   _____

Christians   _____

Jews   _____

Muslims   _____

Asian people   _____

White people

African American people

Latino people

Foreigners

People with physical disabilities

People with developmental
disabilities

Gay people

People you think might be gay

Bisexual people

Straight people

Transgender people

Rich people

Poor people

Republicans

Democrats

People who belong to the
Green Party

People registered as Independent

Beautiful people

Ugly people

Celebrities

People who are HIV+

People who wear suits to work

People who work with
their hands

College graduates

People who have GEDs

People who read a lot

People who are illiterate

People who have AIDS

People from the North

People from the South

People from the Midwest

People from the West

People from New York City

People from California

People who like dogs

People who like cats

People who like birds

People who like snakes

Is there anything you would add to the list?

If you choose, you can share this activity with friends, mentors, classmates, and others you respect. If you choose to discuss it with others, how have your views changed as a result of the discussion?

3. Write the story of how you developed your communication style. How do you communicate? Where does your story start? How old were you? Who influenced you (who were your role models)? How has your style changed throughout your life? Is it working for you? If so, why? If not, why not and what would you change?

For those who do not want to write a narrative, another way to tell your story is through illustration. Make a timeline that has significant dates along it. These dates can include events that happen in your life, such as your first day of school and your first date, as well as events that influenced the development of your communication style and how your communication style has changed throughout your life.

4. Choose an animal other than the ones discussed in the section "Communication Styles Based on Behavior." Describe the characteristics of that animal, and relate these characteristics to how you communicate. The following list of questions may be helpful:

   • How are the general characteristics of your chosen animal humanly expressed?
   • How do these characteristics make it easy for you to communicate?
   • How do these characteristics make it difficult for you to communicate?
   • What misconceptions might others have about your chosen animal type when it comes to communication?
   • What would you like others to keep in mind when communicating with your animal type?

Guidance for Journaling

Often people are unaware of how ingrained their thoughts and behaviors are. They speak and act according to lifetimes of conditioning and subconscious reactions. Journaling is a way to become more self-aware of personal biases, beliefs, and prejudices, and can be a method of discarding old, useless ways of thinking and behaving. By writing down feelings and responses to the information in this chapter, you can see how it applies in your own life, historically and day to day. By journaling, you can track your personal and professional growth and emotional connection with your clients and the massage and bodywork profession.

The journaling can be as long or as short as you wish. Some people may choose to write a few sentences, whereas some may write pages. Journaling is not meant to be a difficult exercise, but one in which readers have, perhaps, an "Aha!" moment, recognizing personal truths and making breakthroughs for healthier communication.

Some key areas to think about while journaling for this chapter are the following:

- The connection between trust and the therapeutic relationship
- The role communication plays in the therapeutic relationship
- What language means to you
- What your personal style of communication is
- How you developed your style of communication
- How your style of communication has been beneficial to you as well as how it has created challenges for you
- What authentic communication means to you
- What you would like to change about how you communicate, and how you would go about it

References

1. Oltmanns, T.F., and Emery, R.E.: *Abnormal Psychology,* ed. 6. Upper Saddle River, NJ, Prentice Hall, 2007, p 540.
2. Mehrabian, F.: Inference of attitude from nonverbal communication in two channels. *Journal of Counseling Psychology* 31:248–252, 1967.
3. Tubbs, S.L., and Moss, S.: *Human Communication: Principles and Contexts,* ed. 10. Columbus, OH, McGraw-Hill, 2006, pp 24–27.
4. Adler, R.B., and Rodman, G.: *Understanding Human Communication,* ed. 10. New York, Oxford University Press, 2009, p 183.
5. Bolton, R., and Bolton, D.G.: *People Styles at Work . . . and Beyond: Making Bad Relationships Good and Good Relationships Better,* ed. 2. New York, AMACOM, 2009.

Professional Presentation of Self

LEARNING OBJECTIVES

After studying this chapter, you will be able to:

1. Explain the impact of first impressions.

2. Discuss how professionalism is reflected in the personal presentation of bodywork practitioners.

3. Delineate the factors involved in creating a therapeutic environment.

4. Explain how societal views of language are not necessarily appropriate for bodywork practitioners.

5. Describe how the pace and rhythm of speech as well as body language affect communication.

6. Explain ways to develop and refine personal and professional verbal and nonverbal language.

7. Discuss appropriate ways in which practitioners should use telephones, e-mail, texting, Web sites, and electronic calendars.

8. Define the components of a mission statement.

9. Outline the different types of written communication necessary in the bodywork profession, and explain how to write each of these.

CHAPTER OUTLINE

First Impressions

Personal Appearance

    Attire

    Personal Hygiene and Grooming

       Oral Hygiene

    Tattoos and Piercings

Therapeutic Environment

Verbal and Nonverbal

Communication

    Accountability and Transparency in Communication

    Word Choice

       Impact of Slang

       Impact of Sexual Innuendo

    Pace and Rhythm of Speech

    Body Language

    Developing and Refining Professional Verbal and Nonverbal Language

Electronic Communication

    Telephones

    E-mail

    Texting

    Professional Web Sites

    Social Networking Web Sites

    Electronic Calendars

    Learning to Unplug

Written Communication

    Mission Statements

    Business Cards

    Brochures and Pamphlets

    Cover Letters, Résumés, and Business Letters

    Intake and Documentation Forms

    Calendar for Client Appointments

Chapter Summary

Review Questions

Activities

Guidance for Journaling

KEY TERMS

Assessment: an evaluation

Chronological résumé: lists employment history in order of dates of employment

Functional résumé: organizes experience by category

Innuendo: hinting at something, but not quite coming out and saying it

Integrity: the quality of transparency and accountability in words and actions

Mission statements: brief statements of the purpose of a company, an organization, a group, or an individual

Presence: the quality of staying focused and centered, specifically during client interactions and treatments (as in being present), but applicable to any interchange

Tactile: relating to the sense of touch

You are a client arriving for your first treatment with a new massage therapist. As you come through the door, you find the massage therapist sitting on the receptionist's desk having a loud and emotional conversation on her cell phone. Her head is turned away, and she does not seem to notice you. You see that she is wearing a tank top, athletic shorts, and flip-flops. You take a seat and wait, feeling awkward and unsure that you are in the right place. Finally, with a string of obscenities, the therapist snaps her cell phone shut and jumps down off the desk. As she looks around, she sees you, nods her head, and says, "You must be my one o'clock. Do you mind if I take a quick smoke?" She brushes past you with her cigarette pack in hand and walks outside.

How you present yourself to your clients and colleagues is a critical aspect of communication. Considering the previous scenario, how likely would you be to stay for a massage with that therapist? How likely is that therapist to have a successful massage practice, given the way she presents herself?

To help you present yourself in as professional a manner as possible, this chapter covers the importance of making a good first impression and how to ensure a professional personal appearance and an effective therapeutic environment.

Another aspect of self-presentation considered in this chapter is verbal and nonverbal communication. Current societal views of language, including slang, sexual innuendo, and outdated terms, and how they affect the bodywork profession are discussed in detail. The pace and rhythm of speech and nonverbal language, or body language, are also covered. Methods to refine personal and professional verbal and nonverbal language are offered for practitioner self-development.

The influence of technology on communication is discussed, as well as how to use telephones, e-mail, Web sites, and electronic calendars effectively. Written communication is also important in the bodywork profession. How to write mission statements, business cards, brochures and pamphlets, cover letters, résumés and business letters, intake forms and documentation forms, and calendars for client appointments to project a professional image rounds out the chapter.

First Impressions

First impressions are just that: the split-second impression made when first looking at someone. It is important that you, as a present or future practitioner, recognize the value of presenting yourself and your treatment space professionally. You need to be aware of the first impressions you are making on others. Clients, colleagues, potential employers, and business contacts, to name a few, will judge you on your appearance and that of your treatment space. Many times they will base their decisions on whether to work with you on their first impressions.

There are many aspects to consider when trying to make a good first impression. One is visual impact. What does the client see when he looks at the practitioner? What does the client see when he looks at the treatment space? There is also an auditory component. What words and tone does the practitioner use when speaking? What kind of music is played during the treatment? Tactile impressions are made as well. How firm is the practitioner's handshake? How soft are the linens used during treatment? What type of pressure does the practitioner use during the treatment?

Just as important as all of these is the energetic aspect of the practitioner. This may also be thought of as the practitioner's **presence.** More than just poise and how the practitioner carries herself, although these are important, presence is the quality of staying focused and centered. It is most often used to describe the quality the practitioner should exhibit during client interactions and treatments (being present). However, it is also important that practitioners exhibit it any time they are engaging with someone else. That way, presence is a sincere part of their personality, not something they "put on" for their clients. By being present, you are perceived by others as being genuine. People respond much more positively to those who are genuine, which will increase your chances of career success in the bodywork profession.

When meeting someone for the first time, a visual **assessment** is usually the first measure taken. An assessment is an evaluation. In the case of bodywork, the client's assessment takes in the practitioner's clothes, hygiene, hairstyle, makeup, skin art (tattoos and piercings), jewelry, complexion, the eyes—color of the whites and clarity (whether they look watery or bloodshot)—posture, gait, body size, and level of fitness, such as whether the muscles look toned. Practitioners, of course, also visually assess their clients using these same criteria but with an eye toward developing the appropriate treatment plan for the client. Potential clients visually assess the practitioner to decide whether they want to receive a treatment from him.

Clients also visually assess the treatment space. This includes the outside of the building such as what building materials were used (brick, wood, or concrete, for example), the color of the building, the surface and surroundings of the parking area, what materials were used for the walkways, what the entryway looks like—what the front door is made of and what color it is, if there are any windows, and how clean and well maintained everything is. Inside, the colors and style of decorating, artwork, cleanliness, degree of clutter, what the furnishings look like, and the general layout of the treatment space are all assessed. The cleanliness and condition of the equipment and supplies are evaluated, as well.

Tactile (relating to the sense of touch) impressions include how firm the practitioner's handshake is, as well as how present the practitioner is. As discussed previously, people instinctively know when someone is not present. The depth of touch with the first massage stroke or other bodywork technique can speak volumes to a new client. The practitioner's confidence level can be felt in the quality of his touch, and his presence, or lack of presence, shows in his touch as well. In the treatment room, how soft the linens are as well as the feel of any lubricant used also make a first tactile impression.

First impressions are also made auditorily. The practitioner's pace of speaking in the initial greeting and when starting the actual treatment, the choice of words, the tone used, how smooth the flow of words is, and how confident the voice sounds all make an impact. Within the treatment space, auditory impressions include how much traffic noise is heard inside, how much noise other practitioners and clients make, how loudly or softly others speak, and any sounds produced by decorations such as fountains and wind chimes. The choice of music played during the treatment also has a big impact: what style of music it is, how loud or soft it is, and how clear it is.

Next, we consider personal appearance, therapeutic environment, and verbal and nonverbal communication in greater depth.

Personal Appearance

Unfortunately, bodywork has long been associated with unsavory professions, such as prostitution. Even today, some consumers still connect it to the adult entertainment industry. This is why practitioners and bodywork organizations have worked hard through the years, and continue to work hard, to educate the public on the legitimacy of the bodywork profession and the benefits of treatments, to increase educational requirements, to set standards for licensing, and to conduct scientific research into the effectiveness of bodywork treatments. They have strived to present themselves as skilled health-care professionals and healing arts practitioners. In short, bodywork professionals have worked hard to be taken seriously.

One way to combat the association of bodywork, especially massage therapy, with sex and to promote a professional image is to take care with your personal appearance. This includes your attire, personal hygiene and grooming, and displaying of tattoos and piercings. It is, of course, important to maintain a professional image while you are working but keep in mind, however, that you are always representing the bodywork profession. The choices you make about your personal appearance when you are not working can affect your bodywork career. For example, you never know when or where you might encounter a potential client. Many practitioners have handed out their business cards after having a casual conversation with someone in line at the grocery store or bank. If such an opportunity arises for you, the chances of the potential client actually scheduling a treatment with you are greatly increased if you appear professional than if you do not.

Attire

Unfortunately, in current Western society, especially in the United States, the latest fashions are not appropriate dress for bodywork practitioners. For women, these fashions include tight tops that show cleavage (in varying amounts), stomachs, and low backs. Pants and shorts tend to be designed to ride low on the hips, with the shorts being very short. For men, current fashion includes loose, baggy pants and shorts that ride low on the hips or even below them. Some fashionable shirts are very baggy, some are tight, and some are cut so that the underarms and the chest are exposed during movement.

Sometimes practitioners argue that because this type of clothing is currently in fashion, it should be considered appropriate to practice bodywork in. Some bodywork students do not understand why their school's dress code prohibits low-cut shirts, low pants, short shorts, or tight clothing. When given information on what proper dress should be, some react with disbelief or anger. These practitioners view being fashionable as being professional, which is not always the case.

A major part of being taken seriously as a legitimate professional is through being professionally dressed. Sometimes being dressed unprofessionally invites uncomfortable situations and outcomes. For example, for women, not only does this type of clothing restrict movement, but as the practitioner moves, greater amounts of cleavage are exposed, and, because of gaps between shirts and the waistband of pants or shorts, either the top of the underwear or the top of the gluteal cleft is exposed. Practitioners who wear this type of clothing may spend time pulling down their shirts and pulling up their pants as they work, but this breaks contact with the client and disrupts the flow of the treatment. It also sends a nonverbal message that certain clients may interpret as, at best, an invitation to make suggestive remarks or, at worst, an indication that sexual services are available.

Male practitioners who wear the type of clothing described as current fashion may find their clothing catching on the massage table (if performing treatments on a massage table) as they move around it, or their pants or shorts slipping down as they move, possibly exposing underwear. Clients can interpret this type of dress as a sign of a lack of professional bodywork skills. They may think, "If he's wearing the clothes of a teenager, did he even bother to learn anything in massage school? I don't want to get a treatment from him." Of course, this message is not what the practitioner intends and is likely very far from how he perceives himself and his skill level. However, despite being highly skilled and having good intentions, a practitioner who dresses unprofessionally can lose prospective clients.

"Clothes make the person" is often quoted in the business world. According to http://www.askandyaboutclothes.com, a Web site devoted to men's clothing advice, "Dressing badly can be taken as contempt for other people or the situation you are in. Clothing is a way to show others that you have respect and consideration for the situation."[1] It is true in the healing arts world of business, as well. Professional practitioners should wear clothes that match the setting in which they work, meaning that they mirror the clothing others in the business or the environment wear.

 Food for Thought

What do think professional dress consists of? Why do you think this is professional? How do you think what you wear affects how you perform treatments?

For example, practitioners working in the spa setting are often required to wear a specific uniform chosen by the employer that is either issued to them or that they must purchase. A practitioner who has a chair massage account at a law firm would look unprofessional providing treatments in jeans and a T-shirt, because the clients will likely be wearing suits, ties, and dress shirts and blouses. A clean, wrinkle-free polo shirt, khaki pants, and clean athletic shoes would be more appropriate. On the other hand, practitioners providing bodywork treatments at an athletic charity event, such as an outdoor walk or run, would be more appropriately dressed in clean, wrinkle-free shorts or casual pants and T-shirts.

Some employers of bodywork practitioners, other than spas, also require practitioners to wear uniforms. Some companies do not have a specific uniform requirement but instead have a dress code that delineates what is acceptable and what is not acceptable for practitioners to wear, and these codes vary in how strict they may be. For example, the dress code of one company may require practitioners to wear scrubs but does not specify what color. For another company, the dress code may specify neat pants and a polo shirt. For yet another company, the dress code may be neat khaki pants or shorts, but not cargo pants or cargo shorts, and a shirt of solid color without advertising. The shirt can be short sleeved or sleeveless, but cannot be a tank top.

Self-employed practitioners have the most freedom in choosing what to wear. But with the freedom of being able to choose what to wear comes the responsibility of being professionally dressed. For some, this may mean scrubs. For others, this may mean neat jeans and nice T-shirts. Some practitioners consider only pants of a solid color (but not jeans) and polo shirts professional.

Consider the following questions when deciding on professional dress:

- Do the clothes fit? They should be loose enough to allow movement while performing treatments. Pants and shorts that are tight enough to outline genitalia and shirts that are tight enough to outline breasts are unprofessional. Shorts that are short enough to reveal the practitioner's gluteals when bending over are unprofessional.
- Do the clothes match? Are they appropriate for the work setting?
- Are the clothes clean? They should never smell of body odor or be grimy in appearance.
- Are there other odors associated with the clothing such as strong scents from essential oils or laundry detergents? Many clients have allergies or chemical sensitivity to scents.
- Do they look neat? Because the bodywork profession is less formal than are other professions, a casual appearance is more acceptable. However, this casual appearance should not include wearing clothes that look like they were picked up off the floor or out of the laundry basket.
- Is the clothing free of advertising slogans, sayings, or logos that are considered offensive by the general public? For example, a practitioner may think that marijuana use should be legalized and is not offended by clothing that has marijuana leaf designs on it. However, most clients would choose not to receive a treatment from a practitioner wearing a T-shirt with a giant marijuana leaf on it.

- Are the clothes thick enough so that undergarments cannot be seen through them?
- Are the footwear and socks clean and in good condition? Some types of bodywork, such as shiatsu and Thai massage, require the practitioner to be shoeless. Practitioners can either wear clean socks or perform the treatments in bare feet. If barefoot, the feet should be clean and odorless.

Figure 2.1 shows examples of practitioners wearing unprofessional dress. Figure 2.2 shows examples of practitioners wearing professional dress.

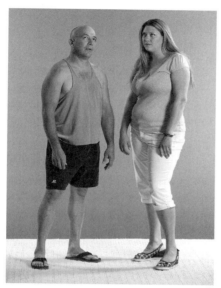

Figure 2.1 Practitioners wearing unprofessional dress.

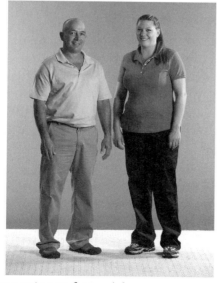

Figure 2.2 Practitioners wearing professional dress.

Part of being professional for women is dressing so that attention is not drawn to the breasts. Women practitioners should wear a bra or some other sort of undergarment that will support the breasts so they do not hang freely or look sexually inappropriate for the professional bodywork setting. It is important for women to be comfortable as they work, so it is worth the time and effort to find the proper-fitting undergarment.

Practitioners should consider the thickness of shirts worn. If the shirt is thin, there is a good possibility nipples will show through, even when wearing a supportive undergarment. Also, it is a physiological fact that breast nipples respond to colder temperatures by becoming more prominent. Women may want to consider using nipple covers or padded bras to prevent the nipples from being noticed.

Part of being professional for men is dressing so that attention is not drawn to the genitalia. In addition to not wearing shorts and pants that are so tight as to outline genitalia, practitioners should wear undergarments that will provide enough support for genitalia so that they are not noticeable or distracting as the practitioner walks, or while the practitioner works. This is especially true for bodywork practitioners who perform treatments such as shiatsu and Thai massage. Because of the nature of the body mechanics involved in these modalities, practitioners' legs and trunk are close to the client, much more so than during massage therapy. This is especially true when treatments are performed on futons on the floor, although it also applies when these treatments are performed on massage tables.

The shoes professionals wear should also support their professional image and provide safety on the job. Closed-toe shoes, such as athletic shoes, are the best choice. They provide support to the practitioner's body during the performance of the treatment, and can protect the toes when practitioners move heavy equipment, such as massage tables and chairs. Because athletic shoes that are worn for everyday use pick up a lot of dirt and grime, practitioners may want to consider designating one pair for professional practice and wear them only while performing treatments. If practitioners prefer open-toe shoes, they should make sure that their feet are clean and that the shoes are odorless.

The height of the shoe is also an important consideration. For proper body mechanics, shoes that are flat and low to the ground are the best option. It is not professional to wear high heels or platform type shoes for bodywork, as it puts the practitioner at risk for injury. Practitioners have even been known to break an ankle giving a massage in platform shoes.

Moreover, clients may make assumptions about the type of massage or treatment they will receive based on the style of shoes the practitioner is wearing. For example, practitioners wearing high heels with open toes and having red-painted toenails may give a client the idea that these bodywork practitioners do more than give a therapeutic treatment. He may think that sexual services are available and all he has to do is ask. Wearing sensible shoes is one way to avoid sending the wrong nonverbal message to clients, and thus avoid unnecessary and perhaps unsafe situations.

Personal Hygiene and Grooming

When choosing to work in the bodywork profession, which requires close physical contact with others, we must recognize that certain actions must be taken to make the experience pleasant for both parties. It is essential that all practitioners be diligent in their hygiene and grooming habits. Daily baths are a must; body odor is detected quickly by clients, especially in the small confines of a treatment room with little or no ventilation. In addition, performing bodywork is a physical activity. Practitioners should check the effectiveness of their deodorant. If they prefer not to use aluminum-based antiperspirants, then they must be sure to wash under their arms between sessions and reapply the deodorant they do use. A treatment that may have been effective otherwise can quickly become an unpleasant experience for clients if the practitioner has body odor.

Fingernails should be short so that they do not scratch the client, and so that they do not become havens for bacteria. Because cracked nail polish provides crevices for bacterial growth, the nails should not be painted. For those practitioners who are barefoot when giving a treatment, the feet must be absolutely clean and odor-free, with no fungus in the toenails. Barefoot practitioners may consider investing in receiving regular pedicures to keep the feet neatly groomed.

Hair must be clean and combed or brushed, kept out of the practitioner's eyes, and not allowed to touch the client during the massage treatment. Therefore, it may need to be tied back. Practitioners should also consider choosing hairstyles that are appropriate for their workplace setting. For example, practitioners who practice in trendy salons may attract more clientele if their hairstyles are in the latest fashion. Conversely, short, spiky, multicolored hair may be off-putting, even frightening, to clients in assisted living facilities, and a more subdued color and style may be more appropriate.

It is also worthwhile for practitioners to inventory all their grooming products to see if they are highly scented. With the increase in clients who are allergic to certain chemicals or have chemical sensitivity, the less scents there are, the better so as to not limit clientele or, more important, cause a client to have an adverse physical reaction.

Oral Hygiene

An important part of personal hygiene is oral hygiene. Practitioners should not only make sure they do not have body odor, but that they are free from mouth odors as well. Sometimes breath mints may be all that is required to cover or eliminate mouth odors. Often, they are not. The best option is to brush the teeth and use mouthwash after eating or drinking beverages such as coffee and tea. There have been many times an otherwise enjoyable treatment has been ruined by a practitioner with bad breath.

Those who smoke and use other products such as chewing tobacco need to pay particular attention to the effects these substances have on the breath and, in the case of cigarette smoking, the smell of the smoke clinging to their clothing. If the person is a particularly heavy tobacco user, nicotine can also emerge from the pores of their skin, adding to the overall unpleasant odor a tobacco user carries around with him or her.

Consider the following:

Robert is a smoker who recently started massage school. The school requires smokers to wash hands, brush teeth, and use mouthwash after smoking and before returning to class. He disagrees with these policies, however.

"I can't smell smoke on myself and my breath mints work better than brushing my teeth," he thinks to himself. He also thinks his cologne is helpful to cover up the smell of cigarette smoke.

After a couple weeks of classes, Robert is having a hard time finding different classmates to pair up with for the hands-on classes. He is able to work only with the two other smokers in the class. He wants to experience other students' skills, but is always being turned down. He also notices that he is not included in the study groups that students have at their homes, and this makes him feel left out. He feels more and more like an outsider in his own class, and he begins to resent the other students.

Out of frustration, Robert approaches one of the women in his class, Liz, and asks her why the class "has it out for the smokers." Liz does not mince words. "Because you all smell like an ashtray. I choose not to smoke. I resent you and the other students coming back from break smelling up the room. I don't like dealing with your secondhand smoke and I don't want to lie on the massage table and have some smoker breathe on me. It's gross! I don't know how you expect to get clients smelling like that. This is a health-care profession. I don't understand why you want to go into this field with a habit that is so destructive to your health, and makes getting a massage horrible for the client. I don't get it."

Robert is stunned. He had never had someone be so blunt with him about smelling like an ashtray nor did he realize that his breath was bad. Liz's feedback was hard to hear, but it got Robert's attention. He decides to contact an organization in town that teaches smoking cessation classes, and starts the long and slow process of kicking the habit.

Tattoos and Piercings

Tattoos and piercings have become a popular form of self-expression in our culture. They are now seen on people from many economic, social, and cultural backgrounds. Despite their increasing prevalence, however, many people still regard them as offensive or as having negative connotations. In the workplace, in particular, practitioners who have them are often viewed as unprofessional.

As a bodywork professional, you should consider how tattoos and piercings will be perceived by your clients. Consider the possibility that upon seeing a bodywork practitioner with multiple piercings on the face, nose, lips, and ears, a client may make the assumption that the practitioner likes to feel pain. The client may be afraid the practitioner will hurt her by using too much pressure during the application of techniques. On the other hand, the client might be very curious and ask the practitioner lots of invasive and personal questions throughout the session, questions that the practitioner may not be comfortable answering.

If you plan on a versatile bodywork career, including working with conservative clientele, then you may choose to have body art on those body parts that can be concealed with clothing. Conversely, if you work exclusively with a clientele who are more accepting of tattoos and piercings, the placement of body art may be a nonissue, as long as you present yourself professionally. Note, though, that tattoos and piercings are not acceptable by many bodywork employers. Depending on the placement of the body art, you may not be hired because of them, or, if hired, be required to conceal them while working. Facial piercings may be required to be removed while the practitioner is at his or her place of employment.

If the tattoos portray violence, pornography, or other objectionable topics, then it might be prudent for those having such emblems to have some work done to make them more presentable within the profession. It is also possible for tattoos to be covered up with body makeup if necessary. Because the makeup can be smeared or transferred to the client's body, it will not be effective for covering tattoos on the hands and forearms of practitioners who use lubricant in their treatments, or the hands, forearms, and legs of practitioners who perform modalities such as shiatsu and Thai massage. However, it can be used to cover up tattoos elsewhere, such as the face and neck. If practitioners wish to remove tattoos permanently, laser treatments are an option to explore.

Be aware of how you physically present yourself to clients, peers, colleagues, employers, and prospective employers. If you are unsuccessful in meeting your professional goals and you suspect it could be due to your appearance, seek out mentors and peers to ask for feedback and suggestions for changes.

Therapeutic Environment

When choosing a location in which to practice, whether it be someone else's business or your own, important considerations are the messages the building and treatment spaces are communicating to clients. The building should be clean and well maintained, both inside and out. Parking areas should be convenient and well maintained, an especially important consideration for disabled or frail clients.

The atmosphere within the therapeutic environment should be warm, welcoming, and tastefully decorated. Granted, not everyone's taste is the same, but the message sent should be one of health and healing. Much research has been done on the impact that colors have on the psyche. Bright colors increase energy, whereas muted colors or earth tones bring about calm and relaxation. A combination can do a little of both, depending on the placement and design. Be mindful of this concept and decorate accordingly to meet the goals of the business.

Some other therapeutic environment factors you should consider include the following:

- Traffic noise should be minimal, as well as noise from other businesses nearby.
- Cigarette smoking should be banned from inside the office as well as at least 20 feet from any doors because of the odor and health risk to clients.
- Heating and cooling appliances should be in good working order and operate quietly.
- Seating in the waiting area should be comfortable and plentiful.
- Bathrooms should be conveniently located and kept utterly spotless.
- Equipment should be maintained and kept in excellent working order to prevent injury to both clients and practitioners.

- Supplies should be clean and fresh.
- If fountains, wind chimes, and other such items decorate the office, the sounds they make should not be distracting.

The treatment room itself should be designed to enhance relaxation and calm. These can be brought about with the use of room colors, subdued lighting (avoid using overhead lights that shine directly into the eyes when the client is supine), and the colors of linens and blankets (avoid using sheets with childish prints on them; they send a message of unprofessionalism). Also, practitioners should consider eliminating as much clutter as possible within the treatment room. This can be a safety issue as well as an aesthetic issue. Figure 2.3 shows an example of a cluttered treatment space and an example of a cleared treatment space.

The art in the room should be tasteful and inspire relaxation. Again, not everyone's taste is the same, but art that is more "edgy" may also make clients more edgy. Music should be soft and mellow for relaxation, or can be more upbeat if a vigorous treatment is being performed or if the client requests it. Songs that have lyrics that are sexually suggestive, political, obscene, or hate filled do not inspire relaxation and should not be played. Sometimes clients bring in their own music; this is fine as long as it does not compromise the practitioner's ability to provide effective treatment.

Verbal and Nonverbal Communication

Your verbal and nonverbal communication with clients and colleagues is another critical aspect of presenting yourself in a professional manner. What follows is a discussion about accountability and transparency in communication, pace and rhythm of speech, body language, and development of professional verbal and nonverbal communication.

As bodywork practitioners, the majority of communication with clients is nonverbal through therapeutic touch. The message that the touch gives to the client will determine how successful the therapeutic relationship will be. Does the touch communicate a sense of compassion and skill? Does it feel uncertain and hesitant? Does the client feel that the practitioner is rushed or just going through the motions without being present?

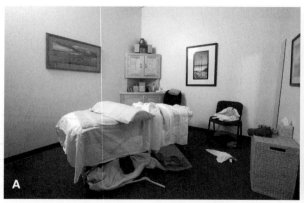 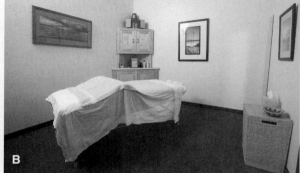

Figure 2.3 Treatment space. (A) Cluttered. (B) Neat.

However, nonverbal communication plays another important role in all of our connections with others. It is the way in which we communicate volumes without saying a word. Consider the steely glare a practitioner gives to a client who is late for an appointment the third week in a row. The client knows immediately that he has crossed a boundary; however, the practitioner may not even be aware that the glare was given.

Much nonverbal communication is performed unconsciously and is directly related to our emotions and how we are feeling about what has just occurred. According to Adler and Rodman, "Nonverbal communication performs the social function of conveying emotions that we may be unwilling or unable to express—or ones we may not even be aware of. Further, nonverbal communication is much better suited to expressing attitudes and feelings than ideas."[2]

Accountability and Transparency in Communication

As a professional, you should strive to be accountable and transparent in your communication with clients and colleagues. When you have made a mistake with a client, be quick to acknowledge the mistake thoroughly and clearly and apologize for it. All too often, when people make a mistake, they may simply shrug it off and the conversation continues without discussing how or why the mistake happened. It is as if accountability for how the mistake occurred, and could be prevented in the future, is not needed as long as there is an acknowledgment, no matter how brief, that someone erred.

If an issue or an incident makes dealing with a client or colleague problematic, it may be tempting not to challenge the person who may be responsible, but to move on. This quick moving on frees both parties from the job of sorting out what happened and how to prevent it from happening again. Conversely, some people, when confronted with some transgression, deny or even deflect responsibility back to the person who is objecting to their words and behavior, sometimes in a threatening manner. Holding others accountable, then, turns into a risky venture. To protect your relationship with your client, however, you should make every effort on your own part to be accountable for your mistakes and ready to apologize for them.

You should also be careful to be transparent in your communication, and not try to purposely cover up or be deceptive about something you have said or done. Too often, people use language to "spin," or create an alternative story about a situation. The speaker tries to backtrack and say something different to make himself appear more favorable to others or to get his expectations met. "That's not what I meant to say"; "You misunderstood what I was saying"; "I didn't mean to say that"; "My words were taken out of context." These are phrases that pepper conversation when expectations are not met in how the message is received. Such attempts to conceal the truth of what one has said can create a barrier to genuine connection, trust, and rapport with others.

Although such lack of accountability and transparency is common in everyday life, it is neither acceptable nor professional for bodywork practitioners. Practitioners should develop the traits of transparency and accountability in words and actions, which is another way of saying that they should behave with **integrity**. Being true to one's word and acting with integrity are the best ways, and the only ways, to develop trust and rapport with clients.

Food for Thought

Think of a time you had a conversation with someone in which their words and actions were clear, but instead of taking responsibility for them, he or she "spun" the situation. How did you feel? What did you think of the person? What would you have liked for him or her to say instead of "spinning"?

Misunderstandings occur all the time. It is how the practitioner handles misunderstanding that can make the difference in whether the therapeutic relationship can be maintained. For example, Max has an appointment scheduled with Ben for 5:30 p.m. on Saturday. When Max arrives at Ben's office at 5:15 p.m., Ben is getting in his car to meet friends for dinner. Ben is surprised to see Max and asks him what he is doing there. Max, equally surprised, says, "I have an appointment with you in 15 minutes."

At this point, Ben has several options: He can tell Max that Max is wrong and should call some other time for an appointment. Max may or may not accept this. If he does not, Ben has lost him as a client. Ben could turn around and give Max the treatment he is expecting. But this requires changing his plans and may make him resentful toward Max. Neither one of these solutions involves accountability or transparency.

In an effort to prevent any harm to the therapeutic relationship, or lose Max's trust and respect, Ben's best option is to acknowledge that there is clearly a misunderstanding, to say that he is not able to give Max a treatment at this time, and to ask how he and Max can work together to resolve this issue. Blame does not have to be assigned to anyone. Ben is being accountable by acknowledging that there is an issue, and he is being transparent by saying that he cannot give Ben a treatment at this time. He is being both accountable and transparent by being willing to discuss the issue with Max and come up with a solution.

Word Choice

In addition to communicating with integrity, it is important to choose the right words when communicating with clients and colleagues. Avoid using slang, sexual innuendo, and outdated terms in your communication, as they can damage your professional presentation of self.

Impact of Slang

Although slang words are a common feature in everyday language, they are not appropriate in your professional communication. For example, although the use of certain words may be quite acceptable to use among friends, they may not be appropriate to use with clients. Keep in mind that your clients may not be familiar with a slang term you use, and therefore might be confused by it. Also, use of slang communicates a level of familiarity with someone that is often inappropriate for formal, professional relationships. Moreover, despite your attempt to be up-to-date and accessible to your clients, they may interpret your use of slang as a lack of professional knowledge or skill. If clients are to trust their bodies to a practitioner, they want to have a good impression of his ability to communicate the needs of the session. For all of these reasons, it is important that you strive to use standard terminology in your professional communication. Be careful to review your use of language, especially if you are prone to using slang in your communication, and make a concerted effort to eliminate any unprofessional terminology.

Consider the following:

Practitioner: Hey gal, how ya doing today?
New Client: Good, I guess.

Practitioner: Fab! What do you want me to work out today?
New Client: Work out? Like at the gym?
Practitioner: No, I mean on your body.
New Client: Um, my back I guess. It's kind of sore.
Practitioner: Snap! I just took a rockin' class on low back work. It will blow you away.
New Client: You're giving me a treatment using rocks?
Practitioner: No, I took a great class on fixing back pain. It rocked! You'll be in nirvana and will forget you ever had a sore back. Feel me?
New Client: What?! I'm not going to feel you!
Practitioner: No, I mean are you straight? Can I use my new tools on your back?
New Client: I don't think it's any of your business if I'm straight and I don't want you using any tools on my body. I'm leaving.

Obviously, the client is not following what is being said by the practitioner, and the practitioner is not picking up on cues that the client is uneasy. Disaster ensues. It is your job to communicate to the client in a fashion that will instill trust, build rapport, and create safety.

Impact of Sexual Innuendo

Another type of language that should be carefully guarded against in professional communication is sexual **innuendo.** Innuendo is hinting at something, but not quite coming out and saying it. Sexual innuendo is particularly harmful in the bodywork profession (massage therapy, in particular), as the profession is still often "joked" about as being part of the sex industry. It is essential that all practitioners correct this image any time they are confronted with, for example, the raised eyebrow or the worn-out jokes about providing happy endings. If practitioners do not take on each and every one of these insults, then they are tacitly telling the "jokester" that it is okay to associate bodywork with sex.

The following are some suggestions on how to become comfortable addressing these types of remarks:

- Practitioners have the right to be treated with dignity and respect.
- Think of addressing the remarks as an opportunity to educate the person or persons making them. Many times people are unaware of how what they are saying can be perceived as offensive.
- Talk about how massage and bodywork are part of the health-care profession.
- Talk about the education and licensing necessary to become a bodywork practitioner.
- Bring up the past connection of massage and bodywork to the sex industry, and mention how it is still perceived that way. Let the person or persons know that by making these remarks, they are applying them to every bodywork practitioner, including the one standing in front of them.
- Most people will get the message the first time. If not, take the risk of sounding like a broken record or limiting contact until they can show respect and understanding for the profession.

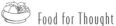

In addition to addressing sexual innuendo from others, you must also be careful not to use sexual innuendo yourself. Sometimes, practitioners inadvertently use sexual innuendo when they use terms that are meant as shortcuts to explaining the work. Examples include the following: "When can I do you?" to mean, "When can we schedule you for a treatment?" or "Can you do me?" to mean asking another practitioner for a treatment. The term "massage virgin" has also been used to describe a client who is receiving a massage for the first time. It is easy to slip into this type of casual language when talking with peers, but sometimes others who are not bodywork practitioners may overhear these conversations and draw the wrong conclusion. Practitioners need to be careful not to compromise their dignity and integrity or those of the profession.

There is also a great responsibility for all practitioners to explain to consumers that the term "massage parlor" is outdated because it implies prostitution. Terms that are much more current include "treatment office," "bodywork office," "bodywork establishment," and so forth. Likewise, the terms "masseuse" and "masseur" need to be addressed. These terms are also outdated. Not only do they have sexual implications, but "masseuse" refers to a female practitioner and "masseur "refers to a male practitioner. Often people do not make this distinction, with the result that male practitioners are sometimes called masseuses. Practitioners should take the opportunity to educate consumers that the current term is "massage therapist." This term is gender neutral and has less of a sexual connotation.

Pace and Rhythm of Speech

In addition to being mindful of the words you use, you should also pay attention to the pace and rhythm of your speech. Speech that is hesitant, stuttering, or stammering, or is peppered with "you know," "um," and "like" gives the impression that the person is not prepared, does not know what to say, or lacks self-confidence and confidence in his or her skills. Speech that is rapid-fire imparts a sense of impatience, and sends a message that the practitioner is not interested in listening, only in talking as fast as possible.

Speaking very quickly may signify that the practitioner is forgetting to breathe. In fact, some clients may be more focused on whether the practitioner is breathing or not than on what the practitioner is saying. Also, practitioners need to be aware that some clients have trouble following speech that is spoken rapidly. If you find yourself speaking too rapidly or your client looking puzzled, try taking a deep, calming breath and slowing down.

Body Language

Body language has a major impact on how people are perceived by others. If practitioners are not mindful of how they are walking, moving, or touching the client outside of the session (such as when walking them to and from the treatment room), then they might be misunderstood and possibly mistreated. For example, if practitioners walk in a suggestive manner and are wearing tight and revealing clothing, they should not be surprised that their roles as professional bodywork practitioners are not taken seriously. The client may misconstrue an innocent touch on the shoulder as a sexual invitation.

When considering physical contact with a client outside of a session, it is important to remember that just because a client comes to you to receive a therapeutic treatment, you should not assume that the client will welcome all touch from you. For example, although the client may have enjoyed receiving the treatment, she may be uncomfortable receiving a hug from you.

Fidgeting involves movements in which a person uses one part of his body to groom, rub, hold, pinch, pick, or otherwise manipulate another body part. The person may be unaware that he is producing these movements, but they can be highly distracting to a person observing him. The client may view the practitioner who fidgets as someone who lacks confidence, as someone who will rush through the treatment, or even as someone who has better things to do than give the client a treatment. If you recognize that you fidget, it would be helpful to develop some strategies to manage it. For some people, using an object to fidget with allows him or her to focus on the task at hand because the need to move has been taken care of by having an object to manipulate.[3] For example, try discreetly squeezing a small rubber ball or rubbing a paper clip while talking to a client.

Conversely, body language can also be used to communicate more effectively and positively with a client. Having a confident bearing can inspire confidence in clients. Having a confident bearing means that the practitioner stands up tall, with shoulders back, and has a stable stance. This body language is considered open, which indicates that the practitioner is welcoming interaction. Figure 2.4 shows a practitioner who does not appear confident and a practitioner who has a confident bearing. In Western culture, a firm handshake, but not one in which the hand is gripped painfully, is also regarded as open body language and an appropriate greeting. Moving gracefully, maintaining eye contact (if culturally appropriate), and smiling are

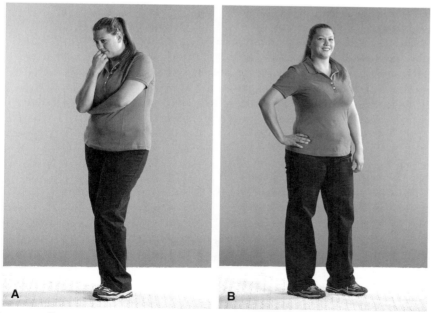

Figure 2.4 Practitioner body language. (A) Not confident. (B) Confident.

other ways to use body language to communicate interest, respect, and kindness to clients.

Practitioners also make an impression in the way they approach the client. Everyone operates in his or her own, internal rhythm, whether it be fast, slow, or somewhere in the middle. Evaluate your individual rhythm and make sure the message sent is the one intended. For example, if you walk quickly, it may be interpreted that you are in a hurry and not focused on the task at hand. Conversely, greeting the client at the last possible minute, while you saunter in talking on your cell phone might communicate that you consider that you are doing the client a favor by showing up at all. Be mindful of the fact that you are being observed and evaluated by your client. Make sure that you are conveying to her that there is nothing else you would rather be doing right now than attending to her needs.

Developing and Refining Professional Verbal and Nonverbal Language

The process of refining a professional image is ongoing and requires you to remain constantly aware of the verbal and nonverbal messages you are sending. Sometimes it is difficult to change behavior because it is what is familiar and therefore feels safe. Sometimes it never occurs to people that changes are possible. The first step is self-inquiry to assess what image you are projecting and whether it matches your intended professional image. The following are some questions to ask yourself:

What am I wearing and what image does it project? Is it the image I want to project?

How do I talk with my clients? Does it sound professional or does it include curse words, slang, or gossip? Am I talking more than they are and taking over the session?

Did I take enough time to prepare for the session so that I look graceful and confident rather than rushed and hurried?

Is there anything else that could be influencing how others react to me?

Seeking information on self-presentation from peers or someone you respect and consider a mentor can help give you an objective viewpoint. For such input to be effective, however, you will need to allow yourself to be vulnerable enough to ask direct questions about your behavior and image. If you do, it can be a huge step in professional development. Some questions you may ask of peers and mentors are the following:

- What has your experience been of my professional behavior/attire/language?
- What have you noticed about how others react to me?
- What information do you have for me that would enhance my professionalism?

Paying attention to how clients respond is another way to assess what image is being projected. For example, if clients ask you out often or behave inappropriately toward you, you may want to consider what messages you are sending to them. If you think you are wearing professional dress and using appropriate professional language and are still getting unwelcome advances from certain clients, then you must be willing to determine what else you may be doing that could prompt such a reaction. This inquiry is best done with friends, peers, supervisors, or clients you trust and who you know can be objective.

If the result of this assessment is that you are doing everything you can to present a professional image, then it might be time to reevaluate the therapeutic relationship with the client. You may need to educate the client clearly on the parameters of the therapeutic relationship or even let the client go.

■ CASE PROFILE

Mickey is a 60-year-old massage therapist. She has been in practice for more than 20 years. Mickey prides herself in being creative and wears colorful cotton clothes that often have bangles and sequins sewn on them, heavily scented essential oils, and flip-flops all year long. She experiments with different hair colors, makeup, and facial piercings. "Just because I'm 60 doesn't mean I have to stop living!" she tells her coworkers and clients.

Mickey's treatments usually begin 10 to 15 minutes past the start of the appointment time but she does not work longer to accommodate the late start. Sometimes Mickey shares with her clients during the sessions her displeasure with the economy, her supervisor at the clinic, or her sister who owes her money.

At a recent staff meeting, Mickey complains that she is very disappointed in the caliber of clients coming to the clinic. She states that she is not getting tipped very often, and that the clients rarely book another session with her, making it clear they are not committed to their own wellness. She says the clinic supervisor should take a look at the office's marketing strategies and see why they are not attracting more sophisticated clients. At this point, the clinic supervisor informs Mickey of the client retention rates of all the office's practitioners, and the overall average amount of tips each practitioner receives. It turns out that the other practitioners on staff are actually doing quite well. Mickey leaves the meeting feeling confused.

List the reasons that Mickey may not be able to maintain a clientele.

Describe Mickey's professional attitude.

If you were Mickey's supervisor, how would you advise her?

If you were Mickey, what steps would you take to change your situation?

Electronic Communication

To truly connect with someone, compassion, empathy, and a genuine interest in the other person as a separate, distinct human being and a willingness to be vulnerable are necessary. This is best accomplished when interacting directly, face-to-face. Fortunately, as a massage practitioner, most of your interaction with your clients will be in person, during sessions. However, your communication with your client will likely extend beyond face-to-face encounters to phone calls, e-mails, and other electronic interactions. Thus, you must also extend your commitment to present yourself professionally in these other media. Next, we consider how to

Words of Wisdom

I believe that a positive attitude is important. Happiness is received much better by clients than grumpiness. But the biggest thing for me is showing up for each and every appointment. I call the day before to confirm with my clients so that there is no confusion about when the appointment is. Clients don't stay around if the therapist cancels a lot. Have a good attitude, show up when you are supposed to, and do good work—that is what works for me.

—LAURA YATES, Massage Therapist since 1991

communicate professionally via the telephone, e-mail, Web sites, and electronic calendars.

Telephones

The telephone is the lifeline for most businesses, and this is especially true of the bodywork business. Telephones are used for a myriad of reasons. Clients use it to contact the business for information and to schedule, change, or cancel appointments. Practitioners use it to communicate with clients and other businesses and to gather information.

Landlines are still the most commonly used telephone service, although many practitioners also have cell phones. Some individual practitioners and businesses are switching to using cell phones exclusively. No matter which type of telephone you use, however, you need to be mindful of communicating effectively when using it. The following are some guidelines for using the phone in a professional manner:

- Record a professional greeting. The voice mail greeting represents you or the business you are a part of. It should be short, yet informative. In today's busy society, many people find it frustrating to have to wait for something to end, such as a song or a long greeting, before recording their message. In fact, many prospective clients will simply hang up and try another business. Also, the greeting should sound professional. Avoid having children record the greeting, having "cute" greetings, or having greetings that sound too casual.

An Example of a Bad Greeting

Thirty seconds of loud music starts the greeting. It is followed by a voice that sounds tired and pauses often between statements:

You have reached Mark Edgers, licensed massage therapist specializing in craniosacral therapy and reflexology. Thank you for calling. I'm sorry I'm not able to take your call right now. All of my calls are important to me. Please leave a message with your name, the time you called, the day you called, and the number for me to call you back. I will try to call you back within 48 hours. If you don't hear from me, please call me again as I may have lost your number. May you have a bright and glorious day.

Fifteen more seconds of music is heard before the tone signaling the caller to speak beeps.

An Example of Good Greeting

The greeting starts immediately. The voice is upbeat and friendly:

Hi. Thank you for calling Tess Catalano at the Wellness Center. Please leave a brief message with your name, phone number, even if you think I have it, and some possible times for me to return your call. I look forward to talking with you soon.

The tone signaling the caller to speak beeps immediately.

- Answer the phone when it rings. As much as possible, answer the phone personally when it rings. Although some practitioners let all their calls go to voice mail and then listen and respond to them all at once, this is not ideal. Most people prefer to talk to a live person, and clients calling for a bodywork appointment prefer to be seen as soon as possible.

- Do not use a business phone as a personal phone. Calls from clients can be delayed or missed while you are on a personal call. This is particularly important if you work as an employee in someone else's business. Often employers will have policies pertaining to personal use of a business phone. If that describes your work setting, be sure to familiarize yourself with phone policies and adhere to them.
- Avoid carrying on personal phone calls around clients. Conducting a personal phone call in the presence of a client can send the message that your personal matters are more important than those of your client. Moreover, you might reveal to your client more about your personal life than you wish to, or than your client wishes to know. Save personal calls for breaks, and make them in a private setting.
- Follow all of the guidelines for verbal communication when on the phone. Avoid using jargon, slang, suggestive language, or outdated terms. Be sure to speak at a pace that your client can follow and understand.
- Turn your cell phone off completely during treatment sessions. Some practitioners think that if they put the phone on vibrate it does not disturb the client. They think they need to know immediately when someone is trying to call them or send them a text message. However, the sound of the vibration is noticeable to some clients. It says that incoming calls are more important to the practitioner than the client he is with. Unless you are expecting an emergency phone call, it is considerate of your client, and professional, to turn off your cell phone during a session to avoid interruption and to focus completely on the client.

E-mail

E-mail can be used to communicate with clients to schedule treatments and send information such as the location of the treatment office, where an onsite treatment is to take place, and what type of treatments are available. As with all other forms of communication, how you communicate via e-mail can affect your professional image.

Even your e-mail address can make a significant impression on your client. For example, "popstar85@nnn.com" does not sound professional. Addresses that reflect your age, gender, or sexual orientation are inappropriate, as well those that are "cute," refer to alcohol or drugs, or contain sexual innuendo.

Also, avoid being overly casual in your e-mail communication. Because e-mail is typically viewed as an informal mode of communication, many people are sloppier and less careful with their messages than they would be otherwise. Avoid using abbreviations that your recipient may not understand, and be careful to double-check your spelling and grammar before sending the e-mail. More suggestions for keeping e-mails professional include the following:

- Never include personal information in business e-mails. You never know who else will be reading them.
- Keep your business contacts separate from your personal contacts by organizing them into different groups. This decreases your chances of accidentally sending information to the wrong people.

- Include a subject in the subject line. Many people organize their e-mails according to subject line and they may miss an important message if the subject line is blank.
- Make sure you attach any attachments. Often, people forget to do this. If you are prone to forgetting, attach the attachment to the e-mail first, then begin writing your message.
- Send only bodywork-related information to your clients. Do not, for example, send jokes, cartoons, or links to video clips you find humorous, or e-mails containing information that reflects your religious or political views. Even if you think you know your clients quite well, you run a high risk of offending one or more of them if they do not share your views.
- Do not inundate your client list and business contacts with e-mails. They may find this tiresome and start regarding your messages as spam.

Develop your thoughts well enough so that the reader does not have to guess at your meaning. Moreover, be careful not to send or respond to an e-mail when you are in an emotionally charged stage, such as being angry or upset, as you may use words or a tone that you may later regret. Take care before pressing Send. Figure 2.5 shows an example of an e-mail conversation gone wrong because of the vast room for error and misinterpretation in e-mail correspondence.

Another consideration is your clients' communication preferences. Some people do not like receiving information by e-mail because they interpret the informality as a lack of professionalism. They might think, for example, that you could not be bothered to communicate other than with a quick, dashed-off note. Also, many people do not check their e-mail inbox regularly, and thus may not receive your messages in a timely manner. If you do choose to communicate regularly with clients, be sure to check your e-mail inbox often (preferably at least daily), so that you do not miss important correspondence.

Texting

Texting is probably the newest form of communication, and it has become a phenomenon. In fact, according to the National Data Book of the U.S. Census Bureau, 110.4 billion text messages were sent in 2008. This is more than twice the number of text messages sent in 2007 (48.1 billion), and almost six times the number sent in 2006 (18.7 billion).[4] It is difficult now to walk down the street or visit a store or restaurant without seeing multitudes of people reading or sending text messages on their cell phone.

Like e-mail, texting is a way to send and receive information quickly and conveniently. It can be even more convenient if practitioners do not always have access to their e-mail account but do to their cell phone. It can be helpful to text clients for a number of reasons. Some examples include the following:

- Confirm appointments
- Let clients know about last-minute openings in your schedule
- Let clients know that they or you are running late
- Send mass business messages out to client lists for such things as treatment options available or a special discount. Practitioners should make sure they do not accidentally send out texts about personal matters to their client lists. They should also make sure they do not send text

From: PatsyQuijada@nnn.com
To: ChristyMorton@nnn.com
Sent: Tue, Jan 8 12:02 pm
Subject: BOUNCED CHECK!

Christy,

Your last check bounced. it cost me $25 in bank fees!!!! Please send me a chx ASAP for the amount of the tx plus the $25 bank fee. What gives? Hope you are OK.

Send the check, lol
Patsy

From: ChristyMorton@nnn.com
To: PatsyQuijada@nnn.com
Sent: Tue, Jan 8 3:04 pm
Subject: Bounced check

Patsy,

Please accept my apology for the inconvenience I caused you by having my check bounce. As you know my unemployment was coming to an end and I apparently miscalculated my balance in my checking account. Although I understand your frustration of having to deal with this, it was simply an oversight on my part. I do not appreciate being yelled at nor do I plan on not paying you as your email indicated. Your lack of sensitivity to my situation is appalling. I will send you your check ASAP.

Christy

From: PatsyQuijada@nnn.com
To: ChristyMorton@nnn.com
Sent: Tue, Jan 8 4:36 pm
Subject: Bounced check

Christy,

Wow! What happened? Of course I understand your situation. I was trying to be funny with my email, not upset you. I am mad at the bank for having such a ridiculous fee, not you. I am sorry I offended you. That was not my intention. There is no hurry on the check. I am sorry for the hurt you are feeling by my email.

Sincerely,
Patsy

From: ChristyMorton@nnn.com
To: PatsyQuijada@nnn.com
Sent: Tue, Jan 8 5:45 pm
Subject: Bounced check

Patsy,

Thank you for your apology. I've already put a check in the mail to you. I'm not sure when I'll be able to come in for another treatment so could you please cancel the ones I've schedule for the rest of the month? Thank you.

Christy

Figure 2.5 An e-mail conversation gone wrong.

messages to their client lists so often that clients start regarding them as spam.

Clients can, of course, also find it convenient to text practitioners. They can, for instance, text to schedule and confirm appointments, and to let the practitioner know if they will be late for their appointments.

However, practitioners should not allow texting to be their primary source of communication with the client. For example, it is unprofessional to text a client if you need to cancel an appointment. A phone call is the better choice because that is communicating more directly with the client.

Texting should not be done at inappropriate times, such as doing personal texting while at work, or texting in front of a client. This sends a clear message to the client that you think he is not as important as whomever you are typing to. Practitioners have even been known to text during treatments. This can involve cradling the relaxed, supine client's head with one hand and texting with the other. Imagine how the client feels, opening his eyes and seeing that the practitioner has better things to do than to focus on his treatment, a treatment that the client is paying for.

Text abbreviations have begun to creep into everyday language. Although those who text regularly may understand these abbreviations, some people, including some clients and colleagues, may not. If you do text, make sure you do not use text abbreviations and lingo in the documentation of your treatments. This may confuse other practitioners, who are expecting standard documentation abbreviations and lingo.

Professional Web Sites

Web sites have become so popular and so much a part of today's world that they are now considered essential to running a business. They are an easy way for people to learn about the business, such as what goods and services the business offers, costs, location, the history of the business, and so forth.

Likewise, Web sites can be a useful marketing tool for bodywork practitioners. Many times potential clients who are in town from another area use Web sites to find out where they can receive treatments. Web sites are used to inform viewers about specials the practitioner or bodywork office is running. They can also be used to let viewers know about other information they may find useful, such as the following:

- Health tips
- Products the practitioner or bodywork office sells
- Bodywork profession press releases
- Upcoming classes
- Community events
- Links to other relevant sites

Web sites are a great way to reach many people quickly. They can be accessed at any time. This is especially convenient for those who want information at times other than normal business hours. In addition, a Web site is a relatively inexpensive way to market your business. You can reach many more potential clients through a Web site than via some other marketing methods, such as sending out brochures and flyers to mailing lists or investing in a television or radio commercial.

However, Web sites do dovetail nicely with other marketing methods such as brochures. Usually brochures contain brief information about your business. Having your Web site listed on your brochures, as well as the rest of your marketing materials, allows readers another avenue to develop a more complete picture of your business or practice. Web sites also let you change prices quickly and offer special discounts for, say, Valentine's Day, without the expense of printing brochures or flyers. If you have an e-mail list of your clients you can simply send them notification of these changes and include a link to your Web site.

If you decide to create a professional Web site or have someone create one for you, the following are some recommendations for presenting yourself in a professional manner:

- The site should look neither too cluttered nor too sparse, and should contain colors and images that welcome the viewer in. The font should be easy to read, and all the decorative images should project professionalism.
- The information should be clear and concise, telling viewers who you are and what you do but it should not be too chatty. Otherwise, viewers will likely simply stop reading and go to another Web site.
- The best type of information to include about yourself is your education, experience, and what types of treatments you perform.
- Be careful regarding any personal information you choose to include on your professional site. Do not include anything that could cause clients or colleagues to question your professionalism. It may be wisest simply not to include any personal information on your professional site, other than your business contact information and, perhaps, a photograph that shows you wearing professional attire.
- The information must be easy to access, and the site easy to navigate. Many times people do not want to spend a lot of time searching through the Web site to find the information they need.
  - Your business phone number, your e-mail address, and the street address of your treatment office should appear on your home page.
  - Everything on your Web site should be no more than three clicks away from the home page.
  - Drop-down menus are also quite useful.
- Keep information updated.
- Set your Web site up as soon as possible. Do not agonize over whether it is perfect from the outset; you can always change it.
- Do not use gimmicks such as flowers bouncing through the screen, butterflies flitting across the screen, a 30-second opening video before the home page comes up, or updates from cartoon animals. They may seem cute or eye-catching but most viewers will find them annoying and unprofessional.

Figure 2.6 shows an example of a professional Web site.

You should also be careful what you include on any separate personal Web sites you have, as clients can easily find these when conducting a basic Internet search. Your professionalism and credibility can be damaged or destroyed by, for example, pictures of you drunk at a bachelor party that a client came across when surfing the Web.

If you are unsure of how to go about setting up a Web site, one of the best resources is to find out who created Web sites that you like and find useful.

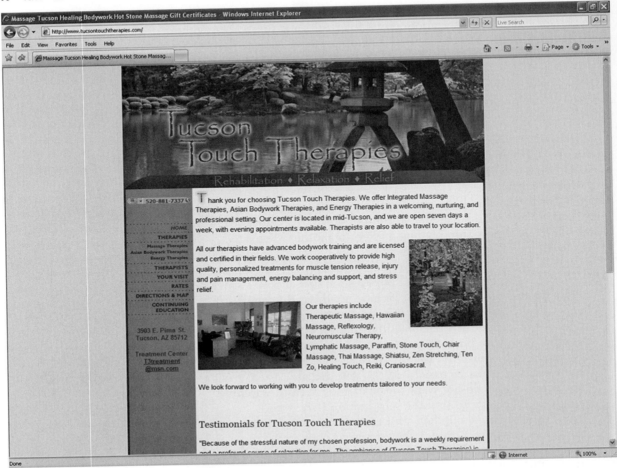

Figure 2.6 Example of a professional Web site.

You can contact the Web site designer to see if he or she is available to create yours. Other resources you can explore include the following:

- Membership organizations. For example, the American Massage Therapy Association (http://www.amtamassage.org) and Associated Bodywork and Massage Professionals (http://www.abmp.com) have free Web site construction packages for their members.
- The site http://www.website-creation.org. This Web site has services for Web site design, content management, webhosting, and Web site maintenance.
- Web site creation software. To help you make an informed choice, http://www.website-creation-software-review.toptenreviews.com is a site that reviews the top 10 software for creating Web sites.

Social Networking Web Sites

In recent years, social networking Web sites such as MySpace, Facebook, and LinkedIn have become wildly popular among people of all ages and backgrounds. These sites are touted as places to meet new people, connect with friends and family, and even network with business colleagues. Even major companies and businesses are setting up pages on these sites to market their businesses and connect with current or prospective customers. If you have your own bodywork business, you may be interested in creating a profile for your business. What follows is a brief description of a few of the most common sites, along with some suggestions for using them to promote a professional image for your business.

In Facebook (http://www.facebook.com), LinkedIn (http://www.linkedin.com), and MySpace (http://www.myspace.com) members design personal Web sites called profiles, which include photos, personal information, and messaging forums. Members can also join networks organized by city, workplace, regions, and even schools to connect and interact with others. Generally, LinkedIn is used more as a professional networking site, whereas Facebook and MySpace are used for both personal and professional networking.

Some practitioners choose to advertise their businesses through these social networking Web sites. If you work with clientele who are Internet-savvy and who perhaps already have accounts set up on these sites, creating an account for your business might be an effective marketing and communication strategy for you.

If you do not have the time, money, or desire to set up a Web site for your business, you can use social networking sites instead. You can create groups on your site and reach a lot of people quickly. It is fast, free marketing for your business. The same types of information you would have on a Web site are appropriate for your social networking site. Also, many practitioners like the convenience and ease of simply creating invitations for events they are having or specials they are running. Their connections can then choose to view the invitation if they want. If you do have a Web site, you can link it to your social networking site so viewers can get more information about your business.

As discussed in the section "Professional Web Sites," if you choose to set up an account with a social networking site, do not mix your personal information with your business information. Not only is it unprofessional, it may also create uncomfortable, unwanted, or even risky situations. For example, a practitioner who states that she is a licensed massage therapist and Reiki practitioner on her site and also has photos of herself in a bikini from her latest vacation in Cabo San Lucas is sending a message that may be construed by certain people that the type of massage she performs is other than therapeutic, or that the term "Reiki" might be a cover for an illicit occupation.

Moreover, even though people can garner a lot of pieces of information and images from these sources, they are not getting a complete picture of who you are and may, in fact, even get a distorted view of you and your practice. Therefore, you should be careful to include in your profile only information and images that you think will create a positive, professional impression of you and your bodywork business.

Electronic Calendars

Electronic calendars are becoming more and more popular for managing busy schedules and can be an excellent tool for bodywork professionals. They

 Food for Thought

Have you visited MySpace or Facebook? If so, choose one of the pages you looked at and describe how you thought of the person whose page it was. Did you want to get to know this person better? Why or why not? How do you think your perception of the person was colored by your own beliefs? Do you think you really knew this person after viewing the person's page?

have several advantages over traditional paper calendars and planners. Electronic calendars, which can be used on a personal digital assistant (PDA, or handheld computer), cell phone, laptop computer, or desktop computer, free you up from having to carry around a potentially bulky paper planner or calendar. Moreover, an individual electronic calendar can be accessed and updated via several different devices at once and by different parties. Therefore, if the calendar is linked to a Web site, clients can see for themselves when appointments are available and schedule themselves in at that moment. Because of this, however, these electronic calendars must be set up so they are easy to use and have clear information about which practitioners, what type of treatments, and what treatment lengths and exact times are available.

Practitioners who use these must be very diligent about checking the calendar for schedule changes, because these can occur quickly. Also, because scheduling can occur without talking directly with the client, there are many opportunities for miscommunication. It is worthwhile for practitioners to confirm every appointment made, changed, and canceled as soon as possible.

Whatever technology you use, be sure to back it up, either electronically or on paper. In fact, it would be wise to have a paper record of names and phone numbers just in case of electronic malfunctions. This duplicate of your client list ensures you will save a great deal of time trying to retrieve their information numbers should something unforeseen happen.

Learning to Unplug

As we have been discussing, it is easy to see that there are more ways than ever before to communicate with others. Unfortunately, the constant bombardment of phone calls, text messages, e-mails, and Internet communication that characterizes modern life can rob us of time to be by ourselves and to think and reflect without interruption. There is a great deal to be said about turning off technology and "tuning out" the noise of modern life.

Being on the go all the time, and having a continued onslaught of information, either through electronic means or other ways, can stimulate the sympathetic nervous system, as well as stimulate the secretion of adrenaline. Being still and quiet allows for the development of internal awareness, which is essential to creating therapeutic relationships with clients. It also provides an opportunity to move from sympathetic mode and to parasympathetic mode. One of the benefits of massage and bodywork can be to assist clients to enter parasympathetic mode. If practitioners do not know what it feels like to be still and quiet, there is a good probability they will not be able to help their clients enter this state. This, in turn, can mean that practitioners may have difficulty listening to their clients, building rapport, and giving a therapeutic treatment.

Therefore, it would be wise and even refreshing for you to consciously limit the time you spend on the phone (talking or texting) and on the computer (sending and reading e-mails and surfing the Internet). Consider scheduling some time in which you turn off your cell phone, shut down your computer, and spend some quiet time by yourself, thinking and reflecting, reading a book, exercising, or pursuing a hobby. Such time can help you recharge, relax, and have more energy to give to your clients.

Food for Thought

What ways do you cultivate stillness in your life? For example, do you like to be out in nature or do you have a quiet hobby such as reading, needlework, or gardening?

Written Communication

Because bodywork is a tactile profession involving physical movement, practitioners sometimes think that written communication is unnecessary or limited in the profession. But writing skills are, indeed, necessary. It is yet another way to present yourself to prospective clients, peers, colleagues, and employers. Effective writing skills are needed in the bodywork profession when composing the following:

- Business cards
- Brochures and pamphlets
- Cover letters
- E-mail
- Résumés
- Business letters to other professionals
- Intake forms
- Documentation forms
- Calendar of appointments

When writing, the first step is to be clear about the intentions behind the piece, because this will determine the audience you will address and the form you choose. You then need to make sure your language is clear, concise, and grammatically correct, and does not contain offensive information. As with verbal communication, use Standard English, avoiding slang, jargon, or trendy expressions. Such language can be offensive to some clients and is subject to misinterpretation by readers, who may get a far different image of you or your business than what was intended.

One place to start in defining your professional image in writing is a mission statement. Once written, the mission statement can serve as a guide for creating your professional image, including how you set up your treatment space and how you create business cards, brochures and pamphlets, cover letters, résumés, business letters, intake and documentation forms, and client appointment schedules.

Mission Statements

Mission statements are brief statements of the purpose of a company, organization, group, or individual. They are valuable because they help define the nature of the business. Another way of thinking of them is that they represent the core principles of the business. They inform and educate potential customers about the character, values, and purpose of the business. Because of this, often the mission statement is used as part of business advertising.

The following elements can be included in a mission statement, and they can appear in any order. It is important, however, to include some tangible goals that support the accomplishment of the mission, so that it is not merely a wish or dream. The state should be clear, concise, complete, and grammatically correct. It should include the following:

- Purpose and values of the organization
- The organization's primary clients or customers

- The responsibilities of the organization toward these clients or customers
- The main objectives supporting the organization in accomplishing its mission

Consider this mission statement: "I want to give massage to lots of different people."

This statement is a wish or a dream. No information is given about how the practitioner intends to do this, or what his responsibilities are in doing this.

The mission statement "Massage Office, Inc., rocks out great treatments to a ginormous bunch of people with practitioners who have lots of training and are licensed" contains more elements essential to a mission statement, such as the purpose ("rocks out great treatments"), primary clients ("ginormous bunch of people"), and responsibilities ("lots of training and are licensed").

However, because the language is casual and "hip," the mission statement can be confusing and possibly offensive. "Rocks out great treatments" could be interpreted by clients to mean that loud music is used, or that the treatments are rushed, or that the practitioners use only deep pressure, or that all treatments include the application of hot rocks. The phrase "ginormous bunch of people" might raise the following question: Are the people themselves large (which is an offensive way to characterize them), or does the office have many clients?

Instead, both these mission statements can be changed as follows:

Massage Office, Inc. delivers treatments designed to fit the needs of diverse clientele through highly skilled, highly educated, licensed massage therapists.

Some other examples of well-written mission statements include the following:

I provide excellent, client-centered wellness care to senior citizens through reflexology.

On the Go Chair Massage provides stress relief to people at work with treatments performed by skilled, licensed practitioners.

The experienced practitioners of Main Street Spa weave together an integrative approach to bodywork and spa services, creating a relaxing retreat for diverse clientele.

I am highly educated and highly skilled in performing craniosacral therapy treatments designed to assist children in self-healing.

Business Cards

A business card is one of the most common and most important ways to market a business. It should contain just enough information to tell others who you are, what your business is, and how to contact you. The card should be easy to read and not cluttered with a lot of information. Some practitioners list every modality that they offer. Although this does give potential clients extensive information on the practitioner's skills, clients may not get past the clutter of words to find the phone number. The card should contain the following details:

- Business and/or practitioner's name
- Credentials that explain the practitioner's training (e.g., CST, for craniosacral therapist)
- Phone number

- Business address
- E-mail address
- Web site information, if relevant
- A *few* of the modalities offered
- A nice touch might be to have a phrase that makes a defining statement about the practitioner's work. As long as it is concise, it will get people's attention and give them a little extra information about the practitioner's work, for example, "Trained in myofascial techniques by the expert in the field!"

Equally important to the written information included are the colors and font used. Make sure that the colors reflect the image of the bodywork practice and that the font is simple. Intricate fonts are much harder to read. It is also worthwhile to determine a budget for creating the business card and deciding what information is essential to include before designing it. Figure 2.7 shows an example of a business card that is hard to read, and an example of a clear, easy-to-read business card.

Brochures and Pamphlets

The purpose of brochures and pamphlets is to provide potential clients a composite of information about the practitioner and the practitioner's business. Brochures can be two-fold or three-fold, depending on how much information they contain. Pamphlets tend to be simpler; they are usually a two-sided sheet of paper and are less expensive to produce than are brochures.

The brochure should have a brief description and summary of the services offered. Some practitioners choose to list prices. However, this requires new brochures every time there are changes in treatment and product prices. Contact and location information should, of course, be included. Depending on space availability, a map may be a nice graphic to include. Individual practitioners may want to include an individual profile, outlining their training, experience, and intentions for their work with clients. Other items to include are as follows:

- Individual practitioner or business mission statement
- Policies
- Guidelines for receiving treatments
- Benefits of the treatments offered
- Testimonials from satisfied clients

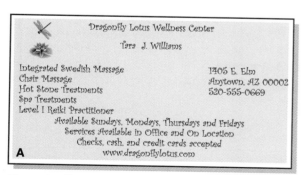
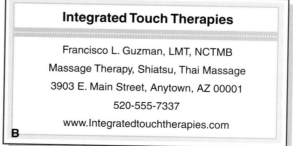

Figure 2.7 Business cards. (A) Difficult to read. (B) Clear, easy to read.

Figure 2.8 shows an example of a clear, easy-to-read brochure.

The information included in brochures should be determined by how and where they will be distributed. For example, at a health fair, the focus could be only on the services offered and contact information to attract new clients. A description of business policies and office guidelines may seem overwhelming and prevent prospective clients from calling.

Equally important to the written information included are the colors and font used. Make sure the colors reflect the image of the bodywork practice and that the font is simple. Intricate fonts are much harder to read. As with business cards, determine a budget, decide what information is essential to include, and plan a distribution area before designing the brochure or pamphlet.

Cover Letters, Résumés, and Business Letters

Several types of written communication are pertinent when seeking employment, including cover letters, résumés, and business letters. Cover letters are used to contact potential employers about applying for a job. One of the most common pitfalls of people applying for a position with a company is the failure to include a cover letter with a résumé. They may think that sending in their résumé is enough. However, the purpose of a cover letter is to ask for an interview for a particular position.

Massage Therapy

Swedish massage plus additional techniques to create an individualized treatment for your needs, ranging from gentle, relaxing sessions to specific, deep tissue work.

Shiatsu

A Japanese form of massage focused on assessing and rebalancing your Qi ("chee"), or vital energy. Therapists use hand and finger pressure, gentle stretches, and joint mobilization to correct imbalances. Shiatsu is performed on a futon on the floor, or on a massage table, without oils or lotions. You wear loose-fitting clothes.

Reflexology

A form of foot massage that affects your entire body. The therapist uses a special pressure technique point on the feet that correspond to different parts of the body. Clients remain fully clothed, with their feet bare. Reflexology can be incorporated into a massage treatment.

Stone Touch Massage

Our Stone Touch is an individual treatment: each therapist has their own style. Stone Touch is catered to your specific needs and is extremely effective for relieving tight and sore muscles. During this treatment, the therapist uses hot (and sometimes cold) stones to facilitate relaxation of your muscle tissue.

Rates

Massage Therapy

◆

Shiatsu

◆

Reflexology

Half hour	$35
1 hour	$65
1½ hour	$90
2 hours	$125

Stone Touch Massage

Half hour	$45
1 hour	$85
1½ hour	$110

Packages

Four 1-hour treatments	$240
Four 1½-hour treatments	$340

Gift Certificates Available

Bodywork Therapies

◆ ◆ ◆ ◆ ◆

Rehabilitation

Relaxation

Relief

◆

520-555-1234

3903 East Center St.
Anytown, AZ 00003

NE corner of Center & Elm

Open 7 Days a Week

www.bodytherapies.com

Figure 2.8 Brochure.

Busy employers do not have the time to scan a résumé in an effort to discover why it has been sent to them. This is especially true of larger companies in which a human resources person is responsible for hiring people for many different areas. For example, a resort can have openings in hospitality, food and beverage, maintenance, and the resort's spa. Unless a cover letter is included letting him or her know in what position the applicant is interested, the human resources person is likely to discard a résumé for an opening for a bodywork practitioner in the spa. In addition, if a company has sites in different parts of the country but résumés and cover letters are sent to only one place, the human resources person will have no idea at what site the person is interested in working.

A cover letter is an opportunity for you to express more of your personality than you can in your résumé. You can mention things that do not fit in your résumé, such as skills and talents that do not speak directly to the job you are applying for but speak to your employability. For example, if a practitioner is applying for a job as a massage therapist at a wellness center, he can say, "Because of my background in nursing, I bring excellent care to clients. I also have an understanding of how the body works and the effects of massage on the different systems."

How a cover letter is written sets the stage for whether employers will read your résumé. The cover letter should express your desire to work for the organization. It should also include a description of the qualities you possess that will benefit the employer. The cover letter should be written in a way that sets you apart from other applicants, but it should be concise, well written, and no more than one page in length.

Cover letters should include the following:

• What position you are applying for
• Your self-introduction, including education and brief work experience
• Why you want to work for the company
• A request for an interview
• A thank you for the employer's time

You should avoid using wildly colored and textured paper, scented paper, or intricate fonts. Do not include a photo of yourself. These are off-putting for busy employers, many of whom dislike gimmicks. Figure 2.9 shows an example of a concise, well-written cover letter.

A résumé accompanies the cover letter. A well-written résumé will include a clear objective related to the position being sought, a summary of education and training reflecting the practitioner's qualifications for the position, and a timeline of work experience that is pertinent to the immediate position available.

Some practitioners who have just graduated from bodywork school may think that employers are not interested in hiring them because they think they do not have relevant experience. However, a résumé can help you get your foot in the door, even if you have no previous professional bodywork experience. Typically, a résumé lists employment history chronologically (in order of the dates of employment). This is called a **chronological résumé**. But if your past jobs are not related to your new career in bodywork, you can organize your experience by category. This is called a **functional résumé.**

Ms. Marina Scheppes, Owner
Greenspring Holistic Center
11245 E. Avenida Strata
Anytown, AZ 00006

Dear Ms. Scheppes,

I recently heard that Greenspring Holistic Center is expanding and plans to start offering massage therapy and bodywork. I have been coming to Greenspring Holistic Center for over three years and have been quite impressed by the quality of treatment and service that I have received. Not only have my physical needs been met, but the professionalism and genuine warmth of the staff and practitioners, especially Norman Johnson, have made me feel very welcome.

Given my three years experience in massage therapy and bodywork, diverse skill set and commitment to client health and healing, I would make a great addition to your team.

During the years I have been operating my private office, Balim Bodyworks, I have come to appreciate how helpful massage therapy, CranioSacral Therapy and Thai massage have been to my clients, both short-term and long-term. However, I think clients could benefit even more through the team approach of Greenspring's acupuncturists, chiropractors, nutritionists, yoga instructors and, soon, bodywork professionals.

I enjoy working with clients of all types and needs. I am in excellent health and can easily perform a great number of treatments daily and weekly.

I would appreciate the opportunity to talk with you about massage therapy and bodywork possibilities at Greenspring Holistic Center. My telephone number is 520-555-6691.

Thank you very much for your time and consideration.

Sincerely,

Tariq Balim

Enclosure

Figure 2.9 Cover letter.

For example, if you have worked as a manager at a fast-food restaurant and as a sales associate for a clothing store, you can organize that information under the category "Customer Service." This way, you can highlight the types of work you did that would make you a desirable candidate for a new position in professional bodywork.

Also, do not underestimate the value of your student clinic work to qualify as job experience. You might write something like the following: "As a student intern, I provided more than 175 treatments to clients in a supervised student clinic setting. I developed a 25% rate of return for clients, compared with the class average of 10%."

Some common pitfalls in writing résumés include the following:

- Failing to put an objective at the top of the résumé. The objective gives the person receiving the résumé instant knowledge about the position you are applying for. If the person is receiving many résumés for many different positions, then the objective immediately tells him or her to what department to send the résumé.
- For professionals who do not have much experience yet, placing bodywork education at the bottom of the résumé instead of just under the objective. Until the practitioner gains more experience, his or her bodywork education needs to be placed in the most eye-catching spot

for the reader. Those practitioners who have many years of experience in the bodywork profession can emphasize that by placing their experience under the objective and moving their education further down the page.

- Including too much information. The résumé needs to be clear and concise.
- Including too much irrelevant information, such as listing all the duties performed as a waitperson when applying for a bodywork position.
- Including outdated information, such as jobs held in college 15 years ago.
- Using small type and not leaving spaces between information. This makes the résumé hard to read and more likely to be discarded.

Practitioners should remember that each employer has his or her own preferences of what he or she looks for in a résumé. For instance, some may want the applicant's creativity emphasized, whereas others may want basic information. You must believe in your résumé and believe in yourself. Being confident in your skills and abilities as a bodywork practitioner will shine through in a professionally written résumé.

It would be beneficial for you to seek out resources if you are uncertain about how to write an effective résumé. There are many resources available on how to write successful résumés, including the following:

- Rockport Institute
  http://www.rockportinstitute.com
  According to the Web site, "Rockport Institute has been a pioneer in developing programs that successfully guide clients through the process of career decision making."
- How to Write a Resume.org
  http://www.how-to-write-a-resume.org
- Membership organizations. For example, the American Massage Therapy Association (http://www.amtamassage.org) and Associated Bodywork and Massage Professionals (http://www.abmp.com) have free Web site construction packages for their members.
- Searching the Internet. Simply type "writing a résumé" in the search area of any search engine, and multiple résumé writing sites will come up.

Figure 2.10 shows an example of a chronological résumé and an example of a functional résumé.

Business letters are used when corresponding with insurance companies, volunteer organizations, medical professionals, and other bodywork practitioners. It is not uncommon for practitioners to be contacted by other health-care professionals to provide information to them. It is important that these letters be concise, accurate, and well written. Figure 2.11 shows an example of a clear, well-written business letter.

Intake and Documentation Forms

Intake forms accomplish two goals for practitioners working with new clients. First, a well-designed intake form allows the practitioner a method to acquire all the pertinent information she needs to make appropriate choices for the client's treatment plan. The intake form should be easy to read and should ask pertinent questions. This allows clients to report accurate information pertaining to their health conditions and health history. Second, the intake form can also act as an informed consent form by including a statement that the client signs, giving the practitioner permission to provide care. The completion of the intake form provides a framework for a mutually agreed-upon treatment session. Figure 2.12 shows an example of an easy-to-read intake form that asks pertinent questions.

Practitioners use documentation forms as records of client treatment sessions. Documentation forms are available in a variety of formats and can be either paper or electronic. Regardless of format, the treatment document should include the following:

- Pertinent information that clients disclose about themselves to the practitioner, such as being involved in a car accident 2 weeks ago, or chronic conditions, such as multiple sclerosis
- Pertinent information the practitioner observes about the client, such as an elevated shoulder or an uneven gait

---

A

Tariq Balim
4250 N. Camino de Oeste
Anytown, AZ 00005
520-555-6691
tballim@nnn.com

Objective

To provide massage therapy, CranioSacral Therapy and Thai massage as a team member of health and bodywork professionals in a wellness center.

Education

December, 2008	Arizona Institute of Healing Arts, Anytown, AZ Certification in Thai Massage
January, 2007	Upledger Institute, Palm Beach Gardens, FL Certification in CranioSacral Therapy Techniques
May, 2006	Arizona Institute of Healing Arts, Anytown, AZ 1000-hour certification in massage therapy. Course program included anatomy, physiology, kinesiology, pathology, massage techniques, massage for special populations, communication and ethics, business, supervised clinical internship

Work Experience

2006 - present	Ballim Bodywork Studio, Anytown, CO Sole owner. Provide massage therapy, CranioSacral Therapy and Thai massage treatments to clients. Manage all aspects of the business including marketing and accounting.
2000 - 2005	Allied Graphics, Inc., Anytown, CO Lead designer. Created graphic designs based on client specifications. Supervised other designers. Managed client accounts.
1997 - 2000	International House of Pancakes, Anytown, CO Shift manager. Supervised wait staff, hosts and cooks.

Professional Affiliations

2006 - present	Arizona state massage therapy license
2006 - present	Member of the American Massage Therapy Association (AMTA)
2006 - present	Nationally Certified in Therapeutic Massage and Bodywork (NCTMB)

References

Available upon request

Figure 2.10 Résumés. (A) Chronological.

B

Francesca Portland
825 E. Pritchard Ave.
Anytown, CT 00003
203-555-4587
fportland@nnn.com

Objective

To provide massage therapy and spa services to guests in a resort setting.

Education

May, 2010   Blue Circle School of Massage, Anytown, CT
750 hour certification in massage therapy
Course program included anatomy, physiology, kinesiology, pathology, massage techniques, hydrotherapy, spa techniques, massage for special populations, communication and ethics, business, supervised clinical internship in both massage therapy and spa techniques

Dean's List all three semesters of program
Received award for highest percentage of return clients in two semesters of supervised clinical internship

Experience

Customer relationship skills: Handled customer complaints in a positive manner. Communicated effectively to help customers find information they needed. Talked with people who were in pain to help put them at ease.

Organizational skills: Developed system that increased office efficiency 25% by streamlining patient record filing system, interoffice communication and telephone callbacks.

Inventory management: Responsible for maintaining back office supplies and product inventory, which supported a high level of customer service and cashier efficiency.

2003 - 2007   Rusty Door Antiques Studio, Anytown, CT
Retail sales clerk and assistant manager
2007 - 2010   Midtown Dental Clinic, Anytown, CT
Receptionist

Professional Affiliations

2010 - present   Connecticut state massage therapy license
2010 - present   Member of the Association of Bodywork and Massage Professionals (ABMP)

References

Available upon request

Figure 2.10—cont'd (B) Functional.

- The techniques the practitioner used on the client and results of the techniques
- Suggestions the practitioner gives the client for self-care
- Any other information relevant to the treatment

Use abbreviations that are standard within the bodywork profession and avoid making up your own, so that other practitioners will be able to understand the documentation notes. Most bodywork students learn the appropriate terms and abbreviations used in documentation during their programs of study. A good resource to have on hand as a reference tool is Diana L. Thompson's *Hands Heal: Communication, Documentation, and Insurance Billing for Manual Therapists,* ed. 3, Lippincott Williams and Wilkins, 2005. The documentation should be clear and concise and easy for other practitioners to read. Figure 2.13 shows an example of a documentation form.

~Massage for Every Body~

February 23, 2011

Lacey Kwan, LAc
Ancient Pathway Acupuncture Clinic
6093 E. Country Club Road
Ocean, MD 00007

Dear Ms. Kwan,

Several of my clients have mentioned that they receive acupuncture from you and that they are pleased with the results. They have also said that you are highly professional and easy to talk to. As a licensed massage therapist and 3rd level Reiki practitioner, I am devoted to my clients' health and well-being and am gratified to hear that your work has benefited them greatly.

I am interested in discussing the possibility of developing a mutual agreement for referrals to better serve both our clients. My treatments provide clients with general relaxation, stress reduction, pain relief, increased flexibility and range of motion, and a sense of calmness and centeredness. I know that acupuncture does all of these, and more, as well.

Because acupuncture and bodywork are a good fit, I believe many of our clients could benefit from our combined services. For example, a client who may see me for Reiki to feel more centered might also need help with insomnia, which your acupuncture treatments could address. Or perhaps a client who comes to you for treatment of frozen shoulder could also benefit from massage therapy techniques to increase range of motion.

I look forward to meeting with you personally to discuss the possibilities. Please feel free to call me at my office, 520-555-8912. Otherwise, I will contact you within the next two weeks to follow up and schedule a time to meet.

Thank you very much for your time.

Sincerely,

Martha Valenzuela, LMT, NCTMB

Enclosures

675 N. Bay Street • Ocean, MD 00007 • 520-555-8912
mvalenzuela@nnn.com
www.massageforeverybody.com

Figure 2.11 Business letter.

One method of documenting treatments is to use SOAP charting:

- S: stands for "subjective," meaning only things the client can feel, such as an upset stomach, headache, or fatigue. The practitioner writes down anything subjective the client reports that is pertinent to the treatment.
- O: stands for "objective," meaning observations that the practitioner can make about the client, such as an elevated shoulder or a limp or what the practitioner feels when palpating and applying techniques to the client. The practitioner writes down anything objective he observes that is pertinent to the treatment.
- A: stands for "assessment," meaning how the client's condition changes, both positively and negatively, as techniques are applied, such as whether a joint's range of motion increased or whether pain levels decreased. The

Bodywork Therapies

Name______________________________ Birthday________________

Address______________________________ City________________

State__________ Zip __________ Home Phone _______________

Referred by______________________ Work Phone ________________

Occupation ____

Health Care Provider____________________ Phone ________________

Emergency Contact ____________________ Phone ________________

Have you ever received professional massage or bodywork treatments? ____Yes ____No.
If yes, please list the types and how often:

Where in your body do you usually feel stress, tension and/or pain?

What type of exercise do you participate in regularly?

Have you had any accidents or surgeries? ____Yes ____No. If yes, please describe them and give the dates they occurred:

Do you have any other medical conditions? ____Yes ____No. If yes, please describe:

Are you currently on any medications? ____Yes ____No. If yes, please describe:

I understand that bodywork treatments are not a substitute for medical care, and that it is my responsibility to let the massage therapist or other bodywork practitioner know of any medical conditions I may have. **I also understand there is a $25 fee for missed appointments and cancellations with less than 24 hours notice.**

____________________________ ________________
Signature Date

Figure 2.12 Intake form that asks pertinent questions.

SOAP Chart

Client Name: Eleanor Whittaker

Practitioner Name: Padma Suresh Date: 11/17/11

S ct: Severe low back/thigh Ⓟ, hurts mostly when sitting or just lying down

O S–HT Ⓑ QL, hams, glutes, IT band and quads

A Stripping, stretching, dsf, elbows, forearms and GSM. Ⓑ HT Δ-QL (L-M), Hams (M^+), Glutes (L^-), IT band (M), quads (M^+, S^-)

P Next treatment recommend heat pack for QL, hams and quads. Showed ct stretches for low back to do daily

Figure 2.13 SOAP chart.

practitioner writes down any assessments that are pertinent to the treatment, as well as which techniques are used during the treatment.

- P: stands for "plan," meaning recommendations for future treatments, such as applying a hot pack to an area to loosen tight muscles or having the client perform certain stretches.

The client's intake form and documentation forms, along with any other relevant forms, such as a list of medications the client takes, should be kept together in one place, such as a file folder. To maintain client confidentiality, client files should be kept in a secure location. How to do this is discussed in more detail in Chapter 7.

Calendar for Client Appointments

Keeping an accurate appointment book is essential for successful client retention. Forgetting an appointment and double-booking clients are both very unprofessional. Choose a method of recording appointments that will keep you informed and on time, that is easy to follow, and that ensures accuracy and consistency. Appointment books are available in a variety of sizes and styles at your local office supply store. Electronic calendars are also an option.

When scheduling clients, be sure to include the client's first and last names, phone number(s), type of treatment, and whether the client is new (and would need to fill out an intake form) or returning (the client's file will need to be read before the client comes in). Figure 2.14 shows an example of a correctly filled out appointment book.

Confirmation calls the night before the appointment are an effective means to reduce the possibility of the client forgetting the appointment. The calls should be brief and include the date and time of the appointment. If you or your employer has a cancellation policy, mention it in the reminder call. For example, add "and don't forget I require 24 hours' notice for cancellation or you will be charged for the appointment" at the end of the call.

Chapter Summary

There are many aspects of professional presentation of self. These include visual, auditory, and kinesthetic impressions of the practitioner and the treatment space. Make sure that your personal appearance, including attire, personal hygiene, and grooming, is professional. If you have or would like to get tattoos or piercings, consider how these will affect your professional appearance as a bodywork practitioner.

You should also pay close attention to your verbal and nonverbal communication and make sure it is professional. If clients have a less than positive response, take the time to evaluate yourself, to ask for feedback from other practitioners and mentors you respect, and to develop and refine your personal and professional verbal and nonverbal language.

Telephones, e-mail, Web sites, and electronic calendars can be very useful in the bodywork profession; always maintain professionalism when using any format. Written communication in the bodywork profession can take the form of mission statements, business cards, brochures and pamphlets, cover letters, résumés, business letters, intake forms, documentation forms, and calendars for client appointments. Be clear and concise in your written communication and make sure it projects your professional image.

April	2009						May	2009					
S	M	T	W	T	F	S	S	M	T	W	T	F	S
			1	2	3	4						1	2
5	6	7	8	9	10	11	3	4	5	6	7	8	9
12	13	14	15	16	17	18	10	11	12	13	14	15	16
19	20	21	22	23	24	25	17	**18**	**19**	**20**	**21**	**22**	23
26	27	28	29	30			24/31	25	26	27	28	29	30

from MAY 18

WEEK 21

MONDAY, MAY 18 138/227	TUESDAY, MAY 19 139/226	WEDNESDAY, MAY 20 140/225
7 Victoria Day (C)	**7**	**7**
:15	:15	:15
:30	:30	:30
:45	:45	:45
8	**8**	**8**
:15	:15	:15
:30	:30	:30
:45	:45	:45
⑨ Lu Markham	**9**	**9**
:15 555-0419	:15	:15
:30 Massage	:30	:30 Miyoki Sasaki
:45 return	:45	:45 555-1411
10	**10**	**10** Reiki
:15	:15	:15 return
:30 Efraim Gonzales	:30	:30
:45 555-0339	:45	:45
11 Thai massage	**⑪** Philip Bronsen	**11**
:15 return	:15 555-6321	:15
:30	:30 Thai massage	:30 Maggie Watson
:45	:45 return	:45 555-8329
12	**12**	**12** massage
:15 Lunch	:15	:15 new
:30	:30	:30
:45	:45	:45 Lunch
① Melissa White	**1**	**1**
:15 555-1019	:15 Lunch	:15
:30 Reiki	:30	:30
:45 new	:45	:45
2	**②** Abe Wu	**②** Lola Ramirez
:15	:15 555-5066	:15 555-9983
:30	:30 craniosacral therapy	:30 Thai massage
:45	:45 new	:45 new
3	**3**	**3**
:15	:15	:15
:30 Molly Kapinski	**:30** Deep Panchu	:30
:45 555-4246	:45 555-7663	:45
4 Massage	**4** massage	**④** Carol Ambrose
:15 new	:15 return	:15 555-7029
:30	:30	:30 massage
:45	:45	:45 new
5	**5**	**5**
:15	:15	:15
:30	:30	:30
:45	:45	:45
6	**6**	**6**
:15	:15	:15
:30	:30	:30
:45	:45	:45
7	**7**	**7**
:15	:15	:15
:30	:30	:30
:45	:45	:45
8	**8**	**8**
:15	:15	:15
:30	:30	:30
:45	:45	:45

Figure 2.14 Appointment book.

Review Questions

Multiple Choice

1. The qualities of staying present and focused are part of the definition of which of the following terms?

   a. Nonverbal language

   b. Verbal language

   c. Presence

   d. Innuendo

2. Which of the following is a factor when considering the therapeutic environment?

   a. Condition of the parking lot

   b. Warm and welcoming atmosphere

   c. Comfortable seating in the waiting area

   d. All of the above

3. Which of the following is a way practitioners should address sexual innuendo in relation to the bodywork profession?

   a. Ignore it and hope it stops

   b. Go along with the joke to show what good sports they are

   c. Talk about the amount of training needed to become a bodywork practitioner

   d. Tell the person in no uncertain terms what a fool he or she is

4. Which of the following is the most professional e-mail address a bodywork practitioner could have?

   a. cutebunny@nnn.com

   b. dmartin@nnn.com

   c. beerchamp90@nnn.com

   d. tanlines@nnn.com

5. Which of the following makes a bodywork practice Web site look professional?

   a. Soothing colors

   b. Fancy font

   c. Practitioner's vacation photos

   d. Lots of information on each page

6. Which of the following should be included in a mission statement?

   a. How long the company has been in business

   b. Purposes and values of the organization

   c. What the company would like to accomplish

   d. What customers do for the company

7. When writing an appointment into a calendar, practitioners should include the client's:

   a. Name

   b. Telephone number

   c. Length of treatment

   d. All of the above

Fill in the Blank

1. Listening to the practitioner's tone of voice and words used is an example of an

   _____ assessment.

2. Three qualities of professional dress are _____ , _____ ,

   _____ , and _____ .

3. A challenge facing practitioners is to be sure that their language matches the _____ they want to project to their clients.

4. In order to truly connect with someone, compassion, _____ , a _____ in the other person as a separate, distinct human being, and a willingness to be vulnerable are necessary.

5. _____ _____ are brief statements of the purpose of a company, organization, group, or individual.

6. Three examples of written communication in the bodywork profession are _____ ,

   _____ , and _____ .

7. Forgetting an appointment and _____ _____ are two of the most unprofessional behaviors that can happen.

Short Answer

1. Explain the impact of first impressions. How can these first impressions affect a bodywork practitioner and bodywork practice?

2. Describe what a confident posture looks like.

3. Explain the impact cigarette smoking can have on a bodywork practitioner's career success.

4. What are four questions that practitioners can ask themselves to see whether the image they are projecting is the same as their intended image?

5. Explain how technology should be used for a successful bodywork practice.

6. Why are written communication skills important in the bodywork profession?

7. Describe the components of a good business card and a good brochure.

Activities

1. Choose a cultural group that you are unfamiliar with. Research what is considered appropriate greetings, both verbal and nonverbal, and compare them with Western cultural greetings.

2. Choose a popular magazine. Take note of the clothing and hairstyles in the photos. What did you discover? Are these styles appropriate for professional bodywork? Why or why not?

3. Role-play a scenario regarding sexual innuendos about bodywork and bodywork practitioners. Have one person make the remarks and the other person address the remarks.

4. Telephone five bodywork offices and ask for information about the treatments they offer. Listen to how the person answers the phone. Did you talk with a person directly, or did you need to leave a message? If you needed to leave a message, how did that feel? How did the person's message sound? If you talked with a person directly, was the person's tone welcoming? Did the person sound professional? Why or why not? Were questions answered patiently or in a hurried manner? Did it seem the practice wanted your business? Would you have felt comfortable scheduling a treatment at this office?

5. Look at five different bodywork business Web sites. What did you like and what did you not like about them? How easy were they to navigate? What messages did you think the look of the Web sites sent about the business?

6. Research online the mission statements of five different companies, at least one of which is devoted to bodywork. Are the mission statements easy to understand and clear in stating the purpose of the company? Do they contain the elements necessary for a mission statement?

7. Look at brochures and business cards of five different bodywork practices. From reading the cards, how do they view themselves? How clearly is the information presented? Are they well written? Do they entice you to want to come in for a treatment?

8. Describe your own treatment space. Include the name, location, layout, décor, furnishings, and any music played. What does it say about you? What does it say about your professional presentation of your space?

9. Write a mission statement for your bodywork practice.

10. Design a business card, brochure, and Web site for your bodywork practice.

11. Write a cover letter and create your résumé.

Guidance for Journaling

Some key areas to think about while journaling for this chapter include the following:

- The impact of first impressions and the messages your personal appearance convey
- How you would create a therapeutic environment
- Cultural views of language and how they affect you in the bodywork profession
- How to refine your personal and professional verbal and nonverbal language
- How you would use different types of electronic communication in your bodywork practice
- How you think writing a mission statement could help you as a professional bodywork practitioner
- What skills you have in terms of written communication necessary for the bodywork profession
- What challenges you have in terms of written communication necessary for the bodywork profession

References

1. Gilchrist, A.: (2009). Clothes DO make the man! *Ask Andy About Clothes* (Web site). Retrieved 16 January 2010 from http://www.askandyaboutclothes.com/Clothes%20Articles/ClothesDOMakeTheMan.htm
2. Adler, R.B., and Rodman, G.: *Understanding Human Communication*, ed. 10. New York, Oxford University Press, 2009, p 136.
3. Ibid, p 147.
4. U.S. Census Bureau, *Statistical Abstract of the United States: 2010,* ed. 129. Washington, DC, 2009. Retrieved 18 January 2010 from http://www.census.gov/compendia/statab/cats/information_communications.html

Communication Skills for Successful Client Retention

LEARNING OBJECTIVES

After studying this chapter, you will be able to:

1. Explain what client retention is.

2. Discuss the factors involved in building and maintaining a client base.

3. Identify appropriate and inappropriate lingo to use with clients.

4. Explain the role that authentic feedback from clients plays in successful client retention.

5. Describe how to give clients permission to give feedback, how to educate them on giving useful feedback, and how to separate useful from non-useful feedback.

6. Explain how to give feedback to clients and to other practitioners.

CHAPTER OUTLINE

KEY TERMS

Client base: a core group of people who see the practitioner on a regular basis

Client retention: keeping a person as a client over a period of time and for repeated treatments as a result of providing satisfactory services

Closed questions: questions that most often result in a yes or no answer

Confidentiality: the safekeeping of clients' personal knowledge. It is considered nondisclosure of privileged information; it may not be divulged to a third party.

Empathy: having an understanding of the feelings or the difficulties another is facing

Feedback: a process in which information is relayed to a person about how his words and actions affect other people

Lingo: vocabulary that is specific to a particular field

Open questions: questions that invite an expanded response

Revolving door syndrome: a situation in which a bodywork business does not have a stable clientele and instead continually relies on new clients for income

---

"Client retention" is the term used to indicate that a client will return to the same practitioner for continued treatments. *Something* happened in the initial appointment that caused the client to feel that her needs were met and she is therefore satisfied receiving treatments from this practitioner. What is that *something*? Is it the phone call that arranged the appointment? Is it the warm and genuine welcome that the client received when greeted by the practitioner? Did the client feel listened to and so trusted that the practitioner was willing and able to focus on the problem area the client discussed? It is likely that *something* is a combination of all of these occurrences. Your ability to inspire trust and confidence in your client begins at first contact, whether it is in person or on the phone.

Client retention is the basis of any successful bodywork business, because it is essential in building a client base that provides stable income. This chapter presents key qualities you need to retain clients, including rapport, trust, credibility, confidentiality, and education. A business that does not have a stable client base and instead continually relies on new clients experiences the "revolving door syndrome." Ways to address this problem are presented, along with methods to build and maintain a client base.

Lingo is a part of almost every profession, including the bodywork profession. However, using massage and bodywork lingo that clients do not understand can have a negative impact on the therapeutic relationship. Ways to be diligent about the use of lingo are presented. Feedback is an important tool you can use to improve your skills and communication with clients. Therefore, encouraging authentic feedback from clients, receiving feedback effectively, and separating useful from non-useful feedback are covered. There are times when it is essential to give clients and other practitioners feedback. Methods to do this in an appropriate and useful manner are also presented.

What Is Client Retention?

The key to any successful business, no matter what type, is customer satisfaction. Customers, or as they are known in the bodywork profession, clients, need to feel appreciated and that the services they receive are worth the money they are paying for them. A major aspect of satisfaction is the therapeutic relationship, as discussed in Chapter 2. Clients also want to receive excellent treatments tailored to their needs in a professional and welcoming space and pay a reasonable fee. When all of this occurs, clients are much more likely to be satisfied and want to return.

Client retention means just that, retaining or keeping clients who return again and again because they are satisfied. It is a goal that business owners work toward by making sure they say and do everything correctly, so that their clients feel they get the best service *from that business and nowhere else.* Client retention creates more security for both individual practitioners and bodywork businesses that employ practitioners because these are clients who can be depended on for repeat business, resulting in a stable income.

In the bodywork profession, client retention is what will make or break an individual practitioner's success. That practitioner is the sole provider of treatments; therefore, he or she is the only person in that bodywork business with whom the client is interacting. Even if the individual practitioner offers other things, such as products for sale or educational information, it is really only the practitioner to whom the client is responding. If clients have positive experiences and enjoyable treatments, it is more likely they will return because they want to repeat that with the same practitioner. If the practitioner does have products for sale, this will also make clients more likely to purchase them. The clients are also more likely to tell their friends about the great practitioner they have seen, and some of the friends may decide that they, too, would like to receive treatments from the practitioner, resulting in a larger clientele for that individual.

However, if clients have bad experiences, it is highly unlikely they will ever return. Furthermore, it is highly likely they will tell all their friends about the practitioner, resulting in a loss of potential new clients for the practitioner.

Client retention can be thought of in terms of a math equation (Fig. 3.1). If the practitioner uses good communication, establishes rapport, exhibits warmth, has a high skill level, and actively listens to the client, and the client has treatment satisfaction, feels heard, feels a connection with the practitioner, and has pain or tension relief, then the result is client retention.

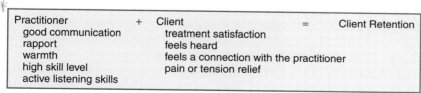

Practitioner	+	Client	=	Client Retention
good communication		treatment satisfaction		
rapport		feels heard		
warmth		feels a connection with the practitioner		
high skill level		pain or tension relief		
active listening skills				

Figure 3.1 Client retention equation.

🦉 Words of Wisdom
Talking with clients before and after the treatment is important. You need to listen to them, and tell them what you're going to do during the treatment and what it will feel like. They will respond to your genuine concern. To have them rebook, you need to be confident enough in yourself and your skills to convey that you're the right practitioner for them.

—David Anderson, NCTMB, licensed massage therapist since 1994

Successful client retention should be every practitioner's goal, including those who work as independent contractors with other practitioners or as employees. Practitioners who work in a setting in which there is a variety of services to offer may have an easier time retaining clients. The client can hear from the practitioner how a combination of services can enhance the wellness goals that the client wants to achieve. Having more choices to offer a client can inspire the practitioner to do more for the client, because it is not just up to one practitioner to do all the work. A team of practitioners is available to create an experience for the client that will be meaningful and satisfactory.

This team approach can be described as a system or a process that allows all practitioners who may work with the client an opportunity to meet and discuss the client's therapeutic needs. Together the team talks about a series of treatments that may benefit the client. When the client is presented with the outcome of this meeting it is evidence that the clinic is committed to providing the best care possible. It also communicates to the client that he or she is cared about and is more than just a source of income for the clinic.

For such a team approach to work, all practitioners must feel ownership in creating a good experience for all clients. Rather than having a territorial attitude of caring only about their own clients, everyone works together for the benefit of *all* clients. This team approach also demonstrates that the employees value collaboration with one another and are committed to the success of the bodywork business as a whole.

When a team approach is not feasible, it is still important for all practitioners to recognize that their work must be consistent and of high quality. The success of an entire bodywork business depends on each individual practitioner's work, creating a whole greater than the sum of its parts. It takes only one practitioner's unprofessional behavior or badly performed treatments to damage the business's reputation as a whole. Such a practitioner may soon be looking for a new job.

Sometimes employees or even business owners may not see client retention as being important. There may be the attitude that, because there are several practitioners, the number of clients the business sees overall is what is important. However, this attitude is short sighted because the work of each individual contributes to the entire business. There may also be the attitude that if a client is not happy with one practitioner, he or she can simply receive a treatment from a different one the next time. Although this is certainly true, the likelihood is that the client will not come back at all.

Some might argue that, if a business is well known, then that is enough to draw clients. Although publicity may bring new clients in initially, of course clients will come back only if they have a positive experience. If a business does not have successful client retention, it will often expend time, money, and energy on marketing methods that businesses with successful client retention do not need. Some bodywork businesses rely on product sales and may think that these sales are enough to make up for income lost through the lack of client retention. However, as discussed previously, clients are more likely to buy products if they have formed a therapeutic relationship with the practitioners in the business.

It should be noted that there are many businesses employing practitioners who realize the importance of client retention. These businesses may give incentives and rewards for clients rebooking with practitioners. For example, practitioners may be paid a higher rate for performing treatments on clients who have requested them. A bonus system may be instituted in which practitioners earn points toward rewards for repeat clients. In some businesses, practitioners must meet a retention quota to stay employed—the practitioner's work performance, and continued employment, is based on his or her client retention rate.

Creating Client Retention

To create client retention, you need to make the right connection with clients. The clients then want to repeat that experience with you. This involves an intimacy that develops between you and the client that transcends the techniques you use to ease pain or bring about relaxation. It is a healthy emotional connection that the client feels during the sessions and that contributes to continued rebooking to see you.

Client retention also involves your ability to consistently give client-centered treatments. The client continues to receive what he or she has asked for. Of course, if you develop a strong relationship with the client, you will also be comfortable suggesting options other than what the client has requested, and the client will likely be receptive to discussing these options.

Client retention can sometimes occur before you even touch the client. Through your skillful presentation, interview, and ability to inform the client about what will happen during the treatment and why, you can set the tone of the interaction as professional, therapeutic, and positive. Initial phone calls should put the client at ease. When the client arrives at your office, your demeanor should be consistent with the tone of the phone call. Your ability to understand the issues the client is having and to tailor a treatment plan to address these issues can help the client feel confident that he or she is seeing the right practitioner.

Several key qualities can be identified as contributing to client retention:

- Rapport
- Trust
- Credibility
- Confidentiality
- Education

Rapport

At times, a chemistry exists between people that makes it easy for them to connect. Sometimes it is felt instantly. For example, in a new work situation when meeting a colleague for the first time, it may feel like reconnecting with an old friend. Or it may happen on an airplane with a seatmate and there is no hesitation in sharing intimate details. An ongoing relationship is more likely to occur in the first situation, but the chemistry is the same in both.

Although establishing rapport with each new client quickly is part of creating the therapeutic relationship and is necessary for the treatment to be

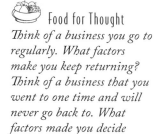

Food for Thought

Think of a business you go to regularly. What factors make you keep returning? Think of a business that you went to one time and will never go back to. What factors made you decide never to return?

successful, it is through building intimacy and strengthening rapport with repeat clients, within the bounds of professionalism, that client retention is developed.

Establishing rapport is an art. It consists of being present in the moment so you can respond to the immediate experience with the client. It requires balance because you must disclose some information about yourself without the treatment session becoming all about you. It requires listening to your client without allowing the pretreatment interview to become lengthy. And it requires pulling back if it seems as though the client is relying too much on you and not enough on his or her own resources.

The art of rapport with clients comes easily for some practitioners and is more difficult for others. Keep in mind that it takes time. You should also be genuine in your interactions. Clients appreciate honesty. Most people instinctively know when comments made are false, so avoid artificial clichés.

Rapport can begin with small talk, which involves talking about safe topics, to break the ice. For example, comments such as, "The weather is certainly getting warmer," or, "How was the traffic on the drive over?" can be a way for you to start conversing with the client. However, some practitioners are not ones to make small talk and may want to state that from the beginning. They can say something such as, "It is very nice to meet you. I am not one for chitchat as I tend to be a little shy," or, "I tend not to talk much because I prefer to be very focused on my work." By acknowledging this up front, the client can understand that the quietness or the "all business" demeanor is the practitioner's nature; it is not about him or her being aloof or unapproachable.

Expressing **empathy** (having an understanding of the feelings or the difficulties another is facing) for what a client is experiencing will strengthen rapport with the client. Psychologists believe that empathy is both an innate ability that can be called upon and refined with conscious effort as well as a skill that can be learned and improved upon through repeated practice.[1] The use of reflective listening skills, such as repeating back key words and phrases that the client says, deepens the connection between the client and the practitioner. Depending on what the practitioner repeats back, the client will either feel understood or correct the practitioner's interpretation. Either way, there is a process of communication between the two that is an opportunity to clarify intention. This helps establish rapport, which increases the strength of the therapeutic relationship.

Yet another skill you can practice to increase rapport with your client is mindfulness. Mindfulness has been described as focusing attention, being aware, being intentional, being nonjudgmental, and being accepting and compassionate.[2] When you notice the sun on your arm as you are driving or the taste of the food you are eating you are in the moment; nothing else matters. When you are truly present from moment to moment, you are in a state of mindfulness. It is this quality of mindfulness that you should bring into all the interactions you have with your clients, whether during the treatment session or during the communication that occurs outside the session. The client perceives the true presence of the practitioner when mindfulness is practiced in the therapeutic relationship as well as in the performance of the treatment.[3] It is this caring and empathy that inspire the client to feel safe and to choose you again and again for his or her practitioner.

Box 3.1 lists Internet resources for learning more about cultivating mindfulness.

When rapport is established, it is actually tangible. It can be felt in the body as a "good feeling" when the practitioner and client are getting along and can be seen in the client's face. Do not get discouraged if rapport does not come easily, however. For some it takes time, patience, a willingness to examine what their challenges to establishing rapport are, and a willingness to work through them.

Examples of ways to build rapport with clients include the following:

- Take note of any hobbies or activities that the client has listed on the intake form. Ask the client about them to show you are interested in the client. You might say, "I noticed on the intake form that you like to hike. Where are some of the places you've hiked?" or "I notice that you marked hiking as an interest on your intake form. How often do you go?" Asking about this particular activity may also give you some insights into what would be helpful for the massage treatment if the hiking has caused the client to seek a session.
- Be approachable and respectful. Have a warm and friendly manner that tells the client that you are genuinely interested in what he or she is sharing.
- Ask follow-up questions about what the client is saying. This demonstrates that you are listening to what the client is saying, and that you want to better understand the client. For example, you might say, "Betty, you say that you love when your grandson visits, but that it's also stressful for you. Can you tell me more about that?"
- Use humor appropriately and wisely. Watch for clues from your client to understand how he or she is responding to your sense of humor. When in doubt, refrain from making jokes. Humor is often misunderstood.
- Be your authentic self. Do not hide behind your expertise or years of experience in the field. It is easier for clients to connect with someone who is gracious and courteous rather than someone who is arrogant and needs to trumpet how good their skills are.

Consider how the following massage therapists, Marcus and Delaney, introduce themselves to a new client:

Marcus: Hi, Joanne. I see on your intake form that you're having trouble with your left shoulder. Well, you came to the right place. I'm known for my deep-tissue work. I know just how to get in there and work out the trigger points I'm sure you have. In fact, I was the best in my class at massage school, and I even

---

| Box 3.1 | **INTERNET RESOURCES ABOUT CULTIVATING MINDFULNESS** |

Insight Meditation: http://www.sharonsalzberg.com
Mindfulness Meditation: http://www.mindfulnesstapes.com
Centering Prayer: http://www.contemplativeoutreach.org
Nonviolent Communication Process: http://www.cnvc.org

show the instructors in the continuing education classes I take a thing or two. Come on back and I'll get started.

Delaney: Hi Joanne. It's really nice to meet you. How was the drive over? I see on your intake form that you're having trouble with your left shoulder. Do you think it might be related to the tennis you've been playing lately? Could you please tell me a little more about that as we walk back to the treatment room?

Which massage therapist, Marcus or Delaney, seems to be more willing to listen? From whom would you rather receive a treatment?

- Encourage the client to ask questions and to provide feedback by assuring him or her that you welcome the input, and that you see it as a way to design the ideal treatment for them. You might say, "If you have any questions or concerns at any point during the treatment, please do not hesitate to speak up. I want to hear from you so that I can be sure I am doing the best job that I can."
- Call or e-mail clients, depending on their preference, within 24 hours of each appointment to follow up on how he or she is feeling from the treatment, and to see if he or she has any questions. You can also use this as a means to express once again your gratitude for the client's business.
- If it is appropriate, contact clients between sessions to offer support or words of encouragement about something that was shared in the treatment. For example, you can wish a client good luck on a job interview, you can let a client know that you will keep him in your thoughts as he awaits results from some medical tests, or you can send a note of good luck to a client on opening night of the play she is directing.

Trust

The Merriam-Webster dictionary defines trust as follows: "assured reliance on the character, strength, or truth of someone; basis of reliance, faith, and hope; confident; to place confidence, depend, entrust, to permit to stay or go or to do something without fear or misgiving, to rely on or on the truth; believe."

Trust is critical to client retention in several ways. The practitioner who inspires trust in clients exhibits character traits such as honesty, being on time, and honoring commitments by keeping client appointments and starting and finishing them on time, cashing client checks for treatment payment promptly, staying within the scope of practice, and making appropriate referrals to other resources.

Of course, trust goes both ways. Practitioners must trust that clients are able to make choices and decisions for themselves regarding their health care. It is not appropriate, for example, for a practitioner to make a client fear that if he does not come to the practitioner, his condition will not get better, or if he does not follow a certain exercise routine or stop seeing particular other health-care practitioners, his condition will worsen. It is ultimately the client's right to choose, with accurate information, what is best for him.

Trust does not develop instantly between a client and a practitioner. It must be earned, just as loyalty is earned. Client trust is the result of offering consistent customer service while providing high-quality therapeutic work that achieves the desired result for the client. It is important to recognize that trust is a dynamic phenomenon in the therapeutic relationship. Not only is it important for the client to trust the practitioner's skills, but the client must also have trust in him- or herself and be able and willing to communicate with the practitioner any information that will enhance the treatment. The practitioner must ensure that the client will be comfortable providing such feedback by creating a trusting and safe environment.

These skills can be broken down into the following formulas:

positive customer service + high-quality care +
customer satisfaction = client trust
client trust in self + willingness to communicate +
honest feedback = practitioner trust

The following are key behaviors and skills that will help you win client trust:

- Upon the initial meeting, display an approachable and confident persona designed to put the client at ease. This persona can be described as being genuinely friendly, easy to talk to, and open-minded about what the client is sharing.
- Answer client questions to the best of your ability. If you do not know the answer to a client's question, say so. It is much better to assure him or her that you will do your best to find the answer than to make up a response to save face.
- Listening attentively while the client speaks and making thoughtful, appropriate responses demonstrate to the client you understand what is being asked of you. This is not to say that you passively agree with everything the client says. Instead, reflect back with your wisdom, experience, and talent as a bodyworker to suggest an appropriate treatment plan based on the client's input. The client is more likely to provide informed consent and be invested in the treatment plan if he or she feels included in the process of developing it. Consider the following as an example of how to suggest an appropriate treatment plan: "I hear that you are tentative about having too much pressure on your low back because you have been experiencing pain in this area for the past 4 weeks. What I would like to suggest is that we start the session with you in side-lying position. This will give me easier access to the deeper muscles while allowing us to have eye contact as we work together to determine a comfortable depth of pressure for you."
- Provide the agreed-upon treatment while being open to modifications according to the client's requests. As the treatment progresses, check in with the client several times to ensure that she is pleased with the session. Sometimes clients have a change of heart once the treatment is under way. They may realize that what they thought was the primary focus area is actually not, or clients may experience discomfort that was not anticipated and want a change in pressure or technique. The client must be able to trust her ability to realize that a change is needed in the treatment as well as feel secure enough to tell the practitioner of any

desired changes. When the client has trust that the practitioner will accommodate her request without judgment, she is likely not to hesitate to express her needs and thus receive exactly the treatment she desires.

- As a way to encourage this trust, you might say, "Mary, thank you for letting me know the work I'm doing in the low back is causing pain in your hip. I'll adjust my pressure and, if it is okay with you, I'd like to explore your hip area to see what may be going on there. What do you think?"

Credibility

Another hallmark of client retention is how credible the practitioner is in his or her skill level. As will be discussed, education is essential. However, knowledge without practice of the various skills and techniques does not go far. Some practitioners are very "cerebral" and like to think about what techniques they can perform to ease a client's discomfort but are not motivated to practice the techniques. As a result, the practitioner's skill level can be low. The client will sense this lack of practice, and he or she will not come back. It is usually disappointing for a client to hear how wonderful a particular treatment plan will be for him and then not experience it.

Credibility is also established through word-of-mouth referrals. If a practitioner does good work and his or her clients get the results they desire, they will talk positively about the practitioner. This is the best marketing and retention tool there is. These practitioners have little trouble keeping clients because the results speak for themselves. Credibility develops over time and is the result of a practitioner's being willing to practice techniques and good communication, and being willing to work on all the clients who come to him or her.

Another aspect of credibility that is important is the practitioner's ability to say, "I don't know, but I will find out," or "That is out of my scope of practice; let me give you a referral." Being honest about limitations and letting clients know that you are willing to find the answers mean much to clients and tend to build trust.

Other ways credibility can be established include the following:

- Publishing an online newsletter on a regular basis. This can be a way to keep your clients informed about, for example, what you are doing professionally, classes you have attended, interesting health and nutrition tips, or recommendations for stretches and exercises. It establishes credibility by giving your clients knowledge about what you do on a day-to-day basis with your business and that you have a genuine interest in the massage profession and health care.
- Having a "brag wall" in your treatment space, where you display all of your credentials, licenses, and certificates of training. Ideally, this is a tasteful display of your achievements that will catch the eye of all clients entering your office. The display shows your accomplishments without you drawing a great deal of attention to them.
- Keeping an ongoing list of all events you have volunteered for and keeping on file any thank-you letters you have received from the organizations you have supported. If you find yourself in a conversation

about any of the organizations, you can mention the work you have done for them.

- Creating a professional Web page that explains your mission statement and goals of your practice. Also include a listing of licenses, credentials, volunteer opportunities, testimonials from satisfied clients, and so forth. Consider having a special section with the list of all the events you have volunteered for. Keep the Web page current and add new information on a regular basis.
- Joining a networking organization that has a high profile in the community

Returning phone calls and talking with people who simply want information but are not yet willing to commit to becoming a client. If you respond to their questions with a warm and friendly tone, and freely give them all the information they require, they are more likely to remember you when they do want a bodywork treatment.

Providing community classes or workshops to demonstrate your body of knowledge as well as your level of skill. Advertise these workshops in prominent places so your name will be recognized.

Confidentiality

Confidentiality is an aspect of trust that deserves its own mention. **Confidentiality** is the safekeeping of clients' personal knowledge. It is considered nondisclosure of privileged information; it may not be divulged to a third party.[4] Keeping confidences is the ultimate requirement for gaining the trust of another person. Often clients share some intimate details of their lives. Practitioners should consider such disclosures as a gift that stays in that treatment room and goes nowhere else. Practitioners should not talk with the client about other clients' issues, as the client will likely wonder whether the practitioner does the same with others about him. This seed of doubt is enough to cause clients to pause and perhaps withdraw from the therapeutic relationship.

You should discuss confidentiality with new clients in the first session so that the client immediately knows his or her privacy is protected. Part of the discussion needs to include the limits of confidentiality. In particular, the client needs to know the following information:

- The practitioner will not discuss the client's identity in social situations or use it in advertising.
- The practitioner will only request information from the client that is relevant to the treatment sessions.
- All client files will be stored and disposed of securely.
- Client information will be released only if requested by the client in writing, if medically necessary, or if required by law.

You can choose to explain your confidentiality policies to new clients during the course of the pretreatment interview. It is also a good idea to give clients a paper copy of these policies, as well as posting them in your treatment space and on your Web site, if you have one. It is also a good idea to revisit the confidentiality policies with your existing clientele, particularly when they disclose issues of a personal nature.

There are several situations in which confidentiality can be waived. The first is when a client signs a release-of-information form granting permission to the practitioner to consult with other health-care providers for the purpose of collaboration. For example, a client with tendinitis may request that documentation of her massage therapy sessions be sent to her physician. The massage therapist and the physician might then work together to resolve her tendinitis.

Confidentiality may be waived in emergencies. For example, a diabetic client may go into insulin shock. You would need to be able to give emergency responders such as paramedics any information you have regarding the client's health history, medications, and contact information to ensure he receives the best care possible.

There is a legal requirement that practitioners report to authorities situations of imminent or life-threatening danger by or to a client or situations in which child or elder abuse is suspected or known.[5] It is important that the practitioner inform the client of such reasons to break confidentiality so that the client can make an informed choice about what to share. This can be a source of concern for some practitioners, because they do not want to cause trouble for a client. However, if there is a situation in which someone could be harmed, and the practitioner knows about it, then the practitioner is required to report it.

However, there are certain situations in which practitioners may want to break confidentiality but it is not necessarily required. Consider the following examples:

- You suspect your client is being physically abused by his or her partner and you fear for your client's safety. An option is to call the local domestic violence hotline, share your concerns, and ask for guidance. If you call the police, be prepared for nothing to happen, as the police may not see it as a case of imminent danger. Conversely, if they do go to the client's home to investigate, a scene may erupt between your client and his or her partner. The client may end up blaming you. When reporting suspected abuse, you must be prepared to face the consequence of losing a client. Domestic violence issues are complex and there is often no easy answer.

- An elderly client who lives alone is showing signs of no longer being able to care for herself. You want to contact the client's children to inform them of what you see. Calling them to report your observations could prevent the client from self-harm but the client may see it as a betrayal of trust. She may refuse to see you again. There could possibly be family conflict that your call adds to, and that you could be blamed for.

- You have a client who is homebound due to a disability. His daughter, who lives in another state, has asked you to keep an eye on her father and call her if you see anything out of the ordinary. You tell her that you cannot do this based on confidentiality issues, but she tells you she will not tell anyone. Your client has shared with you that his daughter does not like the fact that he drinks alcohol at night after dinner. Several months pass, and then your client informs you that he has increased his pain medication at night so that he can sleep better. You have never witnessed your client under the influence of any substances, but he has reported to you that he starts drinking at 6:00 p.m. every night.

How you handle each of these situations is up to you, based on what behaviors you can tolerate in the therapeutic relationship. It is not always an easy decision. With some incidents it may be easy to determine the appropriate course of action; others are not so clear. Spend some time thinking about what your limits are and have a plan of action ready if you are faced with an emergency.

There are other cases in which maintaining confidentiality is even less clear. Because practitioners often hear the stories of others in intimate detail, you must have a code of conduct that includes integrity and inspires trust. Maintaining confidentiality is one of the crucial ways to do this. Earning back trust is extremely difficult once it has been breached.

Confidentiality can be challenging for the practitioner if he or she is working with several members of a family, friends, or coworkers. It can be tempting to relay information that is told in confidence. Sometimes one member of the group inquires about another. It may seem benign to share the information, but it is absolutely unprofessional. A gentle yet firm response in this situation might be, "You will have to ask Eric how his massage sessions are going," or "I know you are concerned about your wife's headaches, but I cannot give you any information without her written permission." By stressing that written permission is needed, you can forestall the inevitable, "Oh, she won't mind if you tell me," or "She doesn't need to know we talked."

You may also have incidents in which one partner will start talking about the other partner in the course of the session and you feel uneasy. It is within your right as a practitioner to kindly ask the client to refrain from such conversations because you do not feel comfortable hearing about the other person when they are not present. An alternative is to inform the client that he or she is welcome to say whatever he or she wants, but you will not be offering any opinions or comments. This will allow the client to feel at ease to talk without the expectation that you will get personally involved.

Education

Practitioners have the responsibility of acquiring bodywork education that can be translated into techniques designed to help clients. The student who is attentive in class, attends classes regularly, participates in discussions, spends extra time practicing techniques outside of class, and studies thoroughly for exams has the profile of a successful practitioner.

Practitioners who choose a high-quality program of study and make the most of their time in school will more likely have good client retention because they have a strong knowledge base and can articulate the art and science of bodywork. They tend not to be anxious with new clients because they will have worked through many client issues while in a supportive school environment, such as a supervised clinic open to the public. Clients will be able to detect the practitioner's confidence and will feel reassured.

After graduating from an entry-level bodywork program, attending continuing education (CE) classes is valuable. In some municipalities it is also

Food for Thought
Think of a time when someone did not keep something you said confidential. How did you feel? How did you react? What would you have done differently?

required as part of maintaining and renewing a license to practice bodywork. Practitioners can use CE classes to stay current with mainstream trends in the profession as well as learn new skills and techniques so that they do not become bored and their work does not become stagnate. CE classes also provide the practitioner with opportunities for professional growth and development. All of this can be translated to career success because, by implementing what they have learned, practitioners can have increased client satisfaction and, therefore, increased client retention.

Often clients are excited for their practitioners to attend classes and want to receive the newly learned modality or technique. It also demonstrates to the clients that they have chosen to work with a practitioner who is committed to furthering skills and education beyond the initial training. In other words, clients can see that their practitioner is serious about being the best professional practitioner he or she can be.

Having the financial means to take CE classes is a challenge that many practitioners face. Some classes are very costly, whereas others can be attended for a nominal fee. A way to start is to decide on the courses you are most interested in taking, as well as those you would benefit from financially by being able to expand your services once you have taken them. Ideally, there will be courses that will meet both these needs.

Once you have decided on the courses that are best for you, determine the costs. Make sure not only to include the cost of the course itself but to factor in travel and hotel expenses (if appropriate), meals, any equipment and supplies you may need to buy for the course, as well as time taken away from your practice. Some businesses pay for their employees to take courses, or some will give time off but not pay the employee while he or she is attending the course. Because independent contractors receive payment directly from clients, they lose income if they take time off to take a course.

Based on all of this information, you can plan which courses you may take the soonest, and which ones require you to have a long-term plan. That way you can start a savings program that makes the most of your economic resources. For example, every month you might put the income from two treatment sessions into a savings account. Setting aside this money each month can assure you that you are working toward your CE goals.

Revolving Door Syndrome

The **revolving door syndrome** is one in which a bodywork business does not have a stable clientele and instead continually relies on new clients for income. The "revolving door" means that new clients come in and they go out. There is nothing in the business to make them interested in returning. Perhaps the treatment was good, but the personal encounter with the practitioner felt flat and lackluster. There might have been a "hurry up and get going" feel to the session, or the practitioner may have made no attempt to connect with the client on a personal level and just spoke in anatomical terms about the treatment.

New practitioners may experience this syndrome until they are able to establish client retention. Sometimes seasoned practitioners experience this syndrome because they become stagnant, have ceased taking continuing education classes, or have gotten complacent in their dealings with clients.

Instead of keeping bodywork fresh and alive for themselves, they have let themselves slide into rote performance. Clients will respond to this accordingly, finding their experience with these practitioners less than optimal. Revolving door syndrome can also occur if the practitioner is distracted and not fully engaged with the client or in the treatment. The client can experience a feeling of disconnect, that he is more a number than a person.

If you notice that you are not getting many return clients, do some self-reflection. Some helpful questions to ask include the following:

- What is similar about the clients who do not come back for a second treatment? Are there commonalities, such as times of the treatments, my mood, day of the week, and so forth?
- What have I been experiencing emotionally, physically, and mentally? Note if there is a pattern of stress and its locus: is it caused by finances, family, relationships, work, illness, allergies?
- How focused am I on my work? Am I bored? Am I genuinely interested in my clients and what they are telling me? Or do I feel they are just another hour out of my day or another treatment fee?
- How is my appearance when I come to work? Do I look professional?
- How is my phone etiquette when I make appointments and confirmation calls? How is my greeting and closing with the client?
- What are my successful colleagues doing differently from what I do?
- Should I seek supervision?

It might be worthwhile for you to look at your marketing plan, where you are getting your clients, what expectations the clients are coming in with, and what outcomes they are experiencing. Perhaps the marketing plan needs to be updated and a different target market determined. Maybe clients are coming in with unrealistic expectations, or perhaps you are not accurately portraying the benefits of the treatments, and the clients are disappointed. It might be time for you to take some continuing education classes for skill enhancement or network with other practitioners for ideas on client retention.

Building and Maintaining a Client Base

Client retention is a very important part of building a **client base.** A client base is a core group of people who see the practitioner on a regular basis. In fact, building and maintaining a client base are the desired outcomes of client retention. Practitioners can choose how large or small they would like their client base to be. Practitioners who practice full-time are more likely to want a large client base because it means a steady and reliable income. Practitioners who practice part-time are more likely to have a smaller client base.

The size of the client base can also depend on other factors, including the practitioner's personality. Practitioners who are more reserved may be more comfortable with a smaller client base. They may prefer not to interact with many different people and personalities so instead develop therapeutic relationships with a select number of people. Practitioners who have more outgoing personalities may tend to like a larger client base because they find interacting with a larger number of clients stimulating.

The size of the treatment space may also affect the size of the client base. A business with one or only a few treatment rooms can offer treatments to fewer clients than can a business with many treatment rooms. In addition, a smaller business may be able to meet its financial needs with a smaller client base. A larger client base would, of course, be required for a larger business to pay expenses and generate income.

To build and maintain a client base, you have to be confident in who you are, how you present yourself, and what services you can offer with skill and expertise. You also need to behave professionally, and put extra effort into working with the client. Box 3.2 has tips for building and maintaining a client base.

The following is an example of how a willingness to work on a variety of clients and having an open, confident attitude can help a practitioner expand her client base.

On a very slow day at the massage clinic, a woman in a wheelchair comes in looking for a treatment. The client, Jayne, has a C-4 injury, a catheter bag attached to her leg, and a caregiver with her who can help with transferring her to the massage table. Although other practitioners are intimidated by working with Jayne, Jordan says, "I'll work with her. I'm sure she'll tell me what she needs and her friend is here to help. I've never worked with a client with these limitations before either, but I'll do my best."

Jordan has a great experience with Jayne. Jayne tells her that she is really enjoying the treatment. During the course of the treatment Jayne asks Jordan if she would be willing to work on some of her friends who also have spinal cord injuries. She mentions that they all play wheelchair (quad) rugby once a week and they could always use a tune-up afterward.

Jayne's friend and caregiver, Maxine, had stayed in the room for the treatment and commented on how great the massage looks. This prompts Maxine to book a treatment with Jordan for the next day. Maxine also tells Jordan that she organizes monthly events for other caregivers and invites Jordan to

---

| Box 3.2 | **TIPS FOR BUILDING AND MAINTAINING A CLIENT BASE** |

- Wear attire that is fitting for a variety of clientele.
- Practice good hygiene at all times.
- Be appropriate in manner and behavior at all times.
- Provide client-centered treatments that show you have listened to the client.
- Call clients the day before their appointments to confirm.
- Arrive at least 20 to 30 minutes before your first appointment starts and honor the time frame of each appointment.
- Do not cancel an appointment unless there is an emergency.
- After each appointment ask the client if he wants to book his next appointment.
- After the treatment, give each of your clients your card with your schedule on it.
- Make a follow-up call within 24 hours after the session to check in with the client.
- Send thank you cards, coupons, and birthday or holiday greetings.
- Return a client's call in a timely manner.
- If you have not heard from a regular client for a few weeks, call to check in.
- Ask appropriate questions that indicate your interest in your client.
- Offer clients a standing appointment for the same day and time each week.
- Offer package deals as a discount, convenience, or incentive.

come to the next one to talk about the benefits of massage therapy and pass out her business cards. By the end of the session, Jordan has learned some effective ways to transfer a client from the wheelchair to the table without putting stress on her low back, she has learned how to work around the catheter bag appropriately so that it does not leak, and she has new groups of potential clients to talk with about massage.

✳Massage and Bodywork Lingo

As with any profession, there is **lingo** associated with massage and bodywork. Lingo is vocabulary that is specific to a particular field. Professionals use lingo as kind of a shorthand when talking their field. By using lingo, fewer words are necessary to communicate a lengthy idea, with the intended meaning still being understood among the professionals.

Categories of Lingo

In the massage and bodywork profession, lingo falls into several categories, including the following:

- Anatomy and physiology. For example, the names of muscles and bones are often shortened: "biceps brachii" becomes "biceps"; "rectus femoris," "vastus lateralis," "vastus medialis," and "vastus intermedius" are shortened to the "quads"; and so forth. Also included under anatomy and physiology are anatomical terms for areas of the body, such as axilla, popliteal fossa, cervical region, thorax, and so forth.
- Directions. These include superior, inferior, lateral, medial, ipsilateral, contralateral, proximal, distal, and so forth.
- Techniques. For example, "forearm and elbow work," "trigger point (or "t.p.") work," "effleurage" (or "gliding"), and "assessments" are technique terms understood by most massage therapy practitioners and do not need to be further explained to them.
- Communication. Terms such as "intake form," "SOAP notes" (or "documentation"), "feedback," "boundaries," and "intent" are common among bodywork practitioners.
- Other. Other lingo that can be used includes terms such as "on-location" and "bolstering" (or "propping").

Using proper terminology helps practitioners present themselves professionally. For example, using the scientific names for the regions of the body, such as "axilla" instead of "armpit" or "patella" instead of "kneecap," demonstrates to clients, other practitioners, and other health-care professionals that you are educated.

Although lingo makes it easier for bodywork professionals to talk to each other, it can be confusing to clients and others outside of the profession. The lingo can, and does, sound like a foreign language. Just as it is disrespectful for people to carry on a conversation in front of someone who does not understand the language being used, it is disrespectful for practitioners to use lingo with or in front of clients who do not understand it.

Some practitioners feel that they present themselves as more professional and knowledgeable when they use lingo without explanation of what the lingo means during interactions with clients who themselves are not part of the bodywork profession. Most often, the practitioner is trying to hide his or her insecurity, which most clients will usually instinctively pick up on. As a result, the client may have a far different impression of the practitioner than the practitioner thinks he is presenting. Instead, the client may be thinking, "Sure, he can throw all these terms around but does he really know anything?" or "He sounds like he's talking down to me, and I don't like that." These impressions definitely work against the practitioner's efforts at client retention.

Clients will be much more impressed by the lingo if it is used as an educational tool. For example, if you say, "I can work on the medial border of the scapula, which is your shoulder blade, to help relieve muscle tension in your rhomboids" and outline the area on the client, then the client has a clearer idea of where you will be applying techniques. It also demonstrates to the client that you are knowledgeable because you know the scientific name for the region and can explain it easily.

Receiving and Providing Feedback

A successful career in the bodywork profession is based on a strong interpersonal connection. As has been discussed, it is important for practitioners to be genuine when speaking and working with clients. An important aspect of this connection is **feedback**. Feedback is a process in which information is relayed to a person about how his or her words and actions affect other people. Feedback is important in the bodywork field because it informs the practitioner about what is working and what is not. Just as it is impossible to get a second chance at making a first impression, it is difficult to get a second chance with a client if the practitioner does not know what the client thought or experienced during the treatment.

Receiving honest feedback is a great learning tool for practitioners. Many times clients who are dissatisfied will not say anything; they just stop going to the practitioner. By encouraging feedback from clients, you can learn on an ongoing basis what is and is not working. This helps you increase treatment satisfaction with current and future clients.

Besides receiving feedback from clients, it is also important that you learn to give feedback to clients and to other practitioners. Feedback is often used during the bodywork education process. It is how students learn from experienced professionals what techniques and skills they have mastered, and which ones they need to improve on. Giving feedback and receiving feedback are both skills. Generally, the better a person is at receiving feedback, the more open people will be to receiving feedback from the person.

Feedback should be given without the intent of hurting the person receiving the feedback. It is about behavior, not the reasons behind the behavior. It should be specific rather than general, and take into account the needs of the receiver. Feedback should be well timed and directed at behavior the receiver can do something about. Questions to ask yourself before giving feedback include the following:

- What did I see, feel, hear, or learn?
- What did I like?

Food for Thought

Have you ever been in a situation in which lingo you did not understand was used in front of you? How did you feel? How would you have preferred to have been communicated with?

- What is the most important part of my feedback?
- Am I too angry or hurt to give feedback?
- What change do I want?
- Can I not be invested in the outcome of this feedback, knowing I do not control another person's response?

Receiving Feedback Effectively

It is important that you understand that feedback (when useful and fair) that clients and other practitioners give you is about your *behavior*, such as your work in the treatment session, how you dress, how you interact with other practitioners, and so forth, and not about you personally. You should not respond in an extremely personal manner, thinking that you are not liked, or that you should just give up on bodywork altogether. This reaction to feedback is extreme, but it points to the necessity to differentiate between professional skills and your value as a person.

A way to differentiate between professional skills and personal attributes is to receive feedback in terms of five sequential gates on a path. A gate has to be open before you can pass through it and move to the next gate. This is illustrated in Figure 3.2. The five gates are as follows:

1. Listen. This means being attentive and using open facial expressions and body language. It does *not* mean being ready to defend oneself or to counterattack.
2. Clarify. To make sure that you heard the feedback correctly, repeat it in your own words. Ask questions that will clarify the feedback, but do not argue with it.
3. Breathe. If you are too upset to breathe evenly, you are too upset to hear feedback. Anxiety may creep in, and it is difficult to stay present and focused, which will manifest as uneven breathing. Ask for a time-out until you can breathe. However, be sure to set a time to come back and listen.
4. Pause. Give the feedback time to sink in; no immediate response is required. Remember the setting and actions of the interaction being talked about; try to picture accurately what happened.
5. Separate. Decide whether the feedback is useful. Decide what is true about the interaction and what is not true; acknowledge that it could be a single person's response to you in the moment. Decide if a change is needed. No defense against inaccurate feedback is needed; take what is necessary and leave the rest.

Receiving feedback about your work is one of the most important tools for career success. Being open to and trusting that the feedback is meant to enhance your skills, and directed toward you personally shows that you are willing to keep learning new things about yourself. It also shows that you are not attached to being a "perfect" practitioner and you are willing to implement new ideas when appropriate.

Another link between success and feedback is being willing to listen to feedback from your supervisor. It shows you are willing to be a team player if you do not take offense and try to make excuses about why the feedback is not accurate. Having an open attitude and willingness to implement the

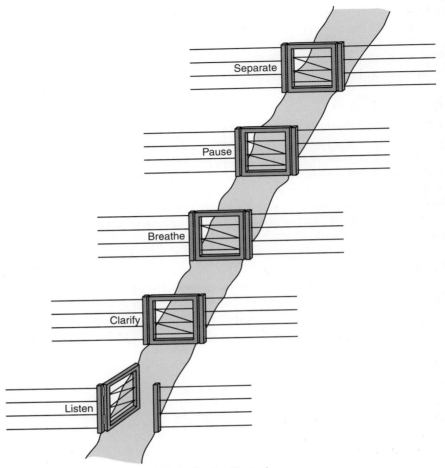

Figure 3.2 Five gates of receiving feedback effectively.

feedback are clear signs that you are open to growth and new ideas. Being willing to listen to only your positive feedback and refusing to admit you have more to learn is a sure way to limit yourself in the bodywork profession, and hamper your ability to build clientele.

Consider the following:

It is Cooper's first day at Healing Hands Clinic. He has been out of school for 3 months but has mostly been working on friends and family. Cooper greets his first client, Sarah, an athletic young woman with an injured hamstring muscle. As Cooper is escorting Sarah to the treatment room his supervisor, Ned, overhears her ask Cooper a question about her hamstring injury. Cooper's response is, "Well, I don't feel comfortable working on your injury, so how about we just avoid that area?" Sarah pauses and looks questioningly at Cooper, then agrees. When Cooper leaves the treatment room so Sarah can get on the massage table after the pretreatment interview, Ned is waiting to speak with him.

> *Ned:* Cooper, I heard you tell your client that you don't feel comfortable working on her injured leg. Why did you say that?

Cooper: I didn't know what to say. I was so surprised she has an injury because she isn't limping. I don't do sports massage so I thought it would be best to avoid massaging the area.

Ned: Cooper, tell me what you know about the hamstrings.

Cooper proceeds to give Ned a very through explanation of the hamstrings, including their attachments, actions, and the best positions in which to place the client's leg to palpate them. He even describes a couple of techniques that he knows would be helpful if Sarah was not injured.

As he is talking, Cooper notices that Ned is smiling and nodding his head. Suddenly, Cooper realizes that he is describing a treatment plan that he could perform on Sarah. He says, "I guess I got freaked about when my client said she has an injury. I didn't trust myself to know what to do. You really helped me focus my attention and calm down. Thanks, Ned."

The key to this feedback session is that Ned is willing to talk with Cooper immediately. Instead of telling Cooper that what he did was wrong, Ned helps Cooper figure out why he responded to Sarah the way he did. He also assisted Cooper in identifying the problem—when Cooper heard the word "injury" he froze and forgot the knowledge that he had. With one simple request ("Cooper, tell me what you know about the hamstrings"), Ned helps Cooper develop a treatment plan for Sarah that she is much more likely to be satisfied with. Instead of being defensive when Ned gives him feedback, Cooper is willing to listen and used the feedback as an opportunity to gain self-confidence and create a better treatment plan for his client. His chances of retaining Sarah as a regular client have now greatly increased.

Inviting Feedback From Clients

One of the best ways you can invite feedback from clients is to ask for it directly in the interview process. You might say, "At any point during the treatment, if you need more or less pressure or if there is anything that you'd like me to change to make this treatment better for you, please don't hesitate to ask. I won't be offended or take your feedback personally. In fact, I welcome it so that I know that you and I are working well together." Giving the client permission at the beginning of the session lets the client know that you are indeed interested in what the client is experiencing, good or bad, and that you are encouraging him to tell you so that you can make the necessary adjustments to meet the client's needs.

Another way to encourage useful feedback from clients is to have a brief feedback session at the end of each treatment. Once the client is ready (e.g., is dressed after receiving massage or has taken a few moments after receiving shiatsu), you and the client can discuss the outcome of the session. This type of closure will give the client an opportunity to say something after each treatment session, which the client might prefer, rather than during the treatment. The drawback is that it does not allow you to make any changes within that treatment; any changes will have to wait for the next treatment.

Even if invited to give feedback, many clients may not feel comfortable doing so. The client may think giving feedback would offend or upset the practitioner. The client may not be in the habit of stating his preferences, so he may not even notice if there is something he would prefer differently in the treatment. The client may feel intimidated by the therapeutic setting and, because he regards the practitioner as the one with all the knowledge, feel too vulnerable to speak up. There is even the possibility that the client is not willing to say something for fear that the practitioner may take it personally and seek some sort of retribution in the session, such as applying unwanted deep pressure, backing off and giving only a general, ineffective treatment, or otherwise behaving inappropriately in response to feeling challenged.

Whether a client will speak up is sometimes a matter of personality. Some people choose to go through life quietly and move on from uncomfortable situations without saying a word to avoid perceived confrontation. Some clients think that because the practitioner has had training in the modality they are receiving, the practitioner should somehow know what the client wants without asking. At the other end of the spectrum, some clients have no problem telling others what they think is right or wrong and what should be done about it, preferably immediately.

When deciding how to invite clients to give feedback, the image of a river may be useful (Fig. 3.3). Certain phrases, such as those in Figure 3.3A, tend to discourage feedback; they essentially dam the river so that only a little water flows through. Other phrases, such as those in Figure 3.3B, tend to encourage feedback, allowing the river of communication to run more freely.

Educating Clients on How to Give Useful Feedback

For the feedback to be useful, it must be specific and focused on a particular treatment. It is helpful to instruct clients to say things such as, "If there is a stroke or stretch I am doing that is not comfortable or if the pressure does not feel like it is meeting your needs, let me know and we can discuss what I can do differently." By giving the client specific cues about what to look for in the treatment that may or may not need adjustments, you are giving a context in which the client can base his or her experience. Simply saying something such as, "Let me know if the pressure is okay," is a bit too vague. In what sense is it okay? What is it being compared to?

Educating clients on what is useful feedback as opposed to non-useful feedback is essential. It is useful to know the desired depth, pressure, and pace that a client likes in his or her massage. It is also useful for the client to be specific if something is not going well for him or her in the treatment. The client should be able to put into words or perhaps express a feeling about what he or she is experiencing. The following are two examples of how the client can express useful feedback: "It just does not feel like you are getting deep enough"; "You seemed rushed today. I didn't feel as relaxed as I normally do." It is your job then to follow up with questions that will help clarify with more information. The following are two examples of follow-up questions: "Did I seem rushed the whole time or just at the end?"; "When did I seem rushed?"

Make sure your questions are open and not closed, to encourage the client to give more information. **Closed questions** most often result in a yes or no answer. They usually begin with phrases such as, "Did you," "Will you," or "Are you." Although the answers to these questions give the practitioner some information, it is limited, unless the client decides to clarify further. **Open questions** invite a more expanded response. Open questions begin with "How," "What," "Who," or "When." Table 3.1 includes examples of closed questions and open questions.

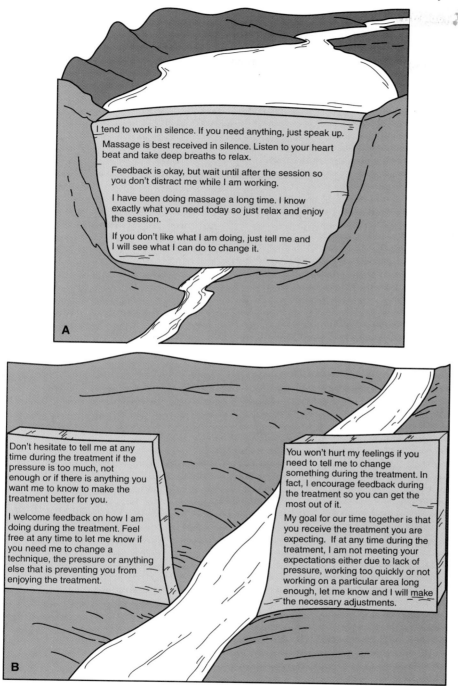

Figure 3.3 Phrases that (A) discourage feedback and that (B) encourage feedback.

Table 3.1	Examples of Closed and Open Questions

Closed	Open
1. Is this pressure deep enough?	1. How does this pressure feel to you?
2. Are you comfortable?	2. What can I do to make you feel more comfortable?
3. Do you feel pain in your low back?	3. Where do you feel pain in your body?
4. Is this music okay for your treatment?	4. What type of music would you like to hear during your treatment?
5. Do your shoulders feel less tight now that I've worked on them?	5. How do your shoulders feel now that I've worked on them?

Be sure to express gratitude after receiving the feedback so that the client knows it was received and taken in. This not only will let the client know that you heard him or her, but also that you consider him or her an equal partner in the therapeutic relationship. You and the client are then working together to achieve optimal results for the client.

Consider the following:

Margo is giving a massage treatment to Glenn. It is clear from Glenn's clenched fists throughout the work on his neck that he is not comfortable. Margo approaches the subject in the following way:

Margo: Glenn, I am noticing that you are clenching your fists every time I massage the sides of your neck. What are you feeling when I work this area?

Glenn: I didn't know I was clenching my fists. Sorry. I'll try to stop.

Margo: No, you don't have to stop. I was just wondering if there's some discomfort for you when I massage that area because I don't want to be causing you any pain.

Glenn: Well, I don't feel any pain, but I do feel like I can't breathe very well when you're doing that.

Margo: How about if I only massage the back of your neck for now and get you comfortable with that sensation. What do you think of that?

Glenn: Will I still get a good massage for my neck? I don't want to get in the way of your work. I am sorry.

Margo: There is nothing to be sorry for, Glenn. I can still give you an effective massage for your neck while not causing you to feel like you can't breathe. You're my main focus here so it isn't about you getting in my way. You're not. I want to help you be comfortable with the massage, so I'm glad you told me. Please tell me at any time when something isn't feeling right so that I can make adjustments. Okay?

Glenn: Okay, I'll let you know.

Non-Useful Feedback

What if the feedback a client gives you is harsh, off the mark, or personal? It is your responsibility to maintain a professional demeanor and not respond by acting offended or defensively with the client. If it seems like the feedback does not match the experience you had or the intention you set forth for the session, you can apologize to the client, saying, perhaps, "I am sorry that you are not satisfied. What would you need to feel better about the session?" Sometimes there is nothing that is needed except for the client to sound off; you may be the target of some misdirected anger. Conversely, there could be something important that you missed during the treatment or some other aspect of the interaction with the client of which you were completely unaware.

Another type of non-useful feedback is client information about something that you cannot change. Perhaps the client wants a spinal adjustment, which is out of your scope of practice. Another example is a client who wants aromatherapy but you have no training in that area and are unable to offer it. Maybe a client complains about the noise from the street outside the treatment space. Sometimes clients are not sure what was not satisfactory, so they are withdrawn after a treatment. This response is difficult to deal with because you gain no information about what did not work well. At these moments, all you can do is ask the client. If, for some reason, the client is not able or not willing to tell you what his or her treatment experience was, then at least you have done all you can do by inquiring.

Depending on the level of dissatisfaction, some clients may want a refund for the treatment. If the opportunity to give feedback was offered and the client chose not to say anything until the end and then asks for a refund, you have a couple of choices to make. You could stem an unpleasant interaction by apologizing for the fact that the client was not satisfied and give the client a full refund. The full refund may satisfy the client, but you have lost the time spent with the client and now have no treatment fee.

Another option is receiving some compensation for the time and effort that you put into the treatment. Yet another option is to offer a discounted or free future treatment. These options may or may not be satisfactory to the client, and you might be faced with an angry client who may decide never to return. You will have to decide for yourself what makes sense in compensating a dissatisfied client. These encounters should be few and far between, as you encourage clients to keep you informed throughout the treatment to ensure that they are receiving client-centered treatments.

The ability to separate useful and non-useful feedback develops over time. As you become more experienced, you will know when you are having an off day and can probably expect to hear about it from certain clients. You will be able to sort out the feedback you receive to find the kernels of useful feedback, take those in, and leave the rest.

Giving Feedback to Clients

It is a given that all of us interact with others with varying degrees of success. We all have needs that we are trying to fulfill, and we are simply moving through the world the best way we know how. In getting these needs fulfilled, we may offend others. Most of the time, it is not deliberate and, much of the time, we may not even be aware of it until it is brought to our attention. When it is brought to our attention, though, we have an opportunity to change our behavior to make our interactions with others better.

 Food for Thought

Think about a time when you were dissatisfied with a service you received. Were you encouraged to give feedback during and after the service? Did you give feedback, whether or not you were encouraged? Why or why not? If you did give feedback, what was the outcome?

All of this applies to giving feedback to clients. They can be saying and doing things that are difficult for practitioners to deal with. Therefore, practitioners should take the time to give clients feedback when it is appropriate to do so. Giving feedback to clients can be useful in several ways. It can educate them, ensure their health and safety, and let them know how their behavior affects the practitioner.

Optimally, feedback is given in a tactful way that is not designed to embarrass or offend the client. The best way to do this, as has been discussed previously, is to focus on the client's behavior, not on the reasons behind it.

Consider the following:

"Stan, I'd like to talk with you before your treatment today. I've noticed that you have been coming here straight from the gym without showering. This is awkward for me to tell you, but your body odor is very strong and causes me discomfort when I am massaging you. What I need is for you to shower before you come for your treatment. For today, I put some washcloths and towels in the bathroom for you to freshen up with before we begin your treatment."

This feedback focuses on the behavior of the client, and how his body odor is a difficult issue for the practitioner. The practitioner makes a request for the behavior to change as well as offering a solution for making today's session comfortable. Being direct can sometimes feel awkward and uncomfortable. However, it shows respect for the client by making him aware of an issue that he may not have been aware of and providing him the opportunity to change his behavior.

"Andrea, I've noticed that when your treatment is about to end, you start making requests for me to go back to an area and spend more time there. I've been accommodating your requests but I'm no longer willing to do that since I've been adding extra time to your session without an increase in fee. I'm happy to provide longer treatments for you as long as we establish the time frame and the fee at the beginning of the session."

This feedback focuses on the practitioner acknowledging that she was willing to accommodate the client's requests in the past, but is being clear with the client why she is no longer willing to do that. In addition, the practitioner lets the client know that the extra time may be possible but it needs to be planned at the onset of the appointment. This client may very well have been unaware of the fact that so much extra time was being added and would have been happy to have paid extra for the added time and attention. However, the practitioner did not speak up until now. This example also illustrates how important it is for practitioners to say something as soon as possible when they are not in alignment with what the client is asking for, and what they are providing, but are going along with the client's request just to be nice.

Some other examples of appropriate feedback to give to clients include the following:

- "Massage therapy does not include spinal manipulations, so I will not be able to perform those on you."
- "You've missed several scheduled appointments without calling. I realize that people get busy, but if you had known you couldn't make the appointments, I could have scheduled another client in that time slot."

• "I have noticed that when you talk a lot about the issues you're having with your boss, your muscles tense up. This makes it difficult for me to help you relax. You might consider simply taking some deep breaths to release the stress and tension while you're receiving the treatment."

No matter how tactfully something is said, clients may still be embarrassed, taken aback, offended, or even outraged. Should this happen, remain calm and professional. Although some clients may want further explanation, you do not have to rationalize your feedback or apologize for making it. You may end up losing a client, but if he or she is unwilling to change behavior that is making your work as a professional bodywork practitioner unmanageable, then you are better off without that client.

Giving Effective Feedback to Other Practitioners

Besides providing feedback to clients, you, as a bodywork practitioner, will also likely need to give feedback to other practitioners. For example, a common occurrence among practitioners who share the same treatment room is that one practitioner may not leave the room as neat as the other practitioner would like. Perhaps during shift changes one practitioner goes over time, cutting into the set up time the next practitioner has. In an office with several practitioners, one or more may try to "steal" clients from other practitioners by disparaging the other practitioners and proclaiming their own skills as better.

You should have a goal in giving feedback, and the feedback should be specific. Changes cannot be made unless the person receiving it has a clear idea about what did and did not work.

Consider the following:

Dale and Mirai have a chair massage business together. They take turns providing the treatments and collecting the payments from the various accounts they have.

One week Dale is surprised to learn that Mirai has not been arriving on time to several of the accounts. Because she is late, some of the employees are not able to get their treatments. A representative for one of the accounts was getting ready to cancel her contract but wanted to talk with Dale to see if she could request him to come each week instead of Mirai. Dale assures the company representative that he would be able to come on a weekly basis and he apologized for any inconvenience.

Dale calls Mirai and asks her to meet him at the office. Mirai agrees, but is 45 minutes late. When she enters the room, Dale says, "Mirai, you are 45 minutes late for our meeting. I was informed today that you have not been arriving on time to our chair massage accounts and have caused some employees to miss their appointments. I don't understand why you are having trouble managing your time and I am angry that you have put our business in jeopardy. What is going on?"

Dale's feedback to Mirai is clear and specific. He states Mirai's behavior and how it is affecting both him and their business. Table 3.2 provides some more examples of unclear and clear feedback to another practitioner.

■ CASE PROFILE

Mark is in his second semester of training at Las Manos Massage Institute. One week Mark's last client is wearing a T-shirt with "Out and Proud" on it. Mark recognizes him as a local activist for gay and lesbian rights who has been on the news lately.

After the pretreatment interview is complete, Mark leaves the treatment room to prepare for the session. In the break room Mark overhears some of the other students, who have realized who his client is, talking. They are making remarks such as, "I'm glad I don't have to massage him"; "I feel sorry for Mark"; "I can't believe they let guys like him come to the student clinic"; "I hope Mark told him he has a girlfriend so he doesn't try to pick him up"; and "I'd show him what to be proud of." Mark cannot believe what he is hearing but he chooses not to address it because it is time for the treatment to start.

Later in the day, at the end of a class, there is time for the students to gather in a group and share with one another their clinic experiences that day. Mark says, "I'm shocked and upset at the behavior and the attitudes of some of my classmates toward my client today. Those of you who made comments about my client being gay and said you were glad that you didn't have to work on him, listen to what you're saying. Your comments were disrespectful, rude, and ignorant. Where is your professionalism? I know we all have the right to our own opinions, but in this setting our personal opinions aren't appropriate to share, especially when they consist of hateful remarks like the ones I heard today. I'm embarrassed, and concerned about the type of attitudes you will bring into this profession when you graduate. Why did you choose to treat my client and me in such a demeaning and humiliating way?"

What do you think of the comments of the students that Mark heard?

How do you think these attitudes will affect their client retention success, and therefore their career success, when these students become professional bodyworkers?

If you were Mark's client and you heard the comments that were made, what would you feel? What would you think? What would you do?

What do you think of the way in which Mark handled this situation? If you were Mark, how would you have handled it?

How much success with client retention do you think Mark will have when he becomes a professional bodyworker?

If you were in this class listening to Mark's comments, how would you respond? Why?

How do you think the clinic supervisor should address the situation with the class? Why?

Table 3.2	Examples of Unclear and Clear Feedback to Another Practitioner
Unclear	Clear
Your forearm work needs to be better.	To improve your forearm work, try slowing down and applying more pressure.
You're dressed unprofessionally.	Professional dress means wearing clean, pressed clothes.
I wish you weren't late all the time.	To make sure you start your first treatment on time, you should be here at least 15 minutes early.
You should think of other people, not just yourself.	Could you please be sure you're out of the treatment room at the designated time so that I have enough time to prepare for my sessions?
You're always so messy.	Could you please be more careful about cleaning up after yourself in the break room?

Chapter Summary

Client retention is essential to the success of your bodywork practice because it is key to building and maintaining a client base. To create client retention, you need to make a connection with clients that is balanced. The key qualities you need to have to retain clients are rapport, trust, credibility, confidentiality, and education. If these are not present, you may experience the revolving door syndrome, in which your business continually depends on new clients for business.

You need to be aware of how using bodywork lingo can affect your interactions with clients. If you use lingo as a way to educate clients, instead of merely to demonstrate your knowledge, it is likely your client base will increase.

Feedback should be given without the intent of hurting the person receiving the feedback. It is about behavior, not the reasons behind the behavior. It should be specific rather than general, and take into account the needs of the receiver. Feedback should be well timed and directed at behavior the receiver can do something about. Educate clients about how to give you feedback concerning the treatment they are receiving so that you can make it a more satisfactory experience for them. Besides receiving feedback from clients, it is also important that you learn to give appropriate feedback to clients and to other practitioners.

Review Questions

Multiple Choice

1. A practitioner who refers a client to another practitioner for services that are beyond her scope of practice is demonstrating what key quality of client retention?

a. Rapport

b. Trust

c. Credibility

d. Education

2. What term describes a bodywork business that lacks a stable clientele and continually relies on new clients for income?

a. Client base

b. Revolving door syndrome

c. Client retention

d. Diversity

3. The terms "deep specific friction" and "contract-relax" are examples of what type of lingo?

a. Technique

b. Anatomy and physiology

c. Communication

d. Directions

4. A client who gives the practitioner information about situations the practitioner cannot change is giving what type of feedback?

a. Closed

b. Useful

c. Open

d. Non-useful

5. When giving feedback it should be:

a. Specific

b. General

c. Personal

d. Indirect

6. Which of the following is the clearest feedback?

a. You need to enhance your bodywork skills.

b. You should schedule clients in the appointment book better.

c. I find it unappetizing to eat my lunch when you leave your dirty linens in the break room.

d. I wish you'd be more considerate when you talk to clients.

7. A way to invite feedback from a client is to ask for it during the:

a. Interview process

b. Treatment

c. Post-treatment discussion

d. All of the above

Fill in the Blank

1. The repeat business of clients is called _____ .

2. A(n) _____ is a core group of people who come to see the practitioner regularly.

3. The process in which information is relayed to a person about how his words and actions affect other people is called _____ .

4. The five steps, or gates, to receiving feedback are to listen, clarify, _____ , and

   _____ .

5. _____ questions most often result in a yes or no answer, whereas

   _____ questions invite a more expanded response.

6. Effective feedback focuses on _____ , not the reasons behind it.

7. Generally, the better a person is at _____ feedback, the more open people will be to listening to feedback from the person.

Short Answer

1. Explain how client retention is crucial to the success of a bodywork practice.

2. List and describe at least five ways to build and maintain a client base.

3. What are at least five questions a practitioner can ask him- or herself if he or she notices that there are not many return clients?

4. Give three examples of unclear feedback and three examples of clear feedback.

5. Explain at least three ways that the practitioner can invite feedback from clients.

6. Describe three situations in which a practitioner needs to give feedback to a client. Write appropriate feedback for the practitioner to give in each situation.

7. Describe three situations in which a practitioner needs to give feedback to another practitioner. Write appropriate feedback for the practitioner to give in each situation.

Activities

1. List at least five original ideas you have for building and maintaining a client base.

2. Think of a treatment you might perform on a client's tight shoulders. In writing, describe what you would do to another practitioner. In writing, describe what you would do to a client who is not a practitioner.

3. Contact at least three professional bodywork practitioners and ask them what their keys to successful client retention are. Ask them what mistakes they have made in building their client base, and what they would have done differently.

4. Contact at least three professional bodywork practitioners and ask them how they encourage clients to give feedback. Also discuss with them situations in which they have had to give feedback to clients and to other practitioners, and how they did it.

5. Research a physical challenge a client may have, such as postpolio syndrome, Parkinson's disease, or multiple sclerosis. Find out the causes, symptoms, and treatments for the condition. Contact an association that advocates for the condition, such as the Parkinson's Disease Foundation, and find out what particular challenges people with the disorder face.

6. List all the derogatory names you know of for the following:

    a. Gay, lesbian, bisexual, and transgender people

    b. Physically challenged people

    Write the answers to the following questions:

    • Which of these terms are intended to be hateful and which are innocent remarks made because of a lack of awareness or education? Does this make a difference to you?
    • What type of environment do you think is created by the use of derogatory comments?
    • How do you think these terms began?
    • Why do you think they are used?
    • How do you think people feel when they are called these derogatory names?
    • How do you think the world would change if these words were no longer used?
    • Were you ever an innocent bystander and heard someone being called a derogatory term? What did you do? How did your choice of action make you feel?
    • If a stranger or good friend made a joke using any of the derogatory terms you listed, would you tell him or her that you did not appreciate the joke he or she told or the words being used?

7. Contact an agency that advocates for the gay, lesbian, bisexual, and transgender community. Find out what would prevent members of this community from receiving bodywork and what would encourage members of this community to receive bodywork.

Guidance for Journaling

 Some key areas to think about while journaling for this chapter include the following:

- Why client retention is important in the bodywork profession
- What you think are ways you can create and maintain a client base
- How you will communicate effectively for client retention
- How lingo is used in the bodywork profession
- How you use lingo as a bodywork practitioner
- What types of feedback you think are important for you to receive, and how you would like to receive feedback
- How you separate useful from non-useful feedback
- When you might need to give feedback to clients, and how you would give it
- When you might need to give feedback to other practitioners, and how you would give it

References

1. Walsh, R.A.: Mindfulness and empathy. In Hick, S.F., and Bien, T. (eds): *Mindfulness and the Therapeutic Relationship.* New York, Guildford Press, 2008, p 73.
2. Ibid, p 5.
3. Ibid, p 41.
4. Salvo, S.: *Massage Therapy: Principles and Practice*, ed. 2. St. Louis, MO, Saunders Elsevier, 2007, p 23.
5. Beck, M.: *Theory and Practice of Therapeutic Massage*, ed. 4. Stamford, CT, Cengage Learning, 2006, p 39.

Communication Gaps and Conflict Resolution

KEY TERMS

Communication gaps: a difference in understanding between two people that causes problems in communication

Homogeneous: a term meaning "the same"

Kanji: the term for Chinese language symbols

Meta-communication: used to describe the hidden or underlying meaning behind spoken words

Personal bias: the tendency to interpret a word, an action, or a person in terms of some personal significance assigned to it

Stay solid: to know oneself and so not be swayed to deny personal feelings or change them because someone disagrees with them

---

Brady is a massage therapist in private practice. Lisa has been his client for 6 months. During this time Brady has not been satisfied with the level of progress being made toward eliminating Lisa's frozen shoulder syndrome. Brady has decided to refer Lisa to another practitioner who has had great success with this condition.

Brady: Lisa, I want to talk with you about the possibility of referring you to another practitioner to work on your frozen shoulder problem.

Lisa: You don't want to work with me anymore? Why not? Did I do something wrong?

Brady: It's not that I don't want to work with you, it's just that I am feeling frustrated that your shoulder hasn't improved more by now.

Lisa: Well, I've done all the exercises you've given me. What am I doing wrong?

Brady: Lisa, you're not doing anything wrong. I'm just saying that I would like to refer you to a practitioner who specializes in neuromuscular therapy because I think she could help you more than I've been able to help you with your shoulder.

Lisa: I think you've helped me just fine. I don't need to go see anyone else unless you are sure you don't want me to come back.

Brady and Lisa both think they are being perfectly clear with each other but, as happens so often, in reality they have a communication gap. Brady is not communicating clearly to Lisa that he believes she would benefit from a different type of bodywork treatment. Lisa interprets Brady's suggestion of a referral as a sign that he is no longer willing to work with her and that she has not been a "good client." Brady did not intend to give Lisa the message that he no longer wants to work with her, but that is what Lisa hears. And no matter how much they think they are clarifying their point of view, they are not understanding each other.

We cannot always know how our clients will interpret our messages. What we can be sure of is making every effort to be clear and succinct in our messages while remaining professional. Consider the outcome if the conversation between Brady and Lisa had gone in the following way instead:

Brady: Lisa, when we started working together 6 months ago, our goal was to eliminate your frozen shoulder syndrome or at least get more range of motion in that joint. As you know, we haven't made much progress even though you've been very diligent in keeping your appointments with me and doing the stretches I've recommended. I have a colleague who specializes in neuromuscular therapy and she has gotten good results working with clients who have your condition. What would you think about seeing her for a few sessions?

Lisa: Do you think it will help?

Brady: I don't know for sure, but I'd like you to consider it.

Lisa: If I don't like it, can I come back to you?

Brady: Of course you can!

Communication gaps occur when people are unable to understand each other because they do not have the same perception of a situation or they are not in agreement about how a situation should be handled. Communication gaps can occur because of generational differences, regional and cultural differences, and personal response styles; all of these are covered in this chapter. How to recognize communication gaps is covered, as well as how to bridge them to ensure client retention. The difficult interactions that practitioners are likely to encounter with clients are presented, along with difficult interactions with coworkers and employers. Methods to manage these difficult behaviors are covered, as well as how to recognize when it is time to end a therapeutic relationship with a client and refer him or her to another practitioner.

Most practitioners will experience unwelcomed or dangerous situations with clients at some point in their bodywork career. These situations can be overt or covert, verbal and/or nonverbal, and are discussed in this chapter. A five-step intervention model that practitioners can use to protect themselves from unwelcomed or dangerous situations is also presented.

Communication Gaps

A **communication gap** is the difference between what is intended to be communicated by the sender of the message and what is actually understood by the receiver. Communication gaps, in general, result when one party or another involved in the communication does not have enough information or makes assumptions. Often, people mistakenly assume that others share their points of view when communicating with them. Then, when misunderstanding occurs, they think that others are being deliberately unhelpful when, in fact, they simply have a different viewpoint.

Differences in age, experience, belief systems, culture, and religion all influence the way people communicate. The words and phrases used; what is considered humorous, taboo, respectful, and disrespectful; and the intonation, pauses between words, and the pace and rhythm of speech also influence the ways in which people communicate. Factor in nonverbal language, such as eye contact, facial expression, and body movements, and it is easy to understand why communication gaps occur so often.

When communication gaps occur, the result is often conflict and a lack of collaboration. People may then experience confusion, annoyance, irritation, and even anger and violence. Whatever the reason for the gap in connecting with one another, it is possible to create a bridge that will reduce misunderstandings and increase collaboration. But before this can occur, we must be able to recognize potential communication gaps and be proactive in resolving them before they start. Because that is not always possible, it is also important to recognize a communication gap as it occurs and change methods to communicate more effectively. And because even *that* is not always possible, it is important to be able to evaluate difficult interactions afterward to see where the communication gap occurred and how it could have been bridged. By learning from the experience, perhaps the same type of communication gap can be avoided in the future.

Recognizing Communication Gaps

Recognizing communication gaps requires being aware that the message given is not being heard or understood as it is meant or that it is being taken out of context. Sometimes, it is not clear that there is a communication gap. In some cases, the person receiving the message acts as though she understands when she actually does not. In other cases, the recipient may think she understands the message but is actually misunderstanding it. Moreover, when a person does express confusion over not understanding a message, the sender of the message may interpret the confusion as uncooperativeness.

Consider the following:

This is Mari's first time receiving a massage. Heidi is the massage therapist who will be performing her treatment.

Heidi: I will step out of the room so that you can disrobe to your level of comfort and get on the massage table. Do you have any questions?

Mari: No.

Heidi returns to the treatment room to find Mari completely clothed and lying on top of the sheets on the massage table.

Heidi: I see that you've left all of your clothes on. Usually clients take off at least their shirts and pants to experience the long, gliding strokes of the massage on their skin.

Mari: Well, I don't want to lie naked on the table.

Heidi: I see. What I failed to explain to you is that there is a top sheet on the table for you to lie under. While the rest of you is covered at all times, I will undrape the area that I will be massaging. Would you like to try the massage that way or would you prefer to stay the way you are?

Mari: I would like to try the draping.

In this case, the communication gap occurred for two reasons. One, Heidi either failed to take into account or forgot that Mari is a client who has never had a massage before. Heidi also failed to explain the draping procedure, even though she thought she was being clear when explaining how to get on the massage table. Two, Mari thought she understood the procedures for getting onto a massage table and made a choice that met her needs for comfort and safety.

Adler and Rodman state that communication gaps occur because not everyone listens to messages in the same way. Our personal listening style will determine what filters are in place when we hear information and how we act on that information. They identify four personal listening styles:

Content-oriented: listens for details and analyzes the quality of ideas in the message; willing to spend time thoroughly exploring and exchanging ideas with others

People-oriented: seeks to understand and support others; concerned with creating and maintaining positive relationships while tuning in to the moods and feelings of others

Action-oriented: appreciates clear, concise messages with the focus on the task at hand; wants to figure out what needs to be done as quickly as possible

Time-oriented: concerned with efficiency, views time as a scarce and valuable commodity; grows impatient with others if time is being wasted[1]

Consider the following examples of how communication gaps can be created through the lens of one's personal listening style:

- Having a continual pattern of misunderstandings with the same person. People-oriented listeners seek to preserve the relationship rather than acknowledge that they did not hear the message.
- Feelings of frustration or anger rather than resolution. Action-oriented listeners do not feel heard and become impatient because of a lack of progress and lack of clarity in the situation.
- Feeling physically constrained or drained, or that the stomach is tied up in knots. People-oriented listeners are overly invested in the emotional aspect of the relationship while not getting their emotional needs met.
- Avoiding certain people because it seems to take too much time and energy to deal with them. Time-oriented listeners are unwilling to meet certain people because it is viewed as a waste of time. They are unable to trust that other people's time frames are just as important as theirs. They also resent the lack of efficiency in the relationship.
- Thinking that no matter how clearly the information is presented, the other person "just doesn't get it." Content-oriented listeners like to stick to their "clear and concise" message, rather than seeking to understand what it would take for the other person to truly understand it.
- Thinking that the other person is just not willing to listen. Action-oriented and time-oriented listeners are unwilling to consider that perhaps no action is necessary or impatient with the amount of time it may take to come to a place of agreement.

We all use each of these listening styles depending on the situation. Being aware of the style you are using will help you make appropriate choices in your interactions with others.

There are many factors that contribute to communication gaps, including the following:

- Use of language that one party does not understand
- Use of language that one party finds objectionable or offensive

- Having a sense of superiority or inflated ego that prevents a person from valuing another's opinion
- Lack of understanding of or respect for another's culture
- Constantly interrupting when in conversation
- Fear-based attitudes about those who are different and a reluctance to learn more about them or accept them as individuals
- Not taking the time to communicate clearly what one's expectations are of the other; being in a hurry
- Assuming that the others know and understand what everyone's expectations are
- Assuming that everyone has the same expectations
- Assuming that they themselves know best, and not being open to other ideas and opinions
- Lacking the confidence to speak up and ask for clarification when confused about what is expected of them
- Lacking self-awareness that personal behavior is preventing a successful connection with others

This is by no means an inclusive list of all the factors that prevent us from engaging in successful communication. What is important to note from the list is that each of the points can be used to learn more about ourselves, what may be preventing us from having fruitful connections with others, and what may lead to ways to increase successful communication.

Generational Differences

One specific type of communication gap is directly related to the age differences between two people. The words used by someone from an older generation can be easily misunderstood or make little sense to someone in his or her twenties, and vice versa. As a practitioner, you will likely work on clients of all ages. Therefore, you should be prepared to communicate effectively with those who may be from an older or younger generation.

For example, as the meaning of words change over time, an older client can innocently use a phrase that meant one thing in his youth, but currently may have a completely different meaning that is no longer innocent and is even embarrassing if heard by others. For example, the client may use the term "gay" to mean "happy" or "joyful."

How do you prepare to communicate with someone who has seen more life than you can possibly imagine? What do you say to the young man who has several facial piercings and wears pants that appear to be falling off of him? Start by being polite, respectful, and inquisitive about what any client needs from a session. Do not assume that an elderly person must be handled as if she were fragile or that the young man with the pierced eyebrows and lip prefers deep tissue techniques. Do not assume that you already know a person based on appearance, age, or dress.

Consider the following:

Candace, a 21-year-old massage therapist, greets her new, elderly client, Harrison Parker, in the lobby. "Are you Harrison? Hi! I'm Candace! I'll be your massage therapist today. So, Harrison, what'll you have today? I could do some hot stones or some barefoot shiatsu. I have some Yamana balls I could use to help you stretch out your shoulders. What's your pleasure, dude?"

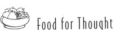 Food for Thought

Think of a time when you had a difficult interaction with someone. How did you feel during this interaction? What was the outcome? Can you identify where the communication gap occurred? How would you have liked the other person to have communicated? What could you have done differently to communicate with this person?

Candace did not even think to adapt her approach with Mr. Parker. She assumed a familiarity with him by using his first name when greeting him. It is a professional courtesy to address an elderly man using Mr. and a woman using Mrs. or Ms. as a sign of respect. As time goes on, he or she may invite you to use a first name, but it should not be assumed that it is all right to do so without his or her permission. Candace also overwhelmed him by reciting a number of modalities, assuming he would know what she was talking about. Consider the outcome if the interaction goes in the following way:

"Mr. Parker?"

"Yes."

"Hi. My name is Candace and I will be your massage therapist today. Shall I take you to the treatment room, Mr. Parker?"

"You can call me Harrison. I'm only called Mr. Parker when I'm in trouble. So where is this treatment room?"

"Right this way, sir. How are you feeling today?"

"Not so good. My back has been giving me trouble."

"I'm sorry to hear that. Have a seat, Harrison, and tell me what you would like to receive from today's massage."

In this exchange, Candace is respectful and professional at all times. She asks an open-ended question that leads Harrison to tell her about his back, and is focused on his treatment needs.

It is good form when working with an elderly person to be mindful of the words you choose to minimize misunderstandings. This does mean that you cannot be completely informal, but that you should always seek to use language that is clear and respectful.

Each generation will have its own jargon and slang that its members accept as part of everyday language. It is the professional's responsibility to make appropriate language choices that will enhance clarity and understanding with our clients.

Regional and Cultural Differences

We live in a multicultural society. The term "culture" is used to describe the beliefs, customs, technological achievements, language, and history of a group of similar people.[2] Our personal thoughts and attitudes are shaped and influenced by our experience of the culture we grew up in. As such, we have a tendency to interpret a word, an action, or a person in terms of some personal significance we assigned to it. This is known as a **personal bias.**

Purtilo and Haddad contend that "personal bias can lead to more favorable or less favorable judgments than are deserved. . . . Understanding the way personal biases influence us and their effect on our attitudes and conduct is important to the health care professional."[2] This understanding starts with becoming aware of any biases you may have and self-assessing to see if these biases limit you in your ability to accept differences in others. Whether you are able to accept differences in others can mean the difference between a successful and unsuccessful career in the bodywork profession.

For example, consider a practitioner at a high-end resort who grew up in a family having little money. Her mother and aunts cleaned houses for little pay. She feels resentment working with wealthy women because they represent the women whose houses her mother and aunts cleaned. Although the practitioner is no longer living in that environment, she still harbors a negative attitude toward the wealthy clients she sees. It would be beneficial for this practitioner to seek supervision or attend diversity training to work through her resentment so that it does not inhibit her ability to be successful at her job.

Communication gaps can also result from regional and cultural differences that the practitioner and client may have. Depending on the area where you practice, you may encounter a clientele that is extremely diverse in regional or cultural backgrounds or one that is relatively **homogeneous,** meaning "the same."

Generally, those practitioners who live in smaller communities may encounter less variety, whereas those in large urban areas may encounter a greater variety, although this is not always true. Given the growing diversity in most regions of the country, however, it is likely that you will interact with at least a few clients who are culturally different from you. Thus, it would be wise for you to be prepared to face communication gaps that may result with such clients.

Consider the following:

A practitioner who grew up in Greece attended a workshop on marketing techniques for the massage therapist in Arizona. During one of the lectures, the speaker made the comment, "For those who would rather not provide direct service and don't mind doing all the legwork, you can set up the accounts and hire employees to do the actual massages." The woman from Greece raised her hand and asked, "Why would I only want to massage the legs and let someone else do the rest of the massage?" In her understanding of English, "leg work" meant massaging the legs, not doing the work of setting up a business via phone calls or office visits to pitch an account.

A massage practitioner is volunteering at a clinic by giving chair massage to predominantly Spanish-speaking clients. She does not speak Spanish and an interpreter is not available, so she decides to "act out" what a client needs to know about receiving the treatment. The practitioner touches her own neck, back, and shoulders to signify where she would be touching the client, and the client nods. The treatment proceeds and the massage therapist thinks everything is going well until she realizes that the client is flinching in pain. This is the only way he knows how to get the practitioner's attention that the pressure is too deep.

The following are examples of cultural considerations you should keep in mind:

- It is considered disrespectful in some cultures for two people meeting for the first time to address each other by first name (this is also true of some elderly clients).
- Some cultures, for example, Japanese and Hispanic, show respect by not making direct eye contact at first.
- Shaking hands when meeting someone for the first time is not acceptable in all cultures.
- Members of certain cultures (including many Muslims) can receive bodywork only from someone of the same gender.

For a good connection with clients, it is important to remember that there are two or more people involved in an interaction. Each has a right to be treated with respect, honesty, and integrity. To ensure that you do this, do not make assumptions about why a client behaves the way she does. The best way a practitioner can find out how a client prefers to be interacted with is to ask in a respectful and tactful manner.

Cultural communication gaps are especially a concern if you plan on practicing in another country. Sometimes individuals choose a career in bodywork because there are opportunities for travel and work in various parts of the country or world. Although this sounds very glamorous, it does require that you make a concerted effort to learn about the region of the world in which you will be living or the cultural expectations of people living in a particular region of the world. Such cultural awareness demonstrates that you:

- Have respect for the people that you will be working with by learning the customs and values of the region
- Are willing to be open to expanding your knowledge and understanding of a new region or culture
- Are aware that you do not expect others to adjust to your mannerisms when you are new to the area
- Are aware that your business can be successful if you do adapt to the local customs and practices

This can be a daunting task to undertake considering how much there is to learn: how to live in a new location, new sets of rules and regulations to practice and live by, and possibly a new language to be able to communicate the simplest information to ensure a safe treatment. In addition, it is likely that you will want to seek out a community of practitioners to receive support from and may need help in advertising that you are open for business and ready for clients. It takes great courage as well as the ability to take risks when the outcome is uncertain.

If you do plan to move to a new area, you must research the region of the country in which you are interested. Planning for your future takes time. It is neither wise nor useful to pick up and move somewhere on a whim and expect to be successful. Make contact with someone in the area who has information and expertise on what it would take to set up a private practice or find gainful employment. It is also a sign of a good professional to be responsible for knowing the licensing requirements and local laws. If you do not use due diligence, then you are running the risk of committing ethical violations or making social mistakes that could stand in the way of a successful transition to a new community.

Response Styles

Another contributor to communication gaps is how the person being spoken to responds to a comment. There are five common response styles that people exhibit when reacting to communication from others: critical, teaching/preaching, supportive, questioning, and clarifying. Some response styles can actually worsen a communication gap, whereas others can help bridge it.

A bodywork client is unhappy with the effects of the massage treatments he has been receiving from Courtney and tells her, "I wish you were better at doing massage." Table 4.1 shows examples of each response style that Courtney could use, along with the intent behind each one.

A critical response from Courtney will not enhance communication with the client. Instead, it will most likely put the client on the defense. When one is critical and judgmental of others, they are essentially being told that their experiences do not matter.

A teaching/preaching response from Courtney will most likely create a gap in communication with her client because this type of response elevates her as being smarter and more experienced than the client. She is telling the client what he should be doing. When the teach/preach response style is used, it can potentially shame and embarrass the client and will likely cause him to go elsewhere for treatment.

The supportive response style is based on Courtney acknowledging the client's efforts in achieving goals as well as assuring him that he is on the right track. Supportive behavior toward the client tends to increase the level of trust. It also motivates both you and the client to continue working toward the same treatment goals.

Table 4.1	**Response Styles and Their Intent**			
Frequency Used	Response Style	Example	Intent	Difficulty Caused to Communication
↑ <é>	Critical	"You shouldn't be upset. I'm a professional bodywork practitioner."	To judge	<ê>
	Teaching/ preaching	"Maybe you should be doing the exercises I showed you."	Give facts, information, "shoulds"	
	Supportive	"I understand that you are frustrated with the lack of progress we're making."	Reassurance	
	Questioning	"It seems like the techniques I've been using haven't been working for you. Is that it?"	Develop a point further	
	Clarifying	"Would you like me to use another approach with different techniques?"	Understanding	↓

Courtney can use the questioning response style to explore with the client information that may not be making sense to him. Asking questions, preferably open ended, allows the client to share more subjective information about his experience. This in turn will provide you with more information about how to proceed with the treatment plan.

The clarifying response style promotes understanding of what the client expects as well as what Courtney expects. The clearer we are and the better we explain what we want, the less room there will be for confusion. Reflective listening is a good skill to refine when seeking clarification from others.

Note that when any of these responses shown in Table 4.1 are used 40% of the time, it results in the speaker perceiving the responder as using that style of response 100% of the time. Also included in Table 4.1 are two factors that affect communication—frequency and difficulty. Frequency means how often a particular response style is used. The level of difficulty corresponds to how easy or difficult the response styles make communication. For example, if your response style to another person is critical, it is likely your intent behind your message is to judge the other person's behavior. Because very few people like to be judged, it will be very difficult to communicate with another person using a critical response. Also, if you frequently respond critically to others, it is likely you have difficulty communicating.

Conversely, if your response is clarification, the intent is understanding. Most people respond more favorably to interactions involving increased understanding. Therefore, the more frequently you seek or offer clarification to others, the more likely you will have less difficulty, or more ease, as you communicate. The key to understanding these response styles and using them effectively is to continually self-assess what your intention is for the communication during all of your interactions.

This is helpful knowledge for the therapeutic relationship because the more you seek to understand what your clients, colleagues, and supervisor are asking for, and the more you seek to make your intentions clear, the more likely you will have clear, comfortable communication. All of these increase your ability to build a clientele and be a successful bodywork practitioner.

Bridging Communication Gaps

Once communication gaps are recognized, it takes time, effort, and energy to bridge them. Sometimes the time, effort, and energy expended are minimal; sometimes there must be a bigger investment. It all depends on how important bridging the gap is to the people involved. In the bodywork profession, success depends on your ability to bridge communication gaps effectively; it is a major part of client retention and building a client base. The practitioner who is unwilling or unable to do this will soon have a reputation in his bodywork community as someone who does not listen to his clients and his colleagues.

One of the barriers to bridging communication gaps is how information is presented in today's fast-paced society. It is given in short bursts using words and pictures designed for maximum impact. The idea is that people will immediately understand the information, then move on to the next piece of information. One has only to look at commercials and news stories, both

 Food for Thought

Looking at various response styles, which style do you tend to use most of the time? Be honest. Think of specific examples in which you have responded to someone critically, teaching/preaching, supportively, in a questioning manner, and to clarify. How did you feel when you responded each of these ways? How did the other person react when you responded each of these ways?

in print and televised, to see this. If something is not understood, then it is immediately discarded and the person moves on to the next message.

Unfortunately, some practitioners may think that bridging communication gaps should come easily and, if it does not, then it is not worth the time to keep working at it. A very common phrase heard is, "She just doesn't get it. Forget her." The assumption is that she should have gotten it right away, and, because she did not, she is no longer worth bothering with. Another assumption is that if there is a communication gap, the problem is with the other person, as the other person "just doesn't get it." Little consideration is given to the reason that the other person "just doesn't get it," or, that if the other person does "get it," maybe she is not in agreement.

Some people will take time to try and bridge communication gaps, but the methods they use are ineffective. For example, saying the same thing over and over, only more loudly and more insistently each time, tends to backfire and widen the gap even more. If someone is not receiving or understanding the message being given, it is usually not because he or she could not hear it. No one appreciates being yelled at, and an angry tone does not foster an atmosphere of collaboration, nor does the phrase, "You're just not listening to me."

What, then, does help bridge communication gaps? Time, effort, and energy are required, as well as the willingness to try delivering messages in different ways and to be very clear about personal feelings and needs.

Feelings and Needs in Communicating With Others

One way that communication gaps can be bridged is by considering your client's feelings and needs. "Communicate from the heart." "Use heart-centered communication." "Listen with your heart." These are all phrases used at various times in bodywork schools to describe the subtle communication that takes place between client and practitioner through touch, silence, or words. The heart becomes a metaphor for the roles that compassion, empathy, and the expression of feelings play in our efforts to connect with our clients.

Clinical psychologist Marshall Rosenberg developed the nonviolent communication (NVC) process as a means of enriching relationships by a "mutual giving from the heart."[4]

The four components of NVC include the following:

- Observe without evaluating what is actually happening in a situation.
- State how you feel when observing this situation.
- State what needs you have in relation to the feelings you have identified.
- Make a specific request that would enrich the relationship for both parties.[5]

NVC's goal is to create the possibility for a flow of communication that embodies compassion while empowering each person to take responsibility for what he or she needs in the relationship. Bodywork practitioners can use NVC strategies with clients who are not forthcoming with what they want from their bodywork sessions or with coworkers who are difficult to work with.

Consider the following:

Brent has been giving Sean, a talkative, easy-going, middle-aged guy, shiatsu treatments every week for the past 2 years. Sean has never missed an appointment without calling in advance to cancel and reschedule. Lately, however, he has started to miss appointments without calling and has not returned phone calls when Brent has left messages about the missed appointments. When Sean does come to his appointments he seems grim and is uncommunicative. When Brent asks for feedback about the treatment, Sean simply says, "Okay," and leaves the office. Brent decides he needs to delve more deeply into what is happening with Sean at his next appointment.

Brent: Sean, I have noticed that over the past 6 weeks you have forgotten your appointment twice without calling and when you do come for your sessions you seem distracted and sad. [observation] I feel concerned for your well-being [feelings stated] and need to know if there is anything I have done to offend you [need stated] or if you are in distress. Would you be willing to tell me what has brought on this change of behavior?

Sean: Nah, I'm all right. It's not anything you did.

Brent: Did something happen that's causing you distress?

Sean: Yeah, but I don't want to burden you with it.

Brent: It's not a burden for me to hear what's caused this change in you. Would you be willing to trust me that I'm open to hearing about what's going on with you without feeling burdened?

Sean: Well, I don't want you to worry about me but I could sure use some support right now.

At this point Sean talks for the next half hour about the loss of his full-time job and the struggle he is having looking for another job. He talks about feeling ashamed at being unemployed and his fear that he will not be able to provide for his family. Brent does not provide any solutions for Sean, yet the compassion and empathy Sean felt by Brent's presence was enough to lift his spirits and not feel so alone.

NVC is a process practitioners can choose to use when they feel unable to connect with a client because of unspoken feelings and needs. Even if the client does not want to disclose what is going on, at least he knows that his practitioner is aware that something is wrong, and is available to help when needed.

Meta-Communication

When needs are not being met, feelings are not being acknowledged or expressed, or assumptions are being made about what one person perceives to be true of the other, the outcome is usually increased frustration to the point of anger. Patterns of poor communication must be examined to find why the intended message is not getting across.

What can be done so that person can be heard? Is the lack of understanding a result of the tone of voice used, the time of day the interaction is taking place, or the words chosen to get the point across? To solve these issues, it may require you to talk with your client about how you talk with each other. This type of communication is called **meta-communication.** Meta-communications[6] are messages that refer to other messages.

 Food for Thought

Think about an interaction in which you expressed your needs and wants clearly. How did the interaction feel? What was the outcome? What would you like to have been different about the interaction? Think about an interaction you had with someone in which you, the other person, or both of you had made assumptions. How did the interaction feel? What was the outcome? What would you like to have been different about the interaction?

Meta-communication encompasses verbal and nonverbal communication factors that add more depth to the message but are often ignored if the receiver is not aware of them. Being aware of meta-communication can help clarify the true meaning of a message, thus minimizing misunderstanding and disconnection between the two speakers.

The focus in meta-communication is on the emotional aspect or the relationship dynamic of the speakers rather than on the content of issues. Having a conversation that places the focus on what is going on emotionally between two people minimizes the chance of a negative outcome. Why? Because meta-communication provides an opportunity for the truth to come out about how well the two parties are relating to one another. If this issue is not addressed adequately, miscommunication will persist.

Consider the following:

Fran is a massage therapist who has recently received training in craniosacral therapy. She is very excited about her new modality and has been incorporating it into her massage therapy treatments. Fran has also been telling her clients how much she loves craniosacral therapy and knows it will help them as well. The following exchange takes place between Fran and Audrey, a client who has been seeing her 5 years.

Fran: How was the treatment for you today, Audrey?

Audrey: Fine. [Shrugs shoulders and sighs.]

Fran: Good! I sensed that you released a lot of tension in your mid-thoracic and pelvic region. What do you think?

Audrey: Well, I'm not sure. I know I was expecting more attention to my shoulders and neck, like you've done in the past. I'm not so sure my pelvic area was having problems. It seems like you just held your hands still a lot and didn't massage much today.

Fran: Well, in craniosacral therapy, the pelvic region is very important in creating a balance for the rest of the body to line up. Trust me, your shoulder and neck did release tension. I could feel the difference between when we started and finished. When should we schedule your next appointment?

Audrey: [Avoiding eye contact] I'm not sure. I didn't bring my calendar and I'm not sure what my schedule is. I'll have to give you a call.

Audrey did not call to schedule another appointment. What did you notice in this interaction about the level of understanding between Fran and Audrey? What message was Audrey giving Fran? What message was Fran giving Audrey? What cues did Fran miss that could have helped her "read" Audrey more accurately?

The communication gap between Fran and Audrey began before the treatment even started. Fran did not ask Audrey if she wanted craniosacral therapy incorporated into the massage; she assumed that Audrey would welcome it. Fran may have lost a long-term client because she was not paying attention to the content or the underlying messages of Audrey's words and actions. It is clear that Fran is very excited to share her craniosacral therapy skills. However, based on Audrey's comment, "you just held your hands still a lot and didn't massage," Audrey is not satisfied with the work. She is saying that she wanted more massage work on her shoulders and not the craniosacral work. Fran did not pick up on this comment and ask for clarification. Instead, she chose to defend her treatment as being just as effective. In essence, she dismissed Audrey's dissatisfaction with her treatment experience.

When expectations are not met, it is often an indication that intentions were not communicated clearly. Not believing or honoring our clients' experience of our work will also create a void in the relationship. Seek to understand why a client makes a certain comment or lets out a deep sigh, for example, when the comment or sigh was not what you were expecting.

Other examples of meta-communication in the therapeutic setting include the following:

- A practitioner who does not listen or respond to client's request because she thinks she knows best
- A practitioner who is very focused in his work and chooses not to respond to a client's comments because he sees doing so as intrusive
- A bodywork clinic employee who is always late or does not attend staff meetings

Guidelines for meta-communication:

- Stay alert! Notice comments, gestures, or silence from your client. These may be ways information is being communicated to you. Some examples include frequent deep sighs, flinching without making any comment, being late for appointments, or not scheduling another treatment.
- Be aware of your own comments, gestures, and use of silence with clients. For example, suppose you are not returning phone calls promptly. Is it because you are too busy? Forgetful? Don't want to talk to this client? Being late for appointments could signal that you have poor time management skills or that you want a certain client to take a hint and stop scheduling with you.
- Seek to understand why a comment was stated or a gesture was made by asking an open-ended question. For example, you might say, "That was quite a series of heavy sighs. Tell me what you are feeling in your body right now," or "I noticed there was a quick movement in your shoulder just now. Tell me what you are experiencing and if what I'm doing is effective."
- Do not get carried away and overthink every interaction you have. Sometimes a sigh is just a sigh. It is the frequency, the tone, and, if it occurs while you are working on a client, the area you are working on when you hear the sigh, that will help you determine how to handle it.

Personal Responsibility

Bridging communication gaps also requires you to have personal responsibility. Personal responsibility is the capacity to be 100% accountable for your thoughts, words, and behaviors. Taking personal responsibility is the hallmark of a mature and grounded individual who does not look to blame others when things do not work out as she had hoped, and takes her share of praise only when she is successful. She is willing and able to reflect honestly on what her part was in an encounter and take ownership of it. Someone who takes personal responsibility will also hold others accountable for their words and their actions. When faced with conflict, distress, or disappointment, this individual will see the situation for what it is: a situation that did not go as planned. She will accept responsibility for her part in it and hold others accountable for their part.

When someone takes personal responsibility for her actions, she is able to **stay solid** (to know oneself and so not be swayed to deny personal feelings or change them because someone disagrees with them) in herself, knowing that she did the best she could with the skills she had. She does not take it personally if someone else ridicules or blames her. Rather, she is able to see beyond the negativity, learn what she can from the situation, and focus on creating positive outcomes in the future.

Taking personal responsibility is essential when working toward resolving communication gaps because it requires each person to focus only on what he or she can contribute rather than telling others how they should do things. This trait implies that each individual trusts that the others are capable of taking care of themselves; no one seeks to rescue the others from mistakes made.

Because you are human, you will have blind spots at times, and not be able to see your part in a difficult situation. However, by sharing honestly with trusted colleagues, mentors, friends, and family members you will be able to grasp sooner rather than later how you can contribute to the greater goal of bridging communication gaps. Also, if you are able to be accountable for your actions, you will also become skilled at asking the same of others. When you hold this value in high esteem, you will often be quick to state preferences and make requests of others for more effective outcomes.

Consider the following key components in taking personal responsibility for your communication:

What was said. This refers to the content of what was said—information, data, and the actual words used. It also means the context—the situation, circumstances, events, and facts surrounding the conversation. Taking responsibility for *what* you said means you are truthful and open about what you said. You do not try to minimize, change the facts, or place blame on others to avoid consequences for your comments.

Why was it said. This refers to the reason, purpose, or motivation for the conversation that took place between you and another person. Taking responsibility for *why* you said what you did means you are able to be honest, first with yourself, and then with others about what you intended your message to convey.

When was it said. This refers to the moment or period of time in which you chose to speak. Were your comments said in the heat of the moment when your emotions were high or did you wait for a period of time to pass before you said what you had to say? Taking responsibility for *when* you said what you did means that you are able to evaluate your words and the impact they can have on others. For example, you do not try to justify saying something inappropriate to another because your emotions got the best of you.

How was it said. This refers to the method of communication you use such as a face-to-face conversation, by telephone, through e-mail, voice mail, or text message. It also means the tone of your communication, such as your attitude; quality of your voice; and communication style, approach, and behavior. Taking responsibility for *how* you said what you did means you are aware of how these communication methods can affect others. For example, if you miss an appointment with a client, you choose to call him to apologize rather than send a text message. A text message is a way to "hide" from the client rather than risk hearing that the client is angry at your behavior.

Putting It All Together

To build a bridge across a communication gap, you must listen. Really listening makes the one being listened to feel worthy, appreciated, interesting, and respected. In the business world, listening saves time and money by preventing misunderstandings, and you can always learn more by listening than by talking. When you listen, you help foster this skill in others by acting as a model for positive and effective communication. **Kanji** are Chinese language symbols. As can be seen in Figure 4.1, the kanji for "to listen" includes the ears, eyes, heart, and undivided attention, which are all the components of effective listening.

Kim Ridley advocates the art of deep listening.[7] She states that when we simply allow another to share his or her story, uninterrupted, and with our full attention, we are bearing witness to another person's view of the world. Ridley identifies four components that will allow you to become a better listener:

1. Be present. Give the other person your full attention while being aware of what you are experiencing.
2. Be open by not acting on assumptions you may have about the other. Listen as a means of understanding what the other is feeling and experiencing.
3. Stay aware of your emotions.
4. Make space. You do this by asking for a few minutes of time to be alone. If you are in the midst of an argument, it will help to take time out to get perspective on the situation.

The following are some tools that aid in listening:

- Restating the speaker's main thoughts and feelings in your own words
- Asking meaningful questions to get more information

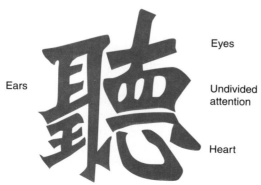

Figure 4.1 Kanji for "to listen."

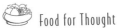

Words of Wisdom

Many of my massage clients have worked with me for nearly 20 years so we have gotten to know each other well and often talk during parts of the treatment. Whether first-timers or regulars I always let the client determine if talking will occur. First-time clients can be nervous and may initially be chatty but I have found that they soon quiet down and relax into the treatment once their questions have been answered calmly and briefly.

I have learned that each treatment session with the same client can be different. They may be very talkative one time and not at all the next three. The focus of their conversation can give you valuable information on where they may be holding stress. It is important to "hear" what they are not saying . . . many clues to tension can be uncovered by topics they avoid or gloss over.

—ANNIE GORDON, MFA, NCTMB, Licensed Massage Therapist since 1991

- Keeping comfortable eye contact and respecting personal space
- Not interrupting the speaker
- Listening patiently without giving advice
- Not changing the subject or talking about yourself

Note that, in particular, asking effective questions to clarify messages or get more information is an important part of actively listening. This shows that you are hearing the speaker's message and are making an effort to understand.

Consider the following conversation between Emilio, a neuromuscular therapist, and John, his client:

John: I don't know why you have to move me around the table so much.
Emilio: What do you mean "move you around the table"?
John: Oh, I don't know. It just seems like I can't lie here and relax when you work on me. I always have to be pushing here or . . .
Emilio: [Interrupts John] That's part of neuromuscular therapy. If you don't follow what I'm doing, you won't get any benefit out of the treatment.
John: Oh.

Was Emilio truly listening to John? Did Emilio ask John for more information? Did Emilio seem as though he was interested in how John experienced his treatment? Do you think Emilio would book another treatment with John? Would you?

What if Emilio had responded to John's complaint in the following way?

Emilio: It sounds like you're not happy with the amount of movement I do in my treatments. What would you prefer?
John: I'm not sure. I just don't want to work so hard while receiving a treatment. You keep me pretty busy!
Emilio: Well, that's true. I'm sorry you didn't enjoy today's treatment. How about next time we decide on the treatment plan in the interview and I make sure to follow it without asking you for assistance? How does that sound?
John: It sounds great. Thank you.

In this case, Emilio did not interrupt John. He restates what John says to make sure he understands, then asks follow-up questions that show he is listening to what John is saying. John is willing and ready to book another treatment with John.

As listening skills are developed, there will be natural pauses in the conversation that are not the same as communication gaps. These can be uncomfortable for some people, especially those accustomed to constant auditory input.

However, being comfortable with silence in another's presence can be a useful trait. One of the major ways bodywork has its effects on the body is through the practitioner simply being there with the client, not saying anything, but providing a focused and reassuring presence. Bodywork is a chance for members of today's fast-paced society; it gives them a chance to have a time-out from the noise and confusion. Practitioners who have developed the skill of being silent and present at the same time are usually the most successful bodywork practitioners.

When responding to a client, choose effective response styles, as discussed earlier in the chapter. Do honest self-reflection to see whether your responses are usually critical, teaching/preaching, supportive, questioning, or clarifying. Most clients appreciate when you want to clarify how the treatment could be made better for them. It shows that you are genuinely interested in the client's experience, and will go a long way toward client retention.

Avoid using vague terms that can mean different things to different people. When you are specific with your choice of words, you lessen, if not eliminate, the chance of being misunderstood by clients. Choose words that are understood by all communicating parties. As discussed in Chapter 3, using bodywork lingo that the client does not understand can lead to frustration on the part of the client. Consider the intention of the questions and choose words wisely. It takes a bit more time and effort to clearly state questions using language that is understood by everyone. However, it is a good investment of time and energy, as it allows you to get the information you need to proceed successfully with your clients.

The following are some examples of vague and specific comments:

Vague: "How is the pressure?"
More specific: "Is the pressure I am using in this area helping to relieve the soreness or would you like me to increase it or decrease it?"
Vague: "Are you comfortable?"
More specific: "Let me know if there is anything I can do to assist your comfort level with this massage. I have a blanket if you get cold, I can change the music if you like, or I can change techniques if you don't like the one I am using. Please don't hesitate to let me know if you are uncomfortable at any time."

Another component of bridging communication gaps is choosing an appropriate time and place to communicate. Talking with the client about her medical conditions in the middle of the busy lobby of the bodywork office is inappropriate. Confidentiality about the client's conditions is not maintained, and the client will be uncomfortable, knowing that others may be listening. The best place to conduct pre- and post-treatment interviews is in the treatment room with the door closed. If you are having a conflict with another practitioner, it is also best if you and the other practitioner interact privately, not in front of other practitioners and certainly not in front of clients.

Managing Difficult Interactions

Unfortunately, difficult interactions with others are always a possibility, no matter how mindful and diligent you are in developing sound communication skills. This section covers how to manage such interactions.

Difficult Client Behavior

The following are some examples of difficult client behavior you may encounter. Difficult clients tend to do the following:

- Have needs that are hard to satisfy no matter what you do
- Tend to push the boundaries or limits of the business policy statements

- Attempt to become friends with the practitioner, even when they have been told that the practitioner does not socialize with clients
- Try to get extra treatment time for free or are malingerers and consistently request more work at the end of the treatment
- Have a negative outlook on life and tend to be draining on the practitioner
- Are not sure what they want and take a long time to describe what they are feeling or needing from you

The last situation can be especially frustrating, as it is difficult for you to come up with an appropriate treatment plan that the client will agree to. This can also result in the client putting all his faith and expectations in you to "fix" him rather than having a mutual working relationship.

Other behaviors that can be categorized as "difficult" are the nonverbal behaviors a client may display, such as heavy sighing, fidgeting on the table, and not being communicative in the intake process. Any behavior from a client that prevents you from connecting in a real and authentic way is difficult behavior. Another hallmark of difficult clients is that you begin to dread seeing them and make up excuses not to book them on a regular basis. You may resent the client because his or her behavior drains you. It is important that you pay attention to these feelings of resentment so that you can explore them and determine if there is a way to resolve the feeling or if it is time to refer the client to another therapist.

Difficult Interactions With Other Practitioners and Employers

You can also experience difficult interactions with other practitioners and employers. These can include the following:

- Practitioners who are habitually late and then need to rush to get ready, expecting you to help them
- Gossiping behind other practitioners' backs
- Maneuvering so that new clients are booked with a particular practitioner rather than by the bodywork business's rotation or seniority system
- "Stealing" clients from other practitioners by downplaying or even criticizing the other practitioners' skills
- Employers scheduling practitioners to work other than mutually agreed-upon times
- Employees not giving practitioners gratuities from the clients they have worked on

Addressing Difficult Behaviors

When addressing difficult behaviors, whether it is from a client, coworker, or employer, the following are useful to keep in mind:

- Be direct; do not beat around the bush.
- Do not wait around and hope the situation goes away without saying anything.
- Use a professional tone of voice when addressing the issues. Do not raise your voice, even if you are angry.
- Take responsibility for your part in the equation of the relationship and then describe to the person how the difficult behavior is affecting you.

- Separate the person from the behavior; bad behavior does not mean that the person is bad.
- Name specific behaviors that are causing the difficulty.
- Discuss possible solutions with the other person to resolve the problems.
- Be honest and respectful.
- Do not ask for something that is not possible to be achieved.

As mentioned before, when managing difficult situations, it is important to explore both the content of the conflict as well as the emotional aspect. The ideal solution to the conflict must be acceptable to both parties.

Consider the following:

Cal, a client of Lani's, enters the office 30 minutes into his treatment time looking visibly shaken and is very apologetic for his lateness. Lani can tell that something is bothering him and abandons her plan to scold him. Instead, she asks what he needs right now and how she can assist. Cal states that he had witnessed a fatal accident on the way to his appointment and it has really upset him. He does not feel up to getting a massage but he wants to honor his commitment to her by coming and explaining what had happened.

Lani suggests that because there is still 30 minutes left in his treatment time, perhaps she could do some gentle craniosacral holds or a scalp massage to help Cal calm down. Cal agrees and expresses much appreciation for Lani's kindness.

Had Lani decided to discuss her office policies regarding late clients with Cal instead of realizing something was wrong, she would have missed the chance to help her client in a meaningful way. The result is that they both had a chance to be heard as well as participate in creating a workable solution. This type of collaboration preserves the integrity of the relationship as well as the longevity of it. Bodywork practitioners must be mindful of how important client retention is and be skilled at creating strategies that will diffuse potential problems and focus on facilitating the success of therapeutic relationships.

Sometimes it may seem to be easier not to address difficult behaviors. If there is not much time and investment in the relationship, or if the parties involved will be interacting for only a short period of time, you may choose to overlook the behavior. There may be cases in which you do not think you have the right to ask for changes in someone else's behavior.

In ongoing relationships, however, not addressing difficult behavior can lead to escalation of the problem, sometimes to the point of explosion and termination of the relationship. In such cases, it is usually much easier to address the behaviors early on, as shown in Figure 4.2.

Conflict Resolution Strategies

Most people approach a dispute with a win and lose attitude because of living in a competitive culture. The reasoning is, "If I let her get what she wants, then I won't get what I want," or "I don't want to be the loser in this disagreement." People often assume that it's an either/or situation: *either* one person wins *or* the other one does. However, instead of competition, solving conflicts can sometimes be reframed in terms of collaboration. Instead of

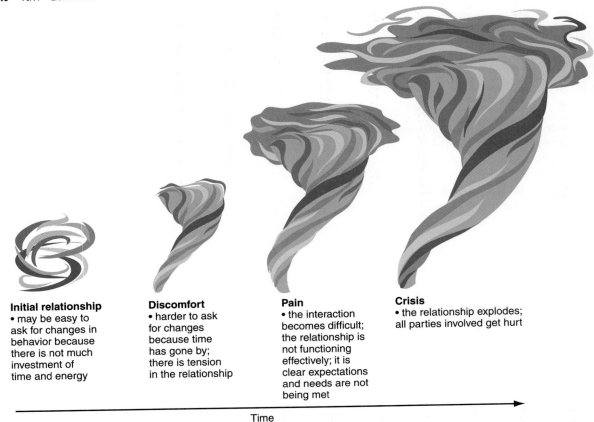

Initial relationship
• may be easy to ask for changes in behavior because there is not much investment of time and energy

Discomfort
• harder to ask for changes because time has gone by; there is tension in the relationship

Pain
• the interaction becomes difficult; the relationship is not functioning effectively; it is clear expectations and needs are not being met

Crisis
• the relationship explodes; all parties involved get hurt

Time

Figure 4.2 Correlation of time and addressing difficult behaviors.

![Food for Thought icon] Food for Thought
What works better for you: being right, or solving a problem? Why did you answer the way that you did?

either/or, the thinking can be changed to, "We can listen to each other and work together to discover a solution that will meet our needs."

Table 4.2 contrasts competition and collaboration approaches to conflict resolution.

Norwegian professor Johan Galtung, one of the founders of modern peace studies, developed a theoretical framework for addressing conflict. Although his work concentrates on global peace and justice issues, the concepts are applicable to interpersonal relationships. Galtung's ABC Theory of Conflict (also known as Galtung's Triangle of Conflict) identifies three dimensions that promote a productive outcome for conflict resolution. The dimensions are the following:

Attitude: the cognitive and emotional assumptions each person has about the issue in question
Behavior: the contributing actions of each person involved in the conflict
Content: the specific issue of the conflict that is causing the disagreement[8]

All three of these dimensions overlap and must be individually dealt with to find a solution that will meet the needs of all involved. When each of these dimensions is considered, each person can generate possible solutions to the conflict.

Table 4.2	Competition Versus Collaboration Approach to Conflict Resolution	
Competition	**Collaboration**
Self-serving	Focus is on the greater good
Focus is on personal interests and goals	Focus is on everyone's needs and goals
Each person wants to be the winner	Each person realizes that they win when everyone wins
Needs can be met only through competing with others	Needs can be met through collaboration
There is much talk but little listening	People listen to each other and work to express ideas clearly
People attack each other verbally and/or physically	People focus their energies on solving the problem
People can be disrespectful through words and actions	People treat each other with respect
Trust is not developed	Trust tends to develop
Issues are brought up that are not connected to the problem at hand	Only specific issues connected to problem are discussed
Relationships may be damaged	Relationships can become stronger
Goal: To be right at all costs	Goal: To understand each other and preserve the relationships

When working to resolve conflicts, Galtung's dimensions can be adapted to determining what the issue is, and then determining honestly what your part is in the conflict. To do this you can then break the issue down into three parts (Fig. 4.3):

- The emotional aspect
- The content of the issue (facts, data)
- The possible solutions to resolve it

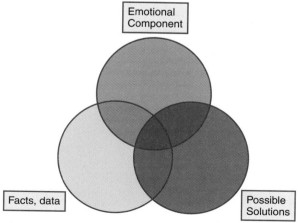

Figure 4.3 The three parts of conflict.

The emotional aspect of conflict is what is not being said because the people involved may not be aware of underlying emotions. For example, Ariel and Mason are partners in a bodywork business. A conflict has arisen because Ariel has promised to update the computer client list but has not done so by an agreed-upon date. She has underlying anxiety because she thinks she has not been building up her clientele enough. She is avoiding updating the list because she can then find out how many clients she has seen, and is afraid to see the actual number. Ariel pretends, even to herself, that she is taking action but, in reality, she is not. Meanwhile, Mason needs the updated client list so that the two of them can plan their next marketing strategy, and is becoming frustrated at the delay.

The facts or data aspect of conflict involves clarity about what the situation is, and what needs to happen. Often it is what is safe to talk about, and what looks like the real issue. However, talking about the facts can also be a way to deflect the emotional aspects of the conflict. In the case of the conflict between Ariel and Mason, the fact is that Ariel has not completed the updated client list. Both Ariel and Mason are clear about this. However, unless the people involved are willing to self-assess and be honest about what they are feeling and then take responsibility for their actions, talking will do nothing but fuel the lack of action. At this point, if Ariel says, "Yes, it is coming along. I know what I have to do. It will be done soon," but still does not complete the task, then it is likely that Mason will grow even more frustrated and start to view Ariel as untrustworthy. Instead of being resolved, the conflict is growing larger.

The possible solutions aspect of conflict can occur only when both the facts and the emotions are aired and discussed. Real action can take place based on what is comfortable for both parties and what is good for the common goals. If Ariel is honest with Mason about why she has not completed updating the client list, then he can have a better understanding of her behavior. Because they are business partners, it is likely he will realize that by offering Ariel support, not only will the list become updated, but they will also be communicating more productively. Their working relationship will become more comfortable, and Ariel may feel more confident about her skills at building a clientele. This will make their business relationship more successful as well. The conflict is resolved.

If you get caught up in one aspect of the conflict and do not openly address or become aware of the other aspects, the conflict cannot be resolved. It may look as though progress is being made, but in reality it is not. The possible solutions that are generated will not last or be successful. The solutions that are successful are the ones that involve both the emotional aspects as well as the facts. In Figure 4.3 these solutions are in the center, where all three aspects overlap.

Ask the other person for a time to discuss the issue. When discussing the issue, each party should decide what is most invested in the relationship and what should be preserved. Each person should express specific behaviors he or she would prefer to see in the other. It is important that the parties involved stay focused on finding solutions and not on placing blame. They should also be prepared to hear something about themselves that is uncomfortable to hear.

Depending on the nature of the conflict, humor may be a useful strategy to defuse an issue. This approach should be used cautiously, because humor is often misunderstood. Conversely, if the people know each other, and each other's sense of humor, humor can sometimes be used to clear up a misunderstanding quickly and comfortably.

Practicing what to say before approaching the other person may be useful. This may help you not get distracted and flustered. Conflict that is left unaddressed leads to stress and tension that could be translated into your work with the client (if that is who you are in conflict with) or stress and tension in the workplace (if the conflict is with another practitioner or an employer). Conflict left unaddressed can even lead to physical illness that could affect your work.

Resolving Conflict With Clients

The three parts of a conflict illustrated in Figure 4.3 can be used to resolve conflict with clients.

Consider the situation between Christine, a Reiki practitioner, and her client Bob. For 3 months Christine has been coming to Bob's home to give him treatments. Bob chats to Christine for 20 minutes before the treatment and takes as long as 20 minutes to get off the table after the treatment.

Christine: Bob, I need to talk with you about how much time I actually spend at your home for your 1 hour treatment. I usually spend no more than 90 minutes at a client's home when providing an hour in home treatment. My appointments with you have been lasting more than 2 hours from the time I arrive until the time I leave. I'd like you to be prepared for your treatment when I arrive so that I can stay on schedule, and I'd like you to get off the treatment table sooner after the session.

Bob: I like to receive a focused treatment, so I wanted to give you some time to rest up before working on me. I'm a little upset you didn't explain to me that you have a schedule to keep. That made it seem like it was okay that you were here so long. In fact, the reason I like having an in-home appointment is so that I don't have to feel rushed like I do at a clinic. If that does not work for you, then I can find someone else to come here. I feel bad that you see me as a selfish person.

Christine: Bob, I don't see you as a selfish person. I appreciate your thoughtfulness about wanting to give me some down time before your session, but I don't need it. I schedule my workdays to allow for enough energy to meet all my clients' needs, no matter what time of day the appointment is. And I can appreciate your need to have a relaxing experience. I apologize and take responsibility for not being clear in explaining the time frame that I was expecting. I'm not opposed to being here for more than 2 hours but I'd need to increase my fee for your session. What do you think?

Bob: Well, I'm glad that you don't think I'm selfish. I really did think I was being helpful. Now that I know what you need from me, I can make some changes in my routine. I can definitely be ready to start the treatment when you arrive if you can come 30 minutes later.

Bob and Christine are able to collaborate to create a solution to the conflict by being honest about how the conflict was affecting each of them and what part they played in creating the conflict. Christine remained professional and did not attack Bob personally nor did she blame him for the problem. She merely stated the facts of his behavior.

They were both able to identify where the breakdown in communication happened. By working through the conflict, they gained a deeper understanding of what each needed in the therapeutic relationship and made a commitment to do their part to ensure success.

The process of conflict resolution does not need to be filled with tension. When done with honesty, integrity, and professionalism, conflict resolution can bring about growth, change, learning, and an increase in understanding among all involved. It can be a transformative experience for both you and the client.

However, conflict resolution with a client does depend on the client's investment in the relationship, his willingness to make an effort to work things out, and his ability to move forward toward to new beginning once a difficult situation has been uncovered and dealt with. Some clients will not be able to tolerate discussion about a conflict and may choose to move on from the relationship. Others may express deep gratitude for the opportunity to change their ways now that they know how it affects others. Yet others may say all the right things in conversation and not have the intention of following through. If this last one describes a situation practitioners have found themselves in with a client, then it may be time to refer the client to another practitioner.

When to Call It Quits

There comes a time in all relationships when the people involved must evaluate whether the relationship is working, whether both parties are getting their needs met in healthy and respectful ways, and whether both parties have a shared desire and commitment for the relationship to continue. At some point, the decision may need to be made that the relationship is just not working out. All that can be done to improve or stay present in the relationship has been done and the amount of time, effort, energy, and interest spent does not equal satisfaction. In the case of employment or working with certain clients, perhaps the financial gain is not worth the feelings of exhaustion and frustration.

Signs that a therapeutic relationship with clients is not working out include behavior patterns persisting even after you have requested that they be changed, or your inability to tolerate the "Oops, I'm sorry I'm late again" clients. If you notice that you are expending a lot of mental and emotional energy trying to figure out how to work with someone, then it may be time for you to refer the client to another practitioner.

Pay attention to the voice inside of you that says, "Enough is enough. I need to make some changes." If this voice is ignored, resentment toward the other person will grow, and it may come out indirectly. One of the worst mistakes you can make is not to address client behavior, and then have resentment toward the client come out somehow during the treatment. Also, stress illnesses can affect you when you are not dealing directly with a situation that is not improving. It is difficult for you to be genuine with your clients if you are not true to yourself. If you conclude that it is no longer appropriate to continue working with a client, it is your responsibility to make a referral. This should be done in a tactful manner, and you should provide appropriate closure. The closure could be as simple as stating that you are making some changes to your schedule and need to refer the client to another practitioner. Give the client at least a month's notice, if possible.

■ CASE PROFILE

Dale is a licensed massage therapist who owns his own bodywork practice. According to Dale's office policy and procedures, if a client is late, he receives only the amount of time left in the treatment session when he arrives for the appointment. The client is still responsible for the full charge of the treatment, regardless of how much time he actually spent receiving the massage.

Luis has been a client of Dale's for 6 months. Initially, Luis was very timely for his appointments and, if he were late, he would call in advance and give Dale an estimated time of arrival.

Luis's work schedule changed, and he asked Dale what time his last appointment time of the day was on Thursdays. Dale informed him that he stopped seeing clients at 8:00 p.m. Luis said, "Great! I'll take your last appointment on Thursday." Dale asked if he still wanted to schedule for the usual 90 minutes and Luis said yes. Dale booked the appointment for 6:30 p.m.

On Thursday, Luis did not arrive for his appointment at 6:30 p.m. Dale figured he was probably running late and was not concerned. When Luis had not arrived by 6:50, Dale called him and left a message on his voice mail stating that he was calling to see if Luis was on the way to his appointment.

At 7:00 p.m., Luis called back, upset, because he understood that his appointment was at 8:00 p.m., Dale's last appointment. He insisted that Dale told him he stops seeing clients at 8 p.m., which was the time for which he made the appointment. In addition, Luis stated that he was in a great deal of pain due to a migraine coming on. He has been anticipating tonight's massage as the only way to keep from getting a full-blown migraine. While Luis was talking, he did not let Dale interject at all into the conversation. Each time Dale tried, Luis talked over him and kept insisting that he needed the massage and that he would be right over.

Define the communication gaps between Dale and Luis.

Describe Luis' behavior. Do you think it is helping or hurting his chances of getting a treatment from Dale that evening?

What should Dale say?

What could have been done differently when the appointment was initially made?

Write out a dialogue between Luis and Dale to resolve this conflict. Have one dialogue be that Luis does not receive the massage. Have the other dialogue result in Luis receiving the massage.

Intervention Model

Most practitioners will experience unwelcomed or dangerous situations with clients at some point in their careers. Certain clients have the idea that sexual services are available, no matter how clearly it is stated otherwise by the practitioner and the bodywork office. Sometimes the behavior is subtle at first. For example, a client may behave appropriately for the first few treatments, then start to ask personal questions of the practitioner. Because the practitioner may think that a therapeutic relationship has been established, she may not think much about this. In subsequent treatments, the questions may become more and more personal, the client may ask the practitioner out, or the client may request no draping be done (in the case of massage therapy) or even come right out and request sexual services. Many practitioners have been caught off guard because the client behaved appropriately at first and then, abruptly, a sexual request is made.

Other times, the client may fidget quite a bit, move the hands over the genital region, or pull the draping off. All of these actions can be disconcerting, to say the least, to the practitioner. Many times, however, clients may make movements and say things that may, in fact, turn out to be innocent.

The following is a strategy you can use to protect yourself from potentially dangerous or unwelcome situations with clients. This strategy is effective because it empowers you to ask for clarifications of what you are experiencing as well as offering the opportunity for dialogue with the client to determine what is going on with him or her during the treatment. It is possible that you can misunderstand the intent of the client, so by asking the client to state his or her intention, you are allowing the client the opportunity to explain. You may then either take the opportunity to educate the client about the purpose of bodywork or tell the client to leave.

The following are the steps to take in such a situation:

1. Stop applying techniques. Redrape if performing massage therapy.
2. State the behaviors you are observing.
3. Ask the client to clarify what his or her intention is for the treatment.
4. Make a decision about whether to stop the treatment or to proceed with it.
5. You may choose to seek supervision to discuss the incident so it does not linger and cause you to be nervous about performing another treatment.

Unless it is unquestionably overt, practitioners must be careful not to assume that all behavior that they consider inappropriate is worthy of using the intervention model. This model is a safety measure for those times that they are unclear about what is going on between them and the client, and if continuing the treatment would cause practitioners undue stress. As practitioners gain experience and confidence, they will trust their ability to interpret a situation and act accordingly. The key to using the intervention model is not to ignore, tolerate, or pretend that something the client is doing does not bother them when it really does. The intervention model gives practitioners a format in which to express what they are experiencing and gain clarification from the client.

Chapter Summary

Communication gaps occur when people are unable to understand each other. There are many reasons communication gaps occur, such as use of language that not all parties understand, assumptions made on the part of the participants, expectations that are not verbalized, generational differences, regional and cultural differences, and personal response styles. Recognizing communication gaps and bridging them ensures client retention. Some of the ways communication gaps can be bridged are through being willing to expend time, effort, and energy to use effective communication; being sensitive to cultural and generational differences; acknowledging that feelings and needs are important in the communication process; using effective listening skills; and using clear language.

You can experience difficult interactions with clients, as when clients have needs that are hard to satisfy, want to cross the line into friendship when you do not, and are emotionally draining. You can also experience difficult interactions with coworkers and employers. When addressing difficult behaviors, be willing to address the situation directly and professionally, take responsibility for your part in the relationship, discuss possible solutions, and create a timeline for follow-up. Sometimes, however, it is time to end the therapeutic relationship with the client and refer him or her to another practitioner, which should be done with tact.

Most practitioners will experience unwelcomed or dangerous situations with clients at some point in their bodywork career. The intervention model is a five-step strategy you can use to protect yourself. It empowers you to ask for clarifications of what you are experiencing as well as to offer the opportunity for dialogue with the client to determine what is going on with him or her during the treatment.

Review Questions

Multiple Choice

1. Which of the following is an indicator that there is a communication gap?

a. Having a continual pattern of misunderstandings with the same person

b. Feelings of frustration or anger rather than resolution

c. Avoiding certain people because it seems to take too much energy to deal with them

d. All of the above

2. Listening for details and analyzing the quality of ideas in the message describes what type of listening style?

a. Content-oriented

b. People-oriented

c. Action-oriented

d. Time-oriented

3. Which of the following is an example of a critical response style?

   a. "You don't know what you're doing; you should leave the expertise to me."

   b. "It sounds as if you'd like me to lessen my pressure during the treatment. Is that true?"

   c. "I understand that you are concerned with how the treatments are progressing."

   d. "Clients usually receive 50% improvement with the techniques I've been using."

4. Which of the following is an example of effective listening skills?

   a. Offering advice to the speaker

   b. Talking about a personal experience that ties into what the speaker is saying

   c. Restating the speaker's thoughts and feelings in the listener's own words

   d. Interrupting the speaker to clarify a point

5. If a practitioner realizes that he is frustrated with a client's behavior, which of the following is the best approach for him to take with the client?

   a. Ignore the client's behavior and hope it stops

   b. Refuse to continue giving the client treatments

   c. Be clear with the client about the effects of the behavior

   d. Immediately refer the client to another practitioner

6. Signs that a therapeutic relationship with clients is not working out include which of the following?

   a. The persistence of client behavior patterns that have been requested to change

   b. Repeated frustration with the client on the part of the practitioner

   c. The practitioner spending much time and energy trying to figure out how to work with the client

   d. All of the above

7. Which of the following is part of the intervention model?

   a. Continue to apply techniques

   b. Ignore the behaviors being observed

   c. Try to forget about the incident

   d. Ask the client his or her intention for the treatment

Fill in the Blank

1. When people are unable to understand each other, this can lead to _____ .

2. A contributing factor to a communication gap is lack of _____ of or _____ for another's culture

3. The intent behind giving facts, information, and "shoulds" to another person characterizes the

   _____ response style.

4. The term used to describe communication about the factors involved in communication is

   _____ .

5. Being concerned with the greater good is an aspect of the _____ approach to conflict resolution.

6. An effective approach practitioners can use to resolve conflict with clients includes creating a(n)

   _____ and scheduling a follow-up conversation.

7. When working to resolve conflicts, the issues can be broken down in the emotional components,

   the facts and data of the issue, and the possible _____ .

Short Answer

1. Explain how communication gaps can occur.

2. Explain why bridging communication gaps is important for client retention.

3. Explain how needs and feelings are intertwined in what and how people communicate with each other.

4. List four examples of cultural considerations practitioners should keep in mind.

5. Explain why taking personal responsibility is essential when working toward resolving communication gaps.

6. Explain useful things to keep in mind when addressing difficult behaviors, whether it is from a client, coworker, or employer.

7. List and explain the three parts of conflict and they can be used to resolve conflicts with clients.

Activities

1. Using the concept of meta communication, have a discussion with a friend or relative about how you communicate with each other. Be sure ask the following questions:

   • Do you understand the messages you give each other?
   • What tone of voice does each of you usually use when talking with each other?
   • Is there a time of day when you communicate the best? The worst?
   • What are some of the words you usually use to get your message across?
   • Do you think the other person really hears you? Does the other person think you really hear him or her?

2. Except for the pretreatment interview and checking in once or twice about the client's comfort, practice being silent while giving a bodywork treatment for an entire hour.

3. If you have traveled to other regions of the country or to other countries, write down what you noticed about the language, customs, food, and the like in these areas. How comfortable were you? Could you make yourself understood easily? Why or why not? Did you get angry or frustrated when you were not understood? Whom did you hold responsible for any communication gaps you experienced?

4. Research another culture in which bodywork is an accepted practice. Describe the customs associated with receiving bodywork in this culture. What is considered polite and what is considered impolite?

5. Write a script of what you would do and say while using the intervention model. Role-play with another person until you feel comfortable using your script.

Guidance for Journaling

 Some key areas to think about while journaling for this chapter include the following:

• Communication gaps you have experienced
• How generational, regional, and cultural differences contribute to communication gaps
• Why bridging communication gaps is important for client retention
• Ways you can bridge communication gaps you are experiencing
• Difficult communication and behaviors you have experienced
• Uncomfortable nonverbal communication you have experienced from clients
• Conflict resolution strategies for career success
• How you have resolved conflicts in the past and ways you can improve your conflict resolution skills
• The intervention model and when you think you might need to use it

References

1. Adler, R.B., and Rodman, G.: *Understanding Human Communication*, ed. 10. New York, Oxford University Press, 2009, pp 111–112.
2. Purtilo, R., and Haddad, A.: *Health Professional and Patient Interaction,* ed. 7. New York, W.B. Saunders, 2007, p 43.
3. Ibid, p 40.
4. Rosenberg, M.B.: *Nonviolent Communication: A Language of Life,* ed. 2. Encinitas, CA, Puddle Dancer Press, 2003, p 1.
5. Ibid, p 6.
6. Adler, R.B., Rodman, G., and Elmhorst, J.: *Understanding Human Communication,* ed. 10. New York, Oxford University Press, 2008, pp 186–187.
7. Ridley, K.: Don't just do something, stand there. *Ode* (July–August): 62–64, 2006.
8. Galtung, J.: Peace by Peaceful Means: Peace and Conflict, Development and Civilization. Oslo, Norway, International Peace Research Institute, 1996.

PART II

Ethics

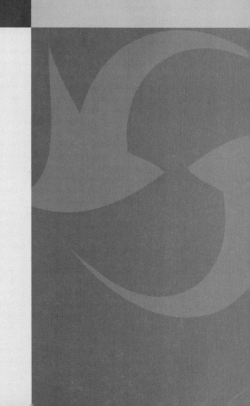

Ethics
The Basics

LEARNING OBJECTIVES

After studying this chapter, you will be able to:

1. Explain the connection between professional work ethics and career success.
2. Explain how ethics, morals, values, and principles are all different concepts yet interconnected.
3. Define and determine your own professional work ethics.
4. Define what a code of ethics is and write your own code of ethics.
5. Explain ethical congruency, codes of conduct, and standards of practice.
6. Explain how to recognize and resolve ethical dilemmas.

CHAPTER OUTLINE

KEY TERMS

Code of ethics: a set of guidelines that delineates the standards of behavior for the members of a group or profession

Codes of conduct: sets of rules listing the proper practices and responsibilities of an individual, organization, or profession

Critical thinking: the process of conscious thought based on weighing all the facts that are known to form an opinion about something

Ethical awareness: self-awareness and willingness to ask, "Am I doing the right thing?"

Ethical congruency: being authentic in both words and actions and having behavior that matches with declared personal ethical standards

Ethical dilemmas: situations that require considering information that requires an opinion, a response, or an action in a situation that challenges a person's ethics

Ethics: a system or set of principles that are used as a framework for choosing between right and wrong behavior and for determining what is good and what is bad

Group ethics: the behaviors and attitudes that a culture, community, organization, or profession determines best reflects its goals and desires

Morals: standards of judgment about behavior and character

Principles: behavioral guidelines based on a person's morals, which can vary widely from person to person

Values: what a person finds desirable

Work ethic: a drive within a person that motivates him or her to arrive at work on time every day, do the best work at all times, work until the work is done, not take excessive amounts of time off, and cooperate with colleagues and supervisors

---

Lindsay has enrolled in a 12-month massage therapy certification program. On the first day of class, as students are introducing themselves, Lindsay says, "I've been giving massages part-time for the past 2 years to make ends meet. Because the state is now requiring all massage therapists to be licensed, I'm here so that I can finally get recognized as a professional."

The instructor responds to Lindsay's introduction by reminding the class that the student handbook states they will have to wait until graduation and completion of the state licensing requirements before they receive payment of any kind. The instructor adds, "When you signed your enrollment contract, you agreed to these terms. If you accept money from practice clients you will be expelled from the program and can't get licensed."

Lindsay is now dealing with an ethical dilemma. Should she continue to work on her clients, accept payment from them, and never tell anyone at the school what she is doing? Should she tell all her clients that she can practice massage on them but can no longer receive payment from them, and find herself another part-time job while she attends school? Should she tell all her clients that she can no longer charge them while she is in school, but if they want to tip her, that would be all right, because she is not asking directly for payment? Should she quit school and build her massage practice without a license, hoping she stays under the radar of the massage licensing board and does not get caught?

Ethical dilemmas like the one Lindsay faces confront bodywork practitioners all the time. The purpose of this chapter is to prepare you to make ethical decisions as a professional practitioner. This chapter begins by defining and differentiating some essential concepts, including ethics, morals, values, and principles. It continues with a discussion of work ethics and how to improve your work ethics as a professional practitioner. Codes of ethics are addressed, which reflect the standards set by a profession. The concepts of ethics and ethical congruency in terms of a solid framework in which to practice as professional bodywork practitioners are also discussed. Because everyone experiences ethical dilemmas, and not everyone has tools to resolve them, ethical dilemmas are defined. Methods to recognize ethical dilemmas are presented, as well as a five-step strategy to assist you in resolving them. Emphasis is also placed on the responsibility you have to report unethical behavior on the part of other practitioners.

Professional Work Ethics and Career Success

Presented below are some essential concepts related to ethics, how to become ethically aware, and how to develop professional work ethics and behaviors.

Definitions

It is common to use the words "ethics," "values," "principles," and "morals" interchangeably. Each word has a thread of similarity but there are differences that will influence how each will be used in this chapter.

Ethics is a system or set of principles used as a framework for choosing between right and wrong behavior and for determining what is good and what is bad. The conduct of individuals, groups of people (from softball teams to entire countries), and professional organizations is governed by ethics. Examples of ethical behavior include abiding by laws and regulations, respecting self and others, and conducting business fairly and honestly.

Morals are standards of judgment about behavior and character. They are measurements of behavior or conduct, when judged by an individual, a society, or a religious standard.[1] Morals tend to be very rigid, not allowing for much interpretation. Two examples of moral behavior include not cheating and telling the truth. Morals are learned; people are not born knowing what is moral behavior.

A person exhibits integrity when his behavior is firmly consistent with his moral values, with an emphasis on being consistent. A person is said to have integrity when everything she says, does, and believes is based on the same set of core values, regardless of arguments or pressure from others. Having actions follow beliefs is an essential component of integrity. The core values may change, as in discarding those that are not useful and incorporating new ones that are, but it is in having values that are consistent with each other and with her behavior that determine a person's level of integrity.

People use their *conscience* to decide whether their actions are right or wrong. They can consult their conscience before saying and doing things to see whether they are conforming to their moral judgments. If they say or do things that go against their morals, they feel remorse. When their words and actions follow their morals, they feel a sense of righteousness and integrity. Unless there is a large issue with which a person is grappling, most often people are not aware that they are allowing their conscience to guide them. They are behaving the way they have learned to behave, which, to them, is the right way to behave.

Most people have said and done things at one time or another that they then regret. Often this is referred to as "speaking or acting before thinking." They did not give themselves time to check in with their conscience before they responded to certain issues. Most people have the capacity for change and can learn from their mistakes. This learning process involves self-reflection and self-inquiry, which may involve asking oneself, "Is what I'm saying or doing in line with my personal morals? If it is, and I'm still feeling uncomfortable or regretting what I've said or done, is it time to change one or more of my morals? If so, what moral do I want to change, and how do I want to change it?" This process can occur so quickly that the person may not be consciously aware of it, or it may take considerable time to evaluate and reconstruct moral values.

Rather than being based on what is right or wrong, **values** are based on what a person finds desirable.[2] Values result from beliefs and experiences and thus can be developed from culture, religion, family, country, age groups, and environment and so can change throughout a person's life. Values can also vary considerably from person to person, situation to situation, and throughout a person's life. For example, a person in his twenties may value highly having enough money to socialize with his friends every Friday night. When that same person is in his forties, his values may have changed to ensuring that his family is cared for financially and having enough money to live on during retirement.

Principles are codes of action to guide our behavior as well as our decision-making process, and they can vary widely from person to person. For example, one bodywork practitioner may choose to charge a wealthy client more for a treatment and charge a client who is not wealthy less for the same treatment. Another practitioner may choose to charge all clients the same amount for treatments, regardless of their financial circumstances.

As you may have realized, ethics can be applied to individuals, groups, and professions. Some examples of ethical standards that we focus on in the bodywork profession include offering client-centered treatments; being respectful to clients, colleagues, and other health-care professionals; working within our scope of practice; following the standards of practice; and carrying liability insurance.

In his book *Do the Right Thing: Living Ethically in an Unethical World*, Thomas G. Plante states that "ethics basically attempts to answer the question, 'How shall I live my life?' Ethics is a set of principles for living and decision making. Ethics is also a discipline of critical reflection on the meaning and justification for moral beliefs."[3]

Plante implies that ethics is an active process and not just theoretical. Every day we make choices about our behavior that will guide us in the direction we want our life to go. These choices are not made at random but are influenced by a set of principles that we believe will get our needs met.

Food for Thought

Can you think of an experience you've had in which you've reevaluated your morals? What prompted you to do this? What was the outcome? How did your morals change or not change? How did you feel throughout this experience?

Defining ethics as "a discipline of critical reflection on the meaning and justification for moral beliefs" addresses the importance of clarifying what we believe and differentiates good from bad and right from wrong behaviors. This knowledge must reside within ourselves if it is to have any true meaning on how we conduct our lives (Box 5.1 and 5.2).

Box 5.1 | **FIVE ETHICAL PRINCIPLES**

Thomas G. Plante identifies the following five ethical principles to guide your behavior and decision-making process in your personal and professional life:

- **Integrity**—following high standards of honesty, justice, and fairness; being complete and consistent in your actions.
- **Competence**—having knowledge, skill, and training that make you qualified for the job you are hired to do.
- **Responsibility**—being accountable and following through on your obligations, promises, and commitments.
- **Respect**—treating others as you would want to be treated; treating others with attention, value, and consideration.
- **Concern**—paying attention and showing interest in the needs of others.[5]

These five principles are not inclusive of all types of principles that you may choose for yourself. However, they do provide a direction in which to begin your exploration and further your understanding of the role they have in defining for yourself what principles you believe are important both personally and professionally.

Make two lists defining what principles you want to have as a set of standards guiding your behavior (1) personally and (2) professionally. Next to each principle state what you would do to demonstrate this principle. Compare the two lists and make note of similarities and differences. Honestly evaluate what this means about differences you have in your personal and professional standards.

Plante, T.G.: *Do the Right Thing: Living Ethically in an Unethical World*. Oakland, CA, New Harbinger, 2004.

Box 5.2 | **WHAT DO YOU THINK?**

You attend a massage school that does not allow students to receive tips or compensation of any kind for massage therapy services. Your school has an active community outreach team that provides sports massage at community events such as bike races, triathlons, and fundraising walks. At any given event, there are typically 15 to 20 students as well as at least 10 graduates who are licensed by the state as massage therapists.

Prior to the start of each event the supervisor makes the following statement to all the volunteers: "As you know, state law as well as school policy forbids students from receiving any money for giving massages. You need to be aware that many of the people participating in the event like to give tips to the therapist who works on them to express their gratitude. Because I can't keep an eye on every student to enforce the 'no tip' policy, there will be a donation jar on the front table. You can let your clients know that this is where to place their tips. The money collected will be donated to the local food bank. Students, you are responsible for monitoring your behavior. I trust that you all will do the right thing. Thanks."

What ethical dilemma are the students faced with? What would your response be if you were a student practitioner at one of this school's events? Why would you respond this way?

Ethical Awareness

Because each person's experiences and beliefs are unique, ethics can sometimes be difficult to define. Sometimes there just is no concrete answer. **Ethical awareness** involves self-awareness and a willingness to ask, "Am I doing the right thing?" Ethics is not something that is just learned once but must be constantly reevaluated. Sometimes the answer is clear; sometimes it is not.

When the answer is not clear, practitioners can develop supporting networks of peers, mentors, and instructors; join professional organizations; and take courses in ethics specific to the massage and bodywork profession. In fact, expanding ethical awareness is so important to this profession that many organizations and some legislative bodies require continuing education courses in ethics as part of the renewal process for membership and licensure.

Besides being a requirement for membership and license renewal, there are many other incentives for practitioners to expand their ethical awareness. These include the following:

- Avoiding potential legal problems
- Avoiding potential public relations problems
- Seeking greater self-knowledge
- Increasing therapeutic skills
- Increasing skills to avoid unethical actions
- Increasing the ability to help others avoid unethical actions

Behaving ethically and professionally can mean something different to each bodywork practitioner. For some, it simply means treating clients with respect and fairness. These practitioners may see behaving ethically as straightforward: do not sleep with clients, charge every client the same treatment rates, always be on time for appointments. For others, it involves more: living life in a way that integrates personal, professional, and spiritual values into every aspect of their lives. Professionals who have this perspective do not make a distinction between how they conduct themselves at work and how they conduct themselves in private. There are those practitioners who are fluid in their ethical behavior. For them, it depends on the situation, the people involved, and what they themselves could gain or lose as a result of their choices.

Each of these ways of thinking and behaving in terms of ethics gives practitioners reward as well as challenges. For example, practitioners who see behaving ethically as straightforward may have this view challenged if a regular client loses her job and is no longer able to pay full price for treatments. A practitioner with rigid ethical guidelines may not consider offering a discount to this client as a way of honoring her many years of loyal business, and may lose the client as a result. By being more flexible, and taking into account the person and the situation, a solution that honors the history of the therapeutic relationship without causing the practitioner to feel as though he or she is violating ethical principles may be the better choice.

At the other end of the spectrum is the practitioner who has no ethical guidelines. For example, she may have several dual relationships with many of her clients, to the point that all clients are considered personal friends. Countertransference issues are a major risk for this practitioner, especially if she is using her bodywork practice as a way to get personal needs met. This practitioner would benefit from receiving supervision to explore these issues.

Then there is the example of a practitioner who works in a treatment office with other practitioners and who chooses to downplay the other practitioners' skills to clients in an effort to gain more clients for himself. Although he has the opportunity to perform more treatments and, therefore, increase his income, other practitioners would likely find out what he has been doing behind their backs. At the very least, he may be made to feel quite unwelcome by the other practitioners in the office. He may be disciplined, then watched very closely by the other practitioners and office manager, or he may even be fired and need to find some other place to work. Depending on how close the network of practitioners is in his community, his reputation for underhanded dealings would spread, perhaps slowly, perhaps quickly, and finding another position could become difficult or, if he is self-employed, fewer practitioners would refer clients to him.

Practitioners who integrate personal, professional, and spiritual values into every aspect of their lives are those who are practicing ethical awareness. The reward for these practitioners is that people are drawn to them because they make decisions based on what would be best for everyone involved, not just for themselves. Their client bases are usually stable. The challenge for these practitioners is that it takes time and effort to keep asking themselves, "What is the best possible decision for me to make? Am I doing the right thing?"

Professional Work Ethics

A professional's values or attitudes provide guidelines for work-related behavior, and are the basis for a person's performance in his work setting. Having a **work ethic** means that there is a drive within a person that motivates him to do the following:

- Arrive at his job on time every day
- Do the best work he can do at all times
- Work until his job is done
- Not take excessive amounts of time off
- Cooperate with his colleagues and supervisors

There are many ways that people can measure their work ethics. Figure 5.1 is a spectrum that can be used as a measurement tool. For example, there are those who have a minimal work ethic (perhaps labeled lazy), those who have a high work ethic (often referred to as motivated), and those who do nothing but work (sometimes called workaholics).

For some, the amount of effort that they put into their work is directly related to personal satisfaction, monetary compensation, or acknowledgment from others. Those who are not invested in the work they do or do not believe anyone cares about the outcome will likely put forth minimal effort. These people tend not to take the initiative and therefore shun the role of leader. They usually wait for someone to give them directions or, if they have completed a task, are not inclined to see what else needs to be done. People without a solid, healthy work ethic tend to look for the easiest way to get a job done, do it incompletely or sloppily, or avoid work entirely.

Conversely, there are those who put 110% of themselves into their work no matter what, who, when, or where. This population tends to be internally

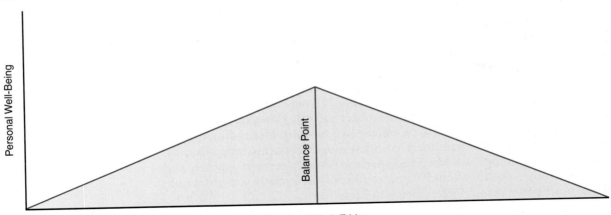

Figure 5.1 Work ethic spectrum.

"Minimal"
- Very little investment of time, effort, energy, money, emotion and so forth in the work
- No accountability
- Chooses to have no control over work outcomes
- Does no delegation nor wants to be delegated to
- Centered around personal issues

- Not goal-oriented

- Unconcerned with work structure
- Is not defined by work
- May or may not have a healthy regard for relationships

"Motivated"
- Appropriate investment of time, effort, energy, money, emotion and so forth in the work
- Accountability
- Chooses to have control over work outcomes
- Able and willing to delegate

- Balances personal and professional concerns
- Goal-oriented

- Sets limits to work structure
- Is not defined by work
- Healthy regard for personal relationships

"Workaholic"
- Huge investment of time, effort, energy, money, emotion and so forth in the work
- Accountability
- Needs absolute control over work outcomes
- Unwilling or unable to delegate
- Centered around professional concerns
- Goal-oriented, but always seeking the next goal ("nothing is ever good enough")
- No limits on work structure
- Defines self only by work
- Work is more important than any relationship

motivated and do not put limits on their efforts. They will work at a project or a task for as long as it takes to get it done right. Often, this individual is an overachiever and sets very high standards for herself. In fact, the standards may be so high that they cannot be met unless a great deal of energy and much time are put in. This may seem like the ideal work ethic. However, there may be some costs for people who become completely wrapped up in their work: stress-related illnesses; lack of free time; and chronic feelings of inadequacy because the goals they set are impossible to meet, which could lead to depression. The challenge such an individual has is finding a balance between what is expected and what is appropriate for her to accomplish, given the time and resources available to her.

In the middle of this work ethic spectrum is the balanced point at which the professional is aware of what she is capable of and is motivated to achieve the most she can from her work by realistic means; reasonable time frames; and a supportive network of friends, family, and colleagues. Finding this balanced point in the spectrum can lead to productive and efficient outcomes. However, it takes self-reflection and a willingness to be honest with oneself about personal attitudes toward work. Everyone has a choice in deciding how much of themselves they are willing to apply in their profession.

Developing Professional Behavior

Employers want employees who have personal characteristics that will enable them to work effectively, productively, and cooperatively within the organization. Their primary concern is to find employees with good work ethics, appropriate social behavior, and self-discipline. It is important for practitioners to learn the professional work ethics and behaviors that will help them obtain and retain employment and advance them in their careers.

Professional behavior describes a person's actions and words while he is in a professional setting. Examples of professional behaviors for practitioners include the following:

- Skilled, consistent treatment performance
- Effective communication skills
- Appropriate appearance
- Reliability, such as being on time for appointments or work shifts, working until the appointments and shift are completed, not taking excessive amounts of time off
- Honesty
- Initiative
- Responsibility
- Enthusiasm for learning
- Adaptability
- Positive attitude
- Cooperation
- Tactfulness
- Respect for the role of authority
- Commitment to quality work and to continually enhancing their skills through continuing education
- Commitment to teamwork, if working in a setting with more than one practitioner
- Commitment to a professional organization, if the practitioner belongs to one
- Commitment to the profession of massage and bodywork
- Respect for self, others, and property

Many work-related values and behaviors are actually the same as those that make someone a productive and valued member of society; they are those of common human decency. They demonstrate integrity, reliability, and empathy. In short, they earn trust and build relationships, which are the cornerstones of career success for bodywork practitioners.

 Food for Thought

The following are some self-inquiry questions that may help you determine your own professional work ethic:

- *What are your earliest memories of work? As a child and adolescent, who were your role models in terms of observing what it meant to "go to work"? Describe the work your role models did.*
- *On the work ethic spectrum, where would you put yourself and why? Are you satisfied with that rating? Explain why. What changes would you be willing to make to change your rating?*
- *Based on your rating, list the things you have lost or gained as a result of having this type of work ethic.*
- *Describe how you think employers, coworkers, friends, and family would describe your professional work ethic. Explain if these reviews are accurate. If so, why? If not, why not?*

■ CASE PROFILE

Manny is a Thai massage therapist working in a clinical setting with 15 other practitioners. All the practitioners are required to fold towels and make sure their treatment rooms are fully stocked before they leave each day.

Case Study Continued to page 170

Case Study Continued from page 169

Manny likes to talk. In fact, his colleagues have noticed that he is most talkative when there are chores to be done around the office, such as cleaning out the break room refrigerator, restocking shelves, or changing out the dirty linen bags. Manny talks about how busy he is with clients all day, as well as all of his personal responsibilities. While he is talking he participates minimally in the work to be done. By the time Manny finishes reporting on all of his activities, he usually needs to dash out to fulfill another important commitment he has made, and simply has not had time to fold a single towel or replace supplies in the treatment room for the next practitioner.

One day, as Manny is getting ready to leave yet again without preparing the treatment room for the next practitioner, his coworkers decide to confront him.

If you were one of Manny's coworkers, what would you say to him? Why?

What behavior, values, and principles is Manny demonstrating?

Has he violated any ethical or professional standards?

What do you think of his overall professionalism?

Practitioners who choose self-employment need these same work ethics and behaviors, as well. A self-employed practitioner may provide treatments in any of the following spaces:

- The practitioner's home or attached structure
- A private office used solely by the practitioner
- Space rented in a massage and bodywork office with other practitioners
- Space rented in another business, such as a hair salon or fitness facility
- Other businesses such as spas, wellness centers, and chiropractic offices as an independent contractor

All of these settings involve working with other people in some capacity. Regardless of the setting, having good work-related values and behavior, appropriate social interaction, and self-discipline are the keys to a successful practice because they are the foundation of ethical and genuine human connection. Without this connection, massage and bodywork are ineffective, client retention decreases, and career longevity is in peril. Also, practitioners, whether they are self-employed or employed by someone else, may choose to join and participate in massage and bodywork organizations in which professional work ethics and behaviors will serve them well.

Humans are not born with an instant understanding of what professional behavior is or how to behave in a professional manner. This is a skill that is learned with the help of teachers who describe and model behavior that is professional, as well as give feedback to others regarding behavior that is not beneficial. These teachers can be parents, other family members, teachers in schools, religious leaders, mentors, and friends.

Professional behavior is also learned by observing people you respect and admire in your chosen field of work. However, the professional behavior being modeled may or may not be appropriate. Because professional behavior varies from person to person, you need to develop a keen sense of what feels right for you, and why. If you do not think that someone is behaving as a positive representative of the bodywork profession, it is your ethical responsibility to give that person feedback. In doing so, you are giving that person the ability to change unprofessional behaviors, especially if he had not realized his behavior was unprofessional. In this way, members of the bodywork profession are holding themselves and others accountable for how they represent the profession.

In some ways, developing professional behavior is a matter of trial and error. Sometimes you must experience a particular situation before you know how to act or react. Once the action is completed, there are feedback cues you can use that will tell you if your actions were appropriate. For example, consider the following questions:

- Did the behavior result in raised eyebrows? If so, why and whose?
- Was the outcome what was expected, or could it have been different?
- Who was affected by the behavior and in what way?
- If there was a chance to behave differently, would you? Why? Why not?

Codes of Ethics

We now turn from an individual's personal ethics to codes of ethics, which apply to whole groups or professions. A **code of ethics** is a set of guidelines that delineates the standards of behavior for the members of a group or profession. The goals of these codes include the following:

- Defining the principles of the professional organization
- Stating the objectives of the profession
- Establishing or improving the profession's identity
- Guiding professional and ethical behavior
- Clarifying members' responsibilities to clients, work settings, and society
- Assisting professionals in making ethical decisions during challenges that arise
- Protecting clients (customers) from incompetent or unethical members
- Providing organizational self-regulating methods
- Protecting members from practices that may result in public condemnation and/or lawsuits

In the massage and bodywork profession, codes of ethics define professional bodywork practitioner behavior and protect the public from unscrupulous practitioners.

Acting ethically can be thought of as "doing the right thing," but determining what "right" is can sometimes be difficult. Generally, groups of people, from entire societies to small organizations, will determine what is right—what is ethical—through questioning, discussing, processing experiences, and assimilating information. Conflicts, doubts, and disagreements are a natural part of this process. Over time, however, a consensus is reached, and ethical behavior is usually codified in some way. Examples include the

United States Constitution, and, of course, the laws that govern communities. Most codes of ethics are developed through group ethics.

Development of Group Ethics

Groups, cultures, and communities have values that most of their members share. These values reflect material objects, characteristics, and conditions that the group considers important. In the United States, for example, values may include competition, wealth, individualism, and freedom. Ancient Romans, conversely, did value athletic competition and wealth, but also valued a strong national identity over individualism.

The development of **group ethics** occurs when members of an established culture, community, organization, or profession gather together to determine what shared values should drive the behaviors and attitudes of the group. When people act as a group, they act with greater strength than they can when acting individually (there is strength in numbers) and take risks necessary to determine what is right because everyone is taking part in how the guidelines are developed.

For example, bodywork practitioners who like working with others benefit from working in a collaborative community setting. This setting provides a supportive environment for keeping morale up, preventing burnout due to isolation, and inspiring creativity by being surrounded by like-minded colleagues or by thought-provoking colleagues who engage in respectful discourse. For a collaborative setting to be most fulfilling for all involved, it is best for the group of practitioners to attend a mandatory meeting to discuss what expectations each individual has for him- or herself, one another, and the business. A good place to start might be a brainstorming session in which everyone feels free to share, and no judgments or restrictions are placed on the ideas shared.

Once everyone has shared what he or she would like to experience, the goals or objectives that are most important for the majority of the group need to be sorted out; the list can then be prioritized. The next step in establishing a group agreement of operation is to put the agreements in writing in the form of a mission statement for the group, develop a plan on how specific ideas will be implemented, and create a time line for the implementation plan so that there is a system of accountability.

Finally, each person in the bodywork group should have a role in making the plan a reality. That may mean creating tasks for each person to do as part of the creation process, or it may mean having the group nominate and vote on leadership positions. These positions may rotate after an agreed-upon period so that each practitioner in the collective has the opportunity to fill a leadership position.

Ideally, the roles will match each person's talents and strengths. If it is apparent that some members are not skilled at leadership, then perhaps there may be other ways for them to contribute so that everyone feels ownership of the bodywork treatment office. To ensure that nothing or no one is overlooked, there should be documentation of the outcome of the planning session with a person's name and the date the task is to be accomplished.

The final step is to establish a regular mandatory meeting schedule so that there are opportunities to communicate and connect, and share ideas or frustrations.

Professional Codes of Ethics

Many organizations have developed a professional code of ethics for their members. Professional massage and bodywork organizations, such as the American Massage Therapy Association (AMTA), Associated Bodywork and Massage Professionals (ABMP), and the National Certification Board for Therapeutic Massage and Bodywork (NCTMB), all have codes of ethics (Fig. 5.2). These codes of ethics are sets of standards each organization has developed and adopted to guide members in making choices that are responsible and professional. But ethics is not just a list of rights and wrongs. Like any set of guidelines, codes of ethics needed to be applied with considered thought, reasoning, and reflection based on experience and learning.

Professional codes of ethics are beneficial for the consumer as well as the practitioner. Consumers are safe and secure when they receive professional services. A professional code of ethics gives the consumer a composite view of what values and attitudes the members in a particular profession should have. A professional code of ethics gives transparency so that consumers know what they can expect from the profession and what professionals are obligated to fulfill as members of the profession. A code of professional ethics provides protection for the consumer should a professional violate the code. Most professions have a grievance committee that hears complaints from consumers. The members of the profession are also expected to report fellow colleagues if they violate the code. If they fail to do so, not only is the consumer harmed, the profession is harmed as well.

Having a code of ethics provides structure and clarity for bodywork practitioners and the profession as well. Regarding the codes of ethics in Figure 5.2, you can see that specifically they:

- Reflect matters important to the profession
- State the goals and aims of the profession
- Clarify responsibilities to clients, their work settings, and to society in general
- Provide guidelines for professional activities
- Provide support for ethical decision making
- Create a framework for ethical and professional behavior
- Help members establish a professional identity
- Protect members from behavior and practices that may result in public criticism or condemnation
- Protect members from malpractice lawsuits
- Enable practitioners and the profession to regulate themselves[5]

From Abstract Concepts to Concrete Behaviors

Ethical principles are, to a great extent, abstract concepts. They are ideas, ideals, conclusions—in short, thoughts. However, they can be translated into concrete behaviors. For example, there are practitioner and client agreements common to all therapeutic work. These include the following:

- The practitioner will do no harm to the client.
- The practitioner will keep confidentiality.

Food for Thought

Do you think developing a code of ethics helps a profession? Why or why not?

Words of Wisdom

Ethical decision making is a process. It is not black or white, but most commonly different shades of gray. Most often there are no simple answers to resolve complex ethical issues. One can never attend too many ethical workshops. Being ethical is a continual, on-going process.

—TEE WILLS, Licensed Massage Therapist since 1991, nationally certified in Therapeutic Massage and Bodywork since 1994, involved with NCBTMB's Ethics and Standards Committee from 1998 to 2009, taught entry-level bodywork education for 12 years

American Massage Therapy Association

Code of Ethics

This Code of Ethics is a summary statement of the standards by which massage therapists agree to conduct their practices and is a declaration of the general principles of acceptable, ethical, professional behavior.

Massage therapists shall:

1. Demonstrate commitment to provide the highest quality massage therapy/bodywork to those who seek their professional service.
2. Acknowledge the inherent worth and individuality of each person by not discriminating or behaving in any prejudicial manner with clients and/or colleagues.
3. Demonstrate professional excellence through regular self-assessment of strengths, limitations, and effectiveness by continued education and training.
4. Acknowledge the confidential nature of the professional relationship with clients and respect each client's right to privacy.
5. Conduct all business and professional activities within their scope of practice, the law of the land, and project a professional image.
6. Refrain from engaging in any sexual conduct or sexual activities involving their clients.
7. Accept responsibility to do no harm to the physical, mental and emotional well-being of self, clients, and associates.

A

As a member of Associated Bodywork & Massage professionals, I hereby pledge to abide by the ABMP Code of Ethics as outlined below.

Client Relationships

- I shall endeavor to serve the best interests of my clients at all times and to provide the highest quality service possible.
- I shall maintain clear and honest communications with my clients and shall keep client communications confidential.
- I shall acknowledge the limitations of my skills and, when necessary, refer clients to the appropriate qualified health care professional.
- I shall in no way instigate or tolerate any kind of sexual advance while acting in the capacity of a massage, bodywork, somatic therapy or esthetic practitioner.

Professionalism

- I shall maintain the highest standards of professional conduct, providing services in an ethical and professional manner in relation to my clientele, business associates, health care professionals, and the general public.
- I shall respect the rights of all ethical practitioners and will cooperate with all health care professionals in a friendly and professional manner.
- I shall refrain from the use of any mind-altering drugs, alcohol, or intoxicants prior to or during professional sessions.
- I shall always dress in a professional manner, proper dress being defined as attire suitable and consistent with accepted business and professional practice.
- I shall not be affiliated with or employed by any business that utilizes any form of sexual suggestiveness or explicit sexuality in its advertising or promotion of services, or in the actual practice of its services.

Scope of Practice/Appropriate Techniques

- I shall provide services within the scope of the ABMP definition of massage, bodywork, somatic therapies and skin care, and the limits of my training. I will not employ those massage, bodywork or skin care techniques for which I have not had adequate training and shall represent my education, training, qualifications and abilities honestly.
- I shall be conscious of the intent of the services that I am providing and shall be aware of and practice good judgment regarding the application of massage, bodywork or somatic techniques utilized.
- I shall not perform manipulations or adjustments of the human skeletal structure, diagnose, prescribe or provide any other service, procedure or therapy which requires a license to practice chiropractic, osteopathy, physical therapy, podiatry, orthopedics, psychotherapy, acupuncture, dermatology, cosmetology, or any other profession or branch of medicine unless specifically licensed to do so.
- I shall be thoroughly educated and understand the physiological effects of the specific massage, bodywork, somatic or skin care techniques utilized in order to determine whether such application is contraindicated and/or to determine the most beneficial techniques to apply to a given individual. I shall not apply massage, bodywork, somatic or skin care techniques in those cases where they may be contraindicated without a written referral from the client's primary care provider.

Image/Advertising Claims

- I shall strive to project a professional image for myself, my business or place of employment, and the profession in general.
- I shall actively participate in educating the public regarding the actual benefits of massage, bodywork, somatic therapies and skin care.
- I shall practice honesty in advertising, promote my services ethically and in good taste, and practice and/or advertise only those techniques for which I have received adequate training and/or certification. I shall not make false claims regarding the potential benefits of the techniques rendered.

B

Figure 5.2 Codes of ethics. (A) American Massage Therapy Association (AMTA) Code of Ethics. (B) Associated Bodywork and Massage Professionals (ABMP) Code of Ethics.

National Certification Board for Therapeutic Massage and Bodywork

Code of Ethics

revised 6/23/2007

Massage and bodyworks therapists shall act in a manner that justifies public trust and confidence, enhances the reputation of the profession, and safeguards the interest of individual clients. To this end, massage and bodywork therapists in the exercise of accountability will:

I. Have a sincere commitment to provide the highest quality of care to those who seek their professional services.

II. Represent their qualifications honestly, including education and professional affiliations, and provide only those services that they are qualified to perform.

III. Accurately inform clients, other healthcare practitioners and the public of the scope and limitations of their discipline.

IV. Acknowledge the limitations of and contraindications for massage and bodywork and refer clients to appropriate health professionals.

V. Provide treatment only where there is reasonable expectation that it will be advantageous to the client.

VI. Consistently maintain and improve professional knowledge and competence, striving for professional excellence through regular assessment of personal and professional strengths and weaknesses and through continued education training.

VII. Conduct their business and professional activities with honesty and integrity, and respect the inherent worth of all persons.

VIII. Refuse to unjustly discriminate against clients or health professionals.

IX. Safeguard the confidentiality of all client information, unless disclosure is requested by the client in writing, is medically necessary, required by law or necessary for the protection of the public.

X. Respect the client's right to treatment with informed and voluntary consent. The certified practitioner will obtain and record the informed consent of the client, or client's advocate, before providing treatment. This consent may be written or verbal.

XI. Respect the client's right to refuse, modify or terminate treatment regardless of prior consent given.

XII. Provide draping and treatment in a way that ensures the safety, comfort and privacy of the client.

XIII. Exercise the right to refuse to treat any person or part of the body for just and reasonable cause.

XIV. Refrain, under all circumstances, from initiating or engaging in any sexual conduct, sexual activities or sexualizing behavior involving a client, even if the client attempts to sexualize the relationship.

XV. Avoid any interest, activity or influence which might be in conflict with the practitioner's obligation to act in the best interests of the client or the profession.

XVI. Respect the client's boundaries with regard to privacy, disclosure, exposure, emotional expression, beliefs and the client's reasonable expectations of professional behavior. Practitioners will respect the client's autonomy.

XVII. Refuse any gifts or benefits that are intended to influence a referral, decision or treatment, or that are purely for personal gain and not for the good of the client.

XVIII. Follow all policies, procedures, guidelines, regulations, codes and requirements promulgated by the National Certification Board for Therapeutic Massage & Bodywork.

Retrieved 20 October 2008 from http://www.ncbtmb.org/about_code_of_ethics.php

C

Figure 5.2—cont'd (C) National Certification Board for Therapeutic Massage and Bodywork (NCTMB) Code of Ethics.

- Both the client and the practitioner will agree clearly on the time, place, duration of the treatment session, and fee.
- The practitioner will receive informed consent from client.
- Both the client and the practitioner will tell the truth to each other.
- Both the client and the practitioner will keep agreements with each other.
- The client will do no harm to the practitioner or the practitioner's property.
- Both the client and the practitioner will not act romantically or sexually with each other.

Table 5.1 shows how these abstract concepts can be translated into concrete behaviors. As you can see, the concrete behaviors require more description because they must be specific and detailed to be as clear as possible.

Table 5.1	**Abstract Concepts and Concrete Behaviors**
Abstract Concept	**Concrete Behaviors**
The practitioner will do no harm to the client.	*The practitioner will:* Work within scope of practice and level of competency and training Use appropriate boundaries and communication skills to avoid emotional stress to client.
The practitioner will keep confidentiality.	*The practitioner will:* Not share private and personal information about the client without signed release form.
Both the client and the practitioner will agree clearly on the time, place, and duration of the treatment session and fee.	*The practitioner will:* Be specific about structure of treatment session, including appointment time, location, length, and cost.
The practitioner will obtain informed consent from the client before performing any treatment.	*The practitioner will:* Fully explain treatment plan to the client including purpose, techniques, benefits, side effects, and expected outcome. Truthfully answer any questions the client has and inform the client of right of refusal. Ask the client for permission to proceed with the treatment, and honor the client's decision.
Both the client and the practitioner will tell the truth to each other.	*The practitioner and the client will:* Speak honestly and directly about the therapeutic relationship. Actively seek to understand what the other is saying, and respond in a truthful and respectful manner.
Both the client and the practitioner will keep agreements with each other.	*The practitioner and the client will:* Fulfill all mutual agreements regarding appointment times, length of treatment sessions, treatment plan, and payment for treatments. Use timely and clear communication to inform each other of any inability to uphold the agreement.
The client will do no harm to the practitioner or the practitioner's property.	*The client will:* Not damage the practitioner or the practitioner's property through misuse, negligence, or deliberate wrongdoing, including slander and libel. Communicate any dissatisfaction to the practitioner in a clear and timely manner. Use legal methods to find a solution, if necessary.
Both the client and the practitioner will not act romantically or sexually with each other.	*The client and the practitioner will:* Maintain a professional, therapeutic relationship at all times. Not engage in sexual contact. If this behavior occurs, the therapeutic relationship will be terminated immediately. Discontinue the professional relationship immediately if mutual romantic or sexual attraction is discovered to preserve dignity and integrity of the bodywork profession.

Ethical Congruency

Ethical congruency means being authentic in both words and actions, and that behavior matches declared personal ethical standards. For example, if the practitioner believes that all clients deserve respect and compassion, these clients are treated that way, regardless of whether they are present or not. If a client calls the practitioner and asks to reschedule an appointment and the phone call becomes complicated and lengthy because of the client's busy schedule, the practitioner may feel frustrated, but she chooses not to let that frustration show, because it goes against her standards of ethical behavior. Professionals find ways to manage frustrating situations without displaying unethical behavior.

Personal ethics is the precursor to professional ethics. Practitioners are not likely to be more ethical in their professional lives than they are in their personal lives. For example, practitioners who are dishonest in their personal financial dealings are more likely to be dishonest in their business accounting methods. Practitioners who cannot keep a friend's secret are likely to put client confidentiality at risk.

Practitioners need to be aware not only of gross violations of ethical principles, but also of subtle ethical violations that occur when the client's well-being is not the practitioner's primary focus. In other words, practitioners need to be aware of subtle breaches in their ethical behavior. One such example is not referring a client to a more qualified practitioner because of fear of loss of income. Professionals can monitor their own behavior by asking themselves often if they are doing what is best for the client and if their behavior is ethical.

Bodywork practitioners are, in general, kinesthetic people. Not only does that mean that they learned best by doing, or through a hands-on approach, but that they also tend to feel emotions physically as well as perceiving them mentally. They can be experts at paying attention to gut feelings. Experiencing such a gut feeling about a particular idea, interaction, event, or action is a major cue for the practitioner to question the ethical ramifications.

The following are questions the practitioner can ask herself to see if there is an issue with ethical congruency:

- Am I having doubts? If so, what are they?
- Is this in line with my personal or professional values?
- Is it against the law, policies, or a professional code of ethics?
- Is this fair to everyone involved, both in the short term and long term?
- What if everyone knew about this? What could their responses be?
- How would I feel if the people I respect knew about this?
- How will I feel about myself afterward?

Professional growth involves changes for the better in the practitioner's knowledge, skills, attitudes, and beliefs. Because situations involving ethical congruency are not always obvious, practitioners are encouraged to use mentoring, supervision, peer support, and continuing education classes (required for license renewal in some areas of the country) as methods to help develop their awareness. Because ethical behavior is an ongoing process, the more tools that practitioners have to assist them, the better.

 Food for Thought

Have you known someone who is personally dishonest? Is that person also professionally dishonest? How do you feel about this person's dishonesty? Do you trust this person? Would you recommend this person to someone else?

Codes of Conduct

Practitioners need more than just being skilled and competent in techniques. They also have the responsibility to be knowledgeable about all aspects of their roles in the profession. Therefore, they must understand all aspects of conduct that embody an ethical practitioner.

Codes of conduct are sets of rules listing the proper practices and responsibilities of an individual, organization, or profession. Although they may seem to be the same as codes of ethics, there is an important distinction. Codes of conduct involve concepts such as honoring client confidentiality and carrying out financial matters with honesty. Codes of conduct are the next step; they outline specific professional behaviors that reflect the code of ethics. Using the code of ethics concept of honoring client confidentiality, a code of conduct might state that practitioners will not share client records with anyone other than the client. The concept of carrying out financial matters with honesty could be stated in a code of conduct as "Practitioners will report all taxable income to the IRS."

Codes of conduct are mutually agreed upon within a community and are often challenged, sometimes resulting in necessary changes. This dynamic process can ensure that the code of conduct remain relevant and not become stagnant. It is expected that persons governed by codes of conduct adhere to them, and there are usually consequences if they do not.

Codes of conduct can be as simple as a short list of agreed-upon behaviors between two work partners to as complex as a formalized document detailing behavior for an organization containing thousands of members. Some examples follow of what can be included in a code of conduct for bodywork practitioners:

- Fulfilling all required licensure and insurance requirements
- Arriving on time for work shifts
- Performing all treatment documentation requirements within a designated time frame
- Displaying a positive and professional attitude toward clients, colleagues, and staff
- Wearing the appropriate attire
- Receiving and implementing feedback openly and willingly to improve techniques, communications skills, or whatever other issues the feedback concerned
- Returning phone calls within 24 hours
- Submitting timesheet and payroll information on time
- Refraining from sexual relationships with clients

Creating and implementing a code of conduct will help you define specifically what behaviors you will accept and not accept from yourself and others. A code of conduct will also help you to set high standards of conduct and practice, and establish a point of reference you can use for self-evaluation. Figure 5.3 is a sample professional code of conduct.

Carefully evaluate the code of conduct that you have written. If you find that how you conduct yourself in your personal life is quite different from what you have written for your professional code of conduct, then you need to honestly evaluate whether you can be a successful professional if you live by a different set of standards outside of your practice.

1. When clients schedule an appointment, I will inform them of the therapeutic intent of the session as well as all business policies and procedures to ensure they are fully aware of what to expect from me and my business.

2. I will uphold safe and hygienic practices at all times by providing clean linens, fresh massage products, well maintained equipment and adequate ventilation in the treatment room.

3. I will return phone calls or emails from my clients within 24 hours.

4. Should a conflict arise between a client and me I will address the issue in a timely manner by meeting with the client, listening to the nature of the complaint and collaborate with the client to find a resolution that benefits both of us.

5. Changes in fees will be communicated to my clients with 6 months advance notice.

6. I will work within my scope of practice and will recognize when I need to refer my client to another practitioner.

7. I will volunteer 3 hours a month providing massage therapy services to promote awareness and education of the benefits of massage therapy.

8. I will honor professional boundaries at all times by conducting myself in a respectful and dignified manner.

Figure 5.3 Sample professional code of conduct.

Scope of Practice and Standards of Practice

There are two different sets of guidelines developed by participants in the profession to define and monitor accepted and appropriate conduct. **Scope of practice** is a set of guidelines that clarifies exactly what the professional can and cannot do based on laws, completion of a course of education or training, and competency of skill and technique. Scope of practice places limits or sets boundaries on services because the practitioner does not have the authority or the training to offer them. **Standards of practice** describe in concrete terms what behaviors are expected, if not guaranteed, by practitioners who are representing themselves as members of a particular profession. They define concepts, attitudes, and behaviors that all professionals are required to abide by, based on their affiliation with a particular profession.

These two sets of guidelines have similar goals but are still considered separate and distinct entities. Both ensure that the professional, as well as the consumer, is well informed and protected from harm if a practitioner does not abide by the standards set forth. In addition, the scope of practice as well as standards of practice overlap in content and expectations with the code of ethics of the profession.

Standards of practice are typically agreed-upon behaviors and attitudes that guide the direction of a profession. These standards are set forth to inform the members of the profession what their fellow peers believe to be representative of ethical conduct and attitudes as well as educate the public on what to expect when they receive services from professionals. Standards of practice create a sense of shared responsibility between the consumer and the professional. If the consumer is aware of what type of care or services she should be receiving but is not, then she can protect herself by discontinuing work with that practitioner. Depending on how severe the violation, the consumer could report the practitioner to a legal authority or a grievance committee established by the profession.

Standards of practice form a stable framework that practitioners can use to ensure that they are acting in the best interests of clients, the profession, and themselves. They are usually more specific than ethical principles, and tell practitioners how to provide care to their clients. Having standards of practice gives practitioners a safety net when they are faced with difficult situations and are unclear how to navigate through them and remain professional. Standards of practice usually delineate the following:

- The services practitioners may provide for clients
- The laws regulating the practitioner's ability to provide these services to the public
- The amount of training that must be completed to ensure a competent delivery of services
- That practitioners must use effective communication skills when interacting with clients
- That practitioners must conduct business in an honest and forthright manner
- That practitioners must set and maintain professional boundaries to ensure the safety of all parties as well as uphold the dignity of the profession and the integrity of the practitioner
- That practitioners should participate in continued education courses to further enhance their skill levels

Following the bodywork field's standards of practice is a good starting point for potential students, current students, or individuals new to the profession who are not fully aware of what it means to be a professional practitioner. Because standards of practice are determined by a group of professionals currently working in the field, it is a good summary of what is expected as well as how the profession presents itself. Having an awareness of expectations and being in alignment with what the profession is asking of its practitioners is the first step toward personal or self-accountability.

Both codes of ethics and standards of practice are enforceable by the membership organizations that create them. Therefore, if a member of the organization is reported to be in violation of a particular statute in a code of ethics or standards of practice by a consumer or another professional, there is a system in place to investigate the allegations and make appropriate recommendations. This system of checks and balances is another layer of protection for both the consumer and the profession. When members of an organization are aware that they will be held accountable for their behavior, they are more likely to follow the expectations set forth for them.

However, there will always be practitioners who believe they do not have to follow such standards and codes and so choose to ignore them. These practitioners may or may not be reported by others. This is where self-accountability comes into play. A committed professional will not require an external influence to keep him within the guidelines of the profession's code of conduct and standards of practice. He makes the choice to abide by set standards because that is the agreement he made with himself and with the profession when he joined.

Recognizing and Resolving Ethical Dilemmas

Ethical dilemmas involve considering information that requires an opinion, a response, or an action in a situation that challenges a person's ethics. Ethical dilemmas require the person to stop and think before proceeding. The pause occurs because the person is faced with a topic or a question, and he wants to be sure that he does the right thing in the eyes of those around him and of people who will be affected by his choice, and in how he sees himself. Ethical issues require people to be clear on their values, know which way their moral compasses are pointing, and what the consequences of a decision to act or not act are.

Ethical issues can be different for everyone. In life we make many choices every day. These may be unconscious decisions for some, but can, in fact, involve conscious ethical decisions for others.

For example, consider the following questions:

- How will I travel today? Do I drive my car so I can get there quickly? Do I take the bus so I don't add to the pollution by driving my car, or should I ride my bicycle?
- How is the food I choose to eat produced? Who gathers the food? Are the workers given a fair price for their labor and safe working conditions?
- Will I buy only products made in the United States, or is it okay for me to buy clothes made in another country, possibly a country that has inhumane working conditions?

Some people may give no thought to how their day-to-day decisions may have far-reaching effects; they may be more concerned with just what is in front of them. Others have a more global perspective and consider that what they choose affects the quality of life of others thousands of miles away. The extent that a person delves into her own value system to consider how her behavior affects others is a personal choice. It is neither right nor wrong to look for these connections with others. The point is to make a conscious choice and to be willing to support that choice if it is questioned.

In the bodywork profession, ethical issues pertain to practitioners making sure they are conducting themselves with honor, upholding the profession with dignity and integrity at all times, being fiscally responsible in all business matters, staying within the scope of practice of the profession, and abiding by the code of ethics of the profession. All of this good and just behavior is geared toward the client's experience, to ensure that no harm is done, and that the client receives a client-centered, therapeutic treatment.

The following are examples of specific ethical issues in the bodywork profession:

- Charging a fee that is incongruent with the practitioner's level of training and expertise
- Representing inaccurately the practitioner's level of knowledge, place of training, and competency of techniques

- Discriminating against or refusing to treat clients who do not meet the practitioner's level of comfort or expectations
- Working without a license
- Disparaging another bodywork modality or type of health care
- Engaging in business activities that undermine the profession
- Breaking confidentiality of the client and discussing him with other clients
- Refusing to do a self-assessment of strengths and challenges so that the practitioner can better meet the needs of clients
- Refusing to take responsibility in the therapeutic relationship when the client disagrees with the practitioner's quality of treatment
- Misinforming the client of the practitioner's policies, then penalizing him for not following the policies (for example, not telling the client that the practitioner bills for missed appointments, then sending the client a bill for appointments he has missed)
- Engaging in sexual activities with a client
- Engaging in illegal business activities with a client (e.g., insider stock trading, selling drugs)
- Sidestepping legal requirements for taxes and income reporting

Some issues seem clear cut and others do not. However, it is essential that the practitioner have a keen sense of her responsibility to be an ethical practitioner. This is where self-accountability is important. The practitioner must have ethical awareness so that she will do the right thing no matter what the consequence. Even if no one ever found out, she would still follow the ethical high road because that is what makes her feel good about herself as well as about her work. It is also what engenders trust from clients, ensures career success, and is what makes the bodywork profession credible.

This can be a challenge for those who have never been self-accountable, or those who have never taken the time to really think about what is ethical. However, the more practitioners do this kind of self-inquiry and self-assessment, the more prepared they will be to make good decisions between what is right and wrong, good and bad, ethical or unethical and the more they will build self-respect.

Recognizing an Ethical Dilemma

An ethical dilemma occurs when a person is faced with a choice and does not know what to do. An ethical dilemma implies that the stakes are high because there is a matter at hand that makes the person pause and think about what the right thing to do for all the parties involved. For example, the list of ethical issues practitioners face in the previous section brings up disparaging another bodywork modality or type of health care. What if the practitioner has personally had a bad experience with acupuncture, and a client asks her opinion about it? Should the practitioner ignore her personal experience, offer no opinion, and suggest the client look on the Internet for information? Should the practitioner disclose her bad experience, but be clear it is her personal experience, and that it should not influence the client's choice about getting acupuncture? If the practitioner's vision of an honest therapeutic relationship includes telling the truth when asked a question, is this a time to suspend that value or is it exactly the right time to share?

Food for Thought

Have you thought about how the choices you make every day can have a global impact? If so, have you made any changes in your choices? If not, do you think you will now?

Ethical dilemmas occur when two or more of the person's values or principles are being challenged. The dilemma is present because the values or principles are in conflict with one another. As the previous example illustrates, ethical dilemmas do not always have straightforward answers. In fact, by their very nature, they require practitioners to be thoughtful, to look at both sides of an issue, and to communicate with others to make a good decision.

The practitioner in the previous scenario holds as a value or principle that she is always honest when her clients ask her a question. Yet she also believes that it is important to be supportive of all healing modalities, even if she personally does not care for one of them. Does she have to forego one value to support another? Can she support both values in having an honest, therapeutic relationship with the client? Of course she can, but she must do so with skilled communication as well as clear intent of what she wants her client to know about her experience. After giving it some thought, the practitioner can reply:

"What do I think of acupuncture? Acupuncture is a very effective means of enhancing health and wellness. I know of several wonderful practitioners in our community. I must be honest with you, though, and please know that this is just my experience, but it was not a good match for me. I needed something more interactive to deal with my stress so I started taking yoga classes. If you think you want to give acupuncture a try, let me know and I will give you some referrals."

In this response, the practitioner is able to uphold both of her principles— she is honest with her client in response to his question, and she spoke favorably about another modality in spite of her personal reservations.

Strategies for Resolving Ethical Dilemmas

Not all ethical dilemmas are easy to resolve. Therefore, practitioners may find it useful to have strategies in place to help them examine dilemmas and to find the best solutions. These involve **critical thinking,** the process of conscious thought based on weighing all the facts that are known to form an opinion about something. Critical thinking involves being willing to be conscious and thoughtful about the topic, being able to see different sides to and opinions about the topic, and being able to keep an open mind before making a final decision or forming an opinion. Sometimes the end result may not be a definite decision or opinion, but rather staying curious or open minded about the topic or situation.

Ethical dilemmas involve the practitioner's ability to be present and aware of how complex the bodywork profession is. Practitioners who do not shy away from such challenges but instead face them with dignity and self-respect are demonstrating professionalism. Every optimal resolution of an ethical dilemma can increase the practitioner's self-confidence, self-respect, and her skill level in dealing with ethical issues. This can result in the respect of colleagues and clients, and contribute to her career success.

Because there are many ways to evaluate an ethical dilemma, Thomas G. Plante makes an argument for becoming familiar with a few of the basic ethical approaches that philosophers and ethicists have been using for centuries to guide us in our decision-making process. Each ethical approach has its own perspective and strategies for framing an issue. The following are basic descriptions of four of the most common approaches:

- **Cultural relativism**—recognizing the role cultural experiences, traditions, and expectations play in creating rules for behavior. Differences in expectations can be based on race and ethnicity, religion, upbringing and socioeconomic and geographic characteristics. For example, a woman who follows the Muslim faith cannot receive a bodywork treatment from a male practitioner because she may be touched only by her husband or other men in her family.
- **Egoism**—making choices based on what will feel good or be in your own best interest. For example, a massage clinic owner knows that her massage therapists would benefit from having at least 20 minutes between sessions but chooses to limit the time to 10 minutes so she can increase the number of treatments her business can provide in a day. She does not ask the massage therapists for their input and offers no additional compensation to them.
- **Utilitarianism**—making choices based on what would please the most people. For example, a shiatsu practitioner chooses to extend her schedule to include evening and weekend appointments because many of her clients are requesting treatments at those times. This may make her clients happy but her partner and daughter will not be pleased.
- **Absolute moral rules**—believing that there are specific rules for behavior that should apply in all circumstances, regardless of the consequences. For example, a massage therapist refuses to work on a client without any discussion because he detects the faint odor of alcohol. Even though there may be a good reason for the odor, he chooses to deny service because it is always contraindicated to massage someone who has been drinking.[6]

There are times when the best choice in an ethical dilemma is based solely on one of these four approaches. More often, however, the best choice is likely based on a combination of these approaches. For example, the massage clinic owner who wants to increase her business by decreasing the amount of time her massage therapists have between appointments could benefit from resolving her dilemma with a mix of these approaches. She could use utilitarianism and ask her therapists what they think of decreasing time between appointments and if they have any other ideas for increasing business. Cultural relativism can come into play in terms of socioeconomic conditions. Perhaps the therapists would want the decrease in time between appointments because they can increase their income by doing more treatments as well.

Having a deeper understanding of the choices available to you when making ethical decisions will allow you to be creative and thorough in your decision-making process. A better understanding of and increased sensitivity to ethical issues may perhaps reduce the tendency to do the easiest thing without taking the time to see if it is the best choice available. Taking the time to seriously evaluate options when making ethical decisions can also lead to clarity about what the long-term effects of the decision will be, not just what seems to be easiest in the moment.

The following five steps are a guide for making ethical decisions:

1. Recognize the ethical issue. Why is it an ethical problem and not just a matter of unprofessional behavior? What are the specific issues involved? Who is involved and who is responsible for what?
2. What are the facts? Get as much information as possible; talk to all parties involved. Define the problem as a breach of values, morals, ethics, the law, or a combination.
3. Examine the alternatives. What if I choose this particular action? What if I choose that particular action? What will happen if I do nothing?
4. Make your decision and take action. What do I need to do? Who do I need to inform?
5. Consider your decision in retrospect. Why did you make the choice you did? What perspective (absolute moral rule, cultural relativism, utilitarianism, egoism) drove that choice? Seek support from someone you trust to discuss the events and bring closure.[7]

Reporting Unethical Behavior

Current culture has an issue with tattletales. It was not "cool" to be the one in school to tell the teacher who was cheating or who was breaking rules. It can get even harder in adulthood to report wrongdoing because sometimes the consequences are high, such as being shunned at work or ignored by friends. However, it is important to report unethical behavior, as it eliminates those people who damage an organization or profession by their behavior.

Human nature causes some people to look for the easy way out or a quick way to get rich. Anything that takes the pressure off them to work hard is tempting. Many know how to resist such temptations. However, there are some who do not take into consideration the profession and organizations they belong to. They may have good reasons in their own eyes for violating ethics, but because they have willingly joined the bodywork profession they are obligated to abide by the code of ethics for the profession or face the consequences. Facing the consequences is not easy, but consequences for ethics violations are essential to stopping unethical practitioners from behaving in ways that damage the profession.

Because the bodywork profession is a fairly new part of the health-care community, practitioners must still sometimes explain bodywork's therapeutic effects for it to be accepted. Therefore, it is essential that bodywork practitioners report practitioners who are breaking the laws or violating codes of ethics, because what they do affects the entire profession. It is a difficult decision to be a whistle-blower, but if the practitioner is sure of the facts, and she is using the correct methods of reporting what she knows, she is having a positive impact on the profession in the long run.

If the practitioner personally witnesses unethical behavior taking place, depending on the behavior, she has several options:

1. Report it as soon as possible to the appropriate authorities.
2. Talk with the offending person to tell him what she observed and that he needs to stop or she will report it to the proper authorities.
3. Ignore it.

The practitioner must make a decision with which she can ultimately live. If she does not have the strength to tolerate what may happen by reporting something, then perhaps talking with the person and expressing her concerns is enough, unless the behavior is illegal. In that case, not reporting the behavior would be tantamount to performing the illegal behavior herself.

The practitioner who ignores another's unethical behavior only perpetuates the problem, and, in some ways, makes herself a part of it. This is an area that requires deep introspection about what is best for the person witnessing the behavior, the person behaving unethically, the people who are affected by the unethical behavior, and the profession. Consider the following:

Joe is concerned about some stories he is hearing about Larry, a massage therapist with whom he went to school. Larry has been bragging about a new marketing plan involving promoting onsite massage therapy services at sorority houses. Larry has reportedly been keeping late hours at the sorority house and has been invited to "spend the night" by a few of the women. The stories fit with Larry's behavior during massage school, which was often inappropriate. Joe regrets that he did not confront Larry on his attitude and actions in school and believes there are now young women who may be at risk of being harmed.

Joe makes an appointment to meet with Larry so that he can find out the truth behind what he has heard. Larry's response to Joe's questions is to laugh and say, "Yeah, can you believe I got so lucky?!" Larry goes on to inform Joe that he has made a lot of money by providing "extra attention" to the clients' inner thighs, and that he is hoping to expand his services to another sorority. "Those chicks have a lot of money to burn," Larry states.

Joe confronts Larry on how unethical his business is. Larry laughs and tells Joe he is jealous because he had not come up with such a great plan. He even offers to introduce Joe to some of the women so he can get into the business with him. Joe declines and tells Larry that he had better be careful.

Two weeks later, the local news reports that Larry has been arrested on sexual harassment charges, with one woman as the complainant, and more women coming forward. The story states that the charges are from Larry's work as a massage therapist in the sorority. The reporter ends the story with a warning for anyone who wants to receive a massage, saying, "You never know what type of person the massage therapist really is, or what he will do."

All the massage therapists in the community are shocked, and are now concerned for their own businesses. They comment on how they knew Larry was not an ethical therapist, but they never thought this would happen. Joe is sincerely regretting that he never filed a letter of grievance with the massage therapy licensing board or contacted the campus director of Greek housing about Larry. The director of Greek housing has now banned all bodywork modality services from sorority and fraternity houses.

Food for Thought

Have you witnessed unethical behavior? What did you do about it? Why did you choose to act the way you did? How did you feel afterward?

Chapter Summary

Ethics, morals, values, and principles are all different concepts, yet they are all interconnected. By having an understanding of each, both their definitions as well as what they mean to individuals, practitioners can increase their chances for career success. Success also depends on having a good work ethic, which includes being prompt, working to the best of one's ability, not taking excessive amounts of time off, and cooperating with colleagues and supervisors. An aspect of a professional work ethic is professional behavior, which includes, among other things, effective communication skills, skilled treatment performance, reliability, cooperation, commitment to quality work and skill enhancement, and commitment to the bodywork profession. Codes of ethics reflect the standards set by a profession, and they develop from group ethics. Many organizations have developed a professional code of ethics for their members, including the AMTA, ABMP, and NCBTMB. Practitioners are encouraged to review these codes of ethics. Ethical congruency means being authentic in both words and actions, and that behavior matches with professed ethical standards. Codes of conduct and standards of practice are written to take the abstract concepts of codes of ethics and ethical congruency and form them into a solid framework so that practitioners know what conduct is expected of them as bodywork professionals. By being able to recognize ethical dilemmas, practitioners can follow a five-step strategy designed to assist them in resolving the dilemmas. Practitioners also have a responsibility to report unethical behavior on the part of other practitioners. Not doing so can harm clients, other practitioners, and the profession.

Review Questions

Multiple Choice

1. What is shown when a person's behavior is consistent with his moral values?

a. Awareness

b. Integrity

c. Standards of practice

d. Code of conduct

2. People who have motivated work ethics are likely to:

a. Focus exclusively on their job

b. Want control over their job outcomes

c. Define themselves exclusively by their job

d. Invest little time and energy in their job

3. Which of the following is professional behavior for practitioners?

a. Honesty

b. Commitment to quality work

c. Reliability

d. All of the above

4. When members of an established culture, organization, or profession determine what behaviors and attitudes best reflect their goals and desires, they are developing:

   a. Ethical awareness

   b. Standards of practice

   c. Group ethics

   d. Conflict resolution

5. Which of the following places limits on services because the practitioner does not have the authority or the training to offer them?

   a. Scope of practice

   b. Code of ethics

   c. Standards of practice

   d. Ethical awareness

6. Which of Thomas G. Plante's ethical principles means having knowledge, skill, and training that makes a practitioner qualified for the job he is hired to do?

   a. Integrity

   b. Competence

   c. Responsibility

   d. Respect

7. Ethical dilemmas occur when a person's principles are:

   a. In conflict with one another

   b. Lacking

   c. Clear

   d. Based on childhood experiences

Fill in the Blank

1. People use their _____ to decide whether their actions are right or wrong

2. Ethical awareness involves self-awareness and willingness to ask _____ .

3. A _____ is a set of guidelines that delineates the standards of behavior for the members of a group or profession.

4. Sets of rules listing the proper practices and responsibilities of an individual, organization, or profession are called _____ .

5. _____ means being authentic in both words and actions, and that behavior matches with professed ethical standards.

6. Situations that challenge a person's ethics and make him stop and consider information before offering an opinion, providing a response, or taking an action in a situation are called _____ .

7. Recognizing the role cultural experiences, traditions, and expectations play in creating rules for behavior is called _____ .

Short Answer

1. Explain the differences and commonalities among ethics, morals, values, and principles.

2. Describe five incentives for practitioners to expand their ethical awareness.

3. Explain what having a work ethic means.

4. Give at least five examples of professional behaviors for bodywork practitioners.

5. Explain eight goals of codes of ethics.

6. List and describe the five steps practitioners can take to resolve an ethical dilemma.

7. Explain why it is important that unethical practitioner behavior be reported.

Activities

1. Create your own personal code of ethics that would guide your personal affairs. Create a professional code of ethics that would guide your bodywork business. Compare and contrast the two. What is similar? What is different?

2. Consider an ethical dilemma that you have encountered. Describe the components of the dilemma: What was the issue; who was involved; what choices did you make; what was the outcome?

3. Describe your work ethic. What and who shaped this work ethic? Are you satisfied with your description? If yes, why? If no, explain why and what steps you could take to be satisfied.

4. When you consider the phrase "career success," what images or concepts appear to you? As a bodywork practitioner, what constitutes a long career? What steps would you recommend to ensure a long and satisfactory career? What are the pitfalls in achieving career success for the bodywork practitioner?

5. What does the phrase "self-accountability" mean to you? How do you measure your level of self-accountability? List factors that influence one's ability to be accountable. List factors that inhibit one's ability or willingness to be accountable? What distinguishes willingness from the ability to be self-accountable?

6. Talk with a professional practitioner who has several years of experience. Ask what ethical dilemmas he or she has faced as a practitioner and how he or she resolved them.

Guidance for Journaling

 Some key areas to think about while journaling for this chapter are as follows:

- What your professional work ethic is and whether your work ethic will contribute to your success
- What your personal ethics, morals, values, and principles are
- Whether codes of ethics have helped promote bodywork as a profession
- Whether you have ethical congruency, and how the answer to this has affected your life
- What codes of conduct and standards of practice are important in the bodywork profession
- Ethical dilemmas you have faced, and what you have done to resolve them

References

1. Corey, G., Corey, M.S., and Callanan, P.: *Issues and Ethics in the Helping Professions,* ed. 7. Stamford, CT, Brooks/Cole Cengage Learning, 2007, p 3.
2. Ibid.
3. Plante, T.G.: *Do the Right Thing: Living Ethically in an Unethical World.* Oakland, CA, New Harbinger, 2004, p 9.
4. Ibid., p 37.
5. Braun, M.B., and Simonson, S.: *Introduction to Massage Therapy,* ed. 2. Philadelphia, Lippincott Williams & Wilkins, 2008, pp 32–41.
6. Plante, *Do the Right Thing,* pp 17–21.
7. Ibid., pp 29–32.

Power Differences

LEARNING OBJECTIVES

After studying this chapter, you will be able to:

1. Define what power is and explain sources of power.

2. Explain how to recognize power differences.

3. Develop strategies for empowering clients in the therapeutic relationship.

4. Explain ways to manage difficult clients.

5. Develop strategies for working within the power differences between employers and employees and among coworkers.

6. Discuss the impact of societal roles of males and females on the bodywork profession, and challenge myths about male practitioners and myths about female practitioners.

7. Discuss the challenges male practitioners face and those female practitioners face in the bodywork profession.

CHAPTER OUTLINE

KEY TERMS

Empower: the process of helping people who do not have power gain it so they can improve their personal or professional circumstances

Power: the capacity to influence the behavior or others and to resist their influence on oneself

Power difference: occurs when, in a relationship, one party has greater control, or power, over the other

Self-empowered: having the means within ourselves to overcome doubts and insecurities rather than relying on an external support system

Status: the position of an individual in relation to another or others; a socially valued quality that a person carries with her or him into different situations, where power and dominance are likely to be seen as a personality trait

M allory visits the We R One Massage center for her very first massage. Her massage therapist is Lena. When asked about her goals for the massage, Mallory states that she just wants to relax and see what it is like to get a massage. Lena says, "Well, I can help you decide what you need from this massage." Lena proceeds to do four assessments of Mallory, ranging from watching Mallory walk down the hallway to assess her gait to having Mallory hold her arms in various positions so Lena can assess the amount of tension in her shoulder region.

Lena offers no explanations during the assessments and Mallory has no idea why she is doing them. In addition, the assessments make her feel uncomfortable and self-conscious but she does not say anything. By the time the assessments are over, there are only 40 minutes left for the actual massage treatment. Afterward, Lena says that Mallory should come back to see her for a series of treatments that would help take care of the problem in Mallory's neck and shoulders.

> *Mallory:* I didn't know I had problems in my neck and shoulders.
> *Lena:* Oh, but you do. It's a good thing you came in when you did because if you don't address those issues soon, you're going to have some real problems down the road. But you're in luck; I specialize in neck and shoulder care so you came to the right person.

By the time Mallory leaves the We R One Massage Center she has spent $280 and scheduled herself for a massage every Tuesday afternoon at 4 o'clock for the next 4 weeks.

At first glance, it appears that Lena does a good job of client retention by promoting her work and educating Mallory about how massage therapy can benefit her. Lena uses her influence and expertise as a professional to inform Mallory how her body is not working as well as it should and she provides Mallory with the means by which to improve. Lena does her job so well that she now has a client who is committed to returning four more times and she has also increased sales for the clinic.

However, looking deeper, did Mallory pay for treatments she does not necessarily need for a condition that she did not know she has? To promote her business, did Lena take advantage of the fact that Mallory did not have any experience with massage therapy? Did Lena misuse her power?

Power differences occur in the bodywork profession and you need to understand how they occur in the client–practitioner relationship, how to empower clients to speak up for their needs, and how to manage clients who want to assume control over all aspects of the treatment.

Presented in this chapter are methods to help you recognize power differences and strategies to work within them, not only during the treatment session with clients, but also between an employer and employee, and among coworkers. In addition, strategies are presented to help you manage difficult client behaviors, such as clients who malinger, clients who talk excessively, clients who are prone to inappropriate emotional outbursts, and clients who "hijack" the session.

Another way power affects us is through traditional societal roles of the genders. These roles have affected the bodywork profession in several different ways, which we explore in this chapter. The challenges that male practitioners and female practitioners each face are presented, along with communication challenges between the genders. Methods to manage these challenges effectively are presented. Finally, myths surrounding male and female practitioners are discussed as well as what the truth really is.

Defining Power Differences

Power. What is it? Who has it? Who wants it? How do people get it? **Power** is defined as the ability to act or produce an effect; a position of ascendancy over others; authority; control. Harvard Business School defines power as "the potential to allocate resources and to make and enforce decisions."[1] Power is also defined as "the capacity to influence the behavior of others and to resist their influence on oneself."[2]

The word "power" elicits a number of reactions from people. Some may conjure up an image of those politicians who misuse their power and harm the political system by being immoral or dishonest. Others may see power as solely related to money; the more money you have, the more power you have. Often power is seen as a negative quality that many want to keep at a distance. Maybe it is because we fear others will not like us or maybe we do not trust ourselves not to abuse the power we have.

In reality, power in and of itself is neither good nor bad. It is what people choose to do with their power that is either beneficial or harmful to others and themselves. Accordingly, bodywork practitioners have a great deal of power, whether they recognize it or not, and they must use this power in a way that earns client trust, creates therapeutic relationships, and builds a stable client base to ensure career longevity.

To understand how to use your power as a bodywork practitioner wisely and ethically, the first step is to look at where power comes from.

Where Does Power Come From?

Some bodywork students and practitioners may be baffled about why power is being discussed, because they deny that they have any power at all. In fact, because the concept of power is often perceived negatively, many will go to great lengths to distance themselves from any conversation about power for fear of appearing aggressive and self-centered.

However, power needs to be discussed for the following reasons:

- It exists.
- It is important that practitioners recognize its existence and their own relationship with power.
- For those who perceive power as evil or wrong, this is an opportunity to broaden their awareness and understanding of power.
- The ethical use of power plays a role in developing successful therapeutic relationships and business strategies.

According to Tubbs and Moss in *Human Communication: Principles and Contexts,* "In the study of communication, power is viewed in relational terms. You do not have power—it is given to you by others with whom you transact. Power has much to do with how we perceive ourselves. Issues about power can occur in all kinds of interpersonal relationships from the most casual to the most intimate."[3] For bodywork practitioners, each time we connect with our clients we have the ability to influence how they perceive our actions, our words, and our intentions.

You must first believe in your own position of power in the therapeutic relationship if you expect your clients to view you as capable of meeting their bodywork needs. Believing that power is a negative quality and does not belong in a therapeutic relationship is not being realistic about the nature of interpersonal relationships. The following are examples of behaviors that describe how clients will perceive you as a person of power:

- When we approach our clients dressed professionally, standing tall, offering a firm handshake and a smile, and making direct eye contact, we have placed ourselves in a position to be perceived as powerful. These nonverbal gestures communicate that we are confident and in a position to offer them something they want—a professional treatment.
- When we speak with clarity and intelligence during the interview and while discussing the treatment plan, we are portraying a position of power because of the knowledge and expertise we are sharing.
- When clients continue to choose us to provide their bodywork treatments, it is because they see our power in being able to develop a healthy therapeutic relationship with them.

Sources of Power

According to *Power, Influence and Persuasion: Sell Your Ideas and Make Things Happen,* five sources of power have been identified. Each of these sources has a set of factors that describes its relationship to power. Note that power is based not only on how we present ourselves, such as the words and behaviors we choose, but also on how others perceive us—from clients, friends, family, colleagues, and acquaintances to society as a whole.

Status—one's place within society. **Status** is defined as the position of an individual in relation to another or others. It is a socially valued quality that a person carries with him or her into different situations in which power and dominance are likely to be seen as personality traits. Factors that determine status include, but are not limited to, level of income, level of education, and ethnicity. Our level of power in society can be limited or enhanced by these factors. For example, in the bodywork profession those who have higher levels of training and education generally are accorded a higher status than those who have just recently completed an entry-level program. A practitioner who owns a large bodywork practice may hold a higher status level in a community than would a sole practitioner. Conversely, if the sole practitioner has a great deal of experience and education, and is nationally known, it is likely he or she will hold a high status level in the community.

Position—one's formal place within an organization or group. Factors that determine position are job titles, a set of responsibilities, level of authority to act, and control of resources within the organization. In bodywork programs, the positions of teachers and administrators hold more power than those of students. In a bodywork membership organization, boards of directors have higher positions, and more power, than do individual members. Within a bodywork practice, your position as a practitioner gives you a set of responsibilities as defined by your standards of practice and scope of practice. The client has given you the authority to provide a treatment using whatever resources, such as a heating pack or essential oils, you deem appropriate.

Expertise—one's level of skill and knowledge. Factors that determine expertise are successful completion of specific training programs, length of time spent developing/practicing/performing skills, and demonstration of competency for a particular level of certification. Completing programs of study, participating in continuing education classes, and working to increase your level of skill give you expertise. This expertise gives clients more confidence in your abilities, which means they perceive you as having the power to give them the treatments they want and need.

Relational—one's connections and relationships with others. Factors that determine how power can emerge from relationships include the level of intimacy, ability to influence others, collaboration skills, and willingness to collaborate with others. Relational power is the foundation of the therapeutic relationship with a client. The practitioner is willing to work with the client to provide a satisfactory treatment experience. The practitioner does not hand over all her power to the client and, for example, allow the client complete control in directing the treatment. Nor does the practitioner take the client's power away by, for example, designing and performing the treatment session without input from the client. Relational power also comes from being able to work well with coworkers, supervisors, colleagues, and other health-care professionals. Having a mentor, working with a support system, and being part of a coalition of bodywork practitioners are other examples of the use of relational power.

Personal—power generated from within. Personal power does not depend on status, position, or relationships. Qualities of personal power include, but are not limited to, self-confidence, trustworthiness, relating well with others, having expertise that others value, and the ability to inspire others. Having personal power means you trust your own judgment when making decisions but are open to the thoughts and ideas of others. As a bodywork practitioner, using your personal power in a healthy and ethical manner means that you discuss the treatment plan with your client, listen to his wants and needs, and

Words of Wisdom

When I get new clients who are also new to massage, I feel it is imperative that they understand that this is a working partnership in their health. I also explain that this appointment is "their time" and we will do what is needed in this time frame to help them realize their goals. I emphasize that it is necessary for them to be proactive in their treatment. This means that they should feel comfortable letting me know if the room temperature is inadequate, if the pressure that I am using is appropriate, if there is an area on their body that they are not comfortable with me working on, if there is any pain or increased tenderness when working a specific area, and if there is any residual pain after the session. I let them know that they are in control of the session. If there is anything that I want for them to realize most, it is that they need to feel comfortable enough with me (or any massage therapist whom they work with) to be able to say, "Stop," or "Ouch." I believe that this empowers my clients to make decisions and requests that will positively affect their health care and maintenance.

—LIL HACKETT, Licensed Massage Therapist since 2001, owner, As You Are Massage and Body Therapy, Tucson, Arizona

perform the treatment and make recommendations, based on your knowledge and expertise, in a way that benefits him. You may choose to consult others about how best to work with clients, but ultimately you decide on the best approach. You are able to offer assistance to coworkers and colleagues when they ask for it, while respecting their thoughts and opinions. Personal power also means that you lead by example—you are on time for your appointments, you dress and act professionally, you treat everyone with dignity and respect, and you ask for help when you need it. [4]

As you may have realized, the most influence we have is on how our personal power is perceived. We have less influence on how our relational power, expertise power, and position power are perceived. Accordingly, the least amount of influence we have is on how our status power is perceived.

Figure 6.1 uses concentric circles to symbolize how much influence we have on how our different types of power are perceived. The way in which others view us plays a bigger role in their perception of our power as the circles move out. The farther from the center we go, the less influence we have on how our position of power is perceived.

Recognizing Power Differences

Power can also be equated with control. The person controlling an outcome or the distribution of information or resources is seen as a powerful person. This is the foundation of **power differences**. A power difference occurs when, in a relationship, one party has greater control, or power, over the other. These relationships can be between family members, such as a parent having power over a child; between those who work together, such as a supervisor

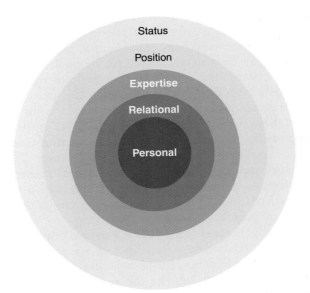

✳ **Figure 6.1** Concentric circles symbolize how much influence we have on how our power is perceived. How others view us plays a bigger role in their perception of our power as the circles move out. Accordingly, the farther out the circles are from the center, the less influence we have on how our position of power is perceived.

having power over an employee; and between those who participate in recreational activities, such as a coach having power over soccer players.

In the bodywork profession, power differences are usually discussed in terms of the therapeutic relationship. By receiving training in bodywork therapies, practitioners are empowered to use the skills learned to help others. Therefore, they can be perceived by clients as having greater power in the therapeutic relationship because, as the expert they must know what they are doing.

Some practitioners do not recognize the power difference and act as if it is necessary for them to make all the decisions about the treatment without consulting the client. They are not practicing client-centered therapy. Instead, they have decided that because someone must be in charge, it should be the practitioner, the person with the skill and expertise. Be mindful of the potential for this dynamic. Accepting power entirely interferes with developing a therapeutic relationship with clients.

Conversely, another dynamic involves clients who want to assume all the power, thus placing themselves in a power position over the practitioner. These are clients who want to control all aspects of the treatment. For example, they may insist on having a treatment only on a particular day and at a certain time, and are inflexible on this point. They will direct the practitioner on what type of techniques to use, how long the technique should be applied, and in what areas of their body. They may even instruct the practitioner on how to do the techniques, or insist the practitioner use techniques in which he has no training. These clients may also insist that only a certain type of music be played, certain color of linens be used, and, in the case of treatments that require lubricant, only a certain one be used. In short, these clients micromanage the entire treatment session because they feel the need to be in control. This can be frustrating because the practitioner's knowledge and skills are being discounted or disregarded by the client, thus potentially resulting in an ineffective treatment for the client.

For a true therapeutic relationship to form, mutual power between the client and practitioner is necessary. The practitioner must share power with the client, because the client is truly the expert on what his body needs. Figure 6.2 shows how the therapeutic relationship cannot form if the client has too much power, or if the practitioner has too much power. Instead, the therapeutic relationship forms through collaboration between the practitioner and the client.

Consider the following potential positions of power within the therapeutic relationship:

The practitioner who does not want to acknowledge her power. Meg limits the amount of information she gives her clients because she does not want to run the risk of being wrong. Even though Meg has received many hours of continuing education and has been a successful practitioner for 5 years, she does not think it is her place to tell the client all that she knows because she is afraid of being seen as pushy.

Meg is actually showing that she is not comfortable with the power she has gained over years of hard work and practice. In this case, Meg is denying her clients her level of expertise and talent. As a result, her practice is mediocre because her clients leave feeling dissatisfied with the lack of information they gained from her. Meg is frustrated with her lack of progress in building a stable client base.

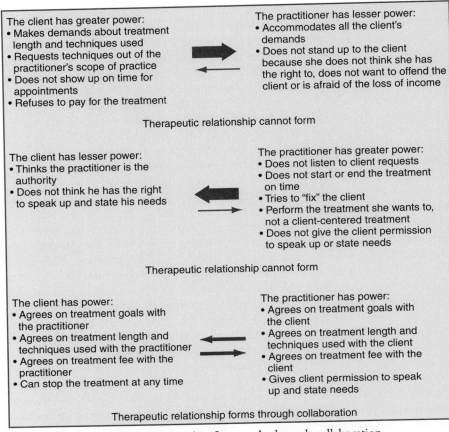

The client has greater power:
- Makes demands about treatment length and techniques used
- Requests techniques out of the practitioner's scope of practice
- Does not show up on time for appointments
- Refuses to pay for the treatment

The practitioner has lesser power:
- Accommodates all the client's demands
- Does not stand up to the client because she does not think she has the right to, does not want to offend the client or is afraid of the loss of income

Therapeutic relationship cannot form

The client has lesser power:
- Thinks the practitioner is the authority
- Does not think he has the right to speak up and state his needs

The practitioner has greater power:
- Does not listen to client requests
- Does not start or end the treatment on time
- Tries to "fix" the client
- Perform the treatment she wants to, not a client-centered treatment
- Does not give the client permission to speak up or state needs

Therapeutic relationship cannot form

The client has power:
- Agrees on treatment goals with the practitioner
- Agrees on treatment length and techniques used with the practitioner
- Agrees on treatment fee with the practitioner
- Can stop the treatment at any time

The practitioner has power:
- Agrees on treatment goals with the client
- Agrees on treatment length and techniques used with the client
- Agrees on treatment fee with the client
- Gives client permission to speak up and state needs

Therapeutic relationship forms through collaboration

Figure 6.2 The therapeutic relationship forms only through collaboration.

The practitioner who takes all the power in the relationship. Louise is very proud of the level of expertise she has gained in her last 5 years as a professional bodywork practitioner. She feels quite comfortable with educating her clients in what will help them, often to the point of dismissing the client's assessment of what he needs in favor of her assessment. She does not hesitate to remind her clients of the number of hours she has spent in training and to trust her when they express hesitation over a particular treatment plan. Louise brags to her colleagues that she has "scared off" clients who are not committed to improving their health or who have blamed her for an injury being exacerbated and not improved.

Louise is actually showing that she is not invested in a collaborative relationship with her clients. By continually reminding her clients of her level of expertise and training, she is creating an atmosphere in which clients do not feel safe to express themselves. In addition, she is harming some clients by not taking their concerns seriously and adapting her approach to the treatment to meet their needs. Louise's comments to her colleagues indicate that she is proud of the power she wields in her practice. However, she is too busy congratulating herself to notice that she has few repeat clients and that none of her colleagues refer clients to her.

The practitioner who does not recognize his responsibility to assert his power. Anju is very social with his clients. He loves them all and enjoys hearing about their families, their jobs, and any other topic that comes up during the treatment. When clients come in with a specific issue on which to focus, Anju listens intently and shares in their frustration that they are experiencing pain and discomfort. When these clients press Anju for more information about what could be going on, he shrugs his shoulders and says, "I don't know. What do you think?" Sometimes a client is compliant with this nondirective approach because she thinks Anju is a nice person. Others, however, decide to look for another practitioner who offers more input and assesses for what could be contributing to their pain and discomfort.

Anju is actually showing that he is oblivious to the power he has to improve his clients' conditions when they come to him. Although he is client centered, as evidenced by listening to and being empathetic with his clients, he does not assume his role as the professional with expertise who can share with his clients. Anju has underestimated his talent and skills and therefore is denying his clients the opportunity to benefit from them. It may also be that Anju is using his practice as a means to socialize with his clients rather than focusing on performing skillful treatments that benefit them. Anju is becoming bored with doing the same things over and over in every treatment, which is coming through in his touch. He has noticed that, while he still has his regular clients, few new clients reschedule with him and he does not understand why.

The client who takes all the power in the relationship. Tyler has a client, Pat, who has had a great deal of previous massage therapy experience. Pat receives a massage every week and does not hesitate to let Tyler know what needs to be done for the session. Each time Tyler suggests a particular treatment plan or incorporates a new technique, Pat objects and insists that Tyler follow the same plan as usual. Tyler reluctantly abides by Pat's demands but he feels resentful and bored working with her.

This situation can become complex. Tyler is actually telling Pat that she has more knowledge and expertise than he does. He is agreeing with her that because money is being exchanged she therefore has the right to direct the session. Tyler can be more assertive, to a point. However, if his income is dependent on having a certain number of weekly appointments, then he may choose to allow Pat to continue to have all the power. Conversely, if he is resentful toward Pat, and bored with the treatments he is required to perform on her, he may not be delivering quality work. He has to weigh his needs against hers and decide whether to keep things the way they currently are, strive to create a situation that is satisfactory to both of them, or terminate their therapeutic relationship and refer her to another practitioner. No matter which he chooses, it will require effort on his part.

The client who takes no power in the relationship. Rachel has seen Ethan for three treatment sessions. During each pretreatment interview she asks Ethan what he needs from the session. He always says, "You decide. You're the expert." No matter how much Rachel tries to engage Ethan with open-ended questions, he has no input for her. As a result, the treatments she performs on him vary, depending on her best guess about what he needs. Ethan ends each session by saying, "That was good. See you next week." Rachel is feeling uneasy with these sessions because she does not know if she is accomplishing anything for Ethan. Even though he seems satisfied, Rachel would rather work on someone who is more invested in the therapeutic relationship. She is contemplating referring Ethan to another practitioner.

This situation is as complex as that of the client who takes all the power in the relationship. Rachel is actually telling Ethan that he does not need to contribute anything to the therapeutic relationship. The result is that, because of Ethan's lack of engagement and participation, there is now a huge power difference. Rachel recognizes this and is frustrated by it. If her income depends on Ethan's appointments, then she may choose to allow Ethan to continue denying his power in the therapeutic relationship. Conversely, Rachel's ethics make her question whether she is performing beneficial treatments for Ethan. Like Tyler in the previous scenario, she needs to weigh Ethan's needs against hers and decide whether to keep things as they currently are, strive to create a situation that is satisfactory to both of them, or terminate their therapeutic relationship and refer him to another practitioner. No matter which she chooses, it will require effort on her part.

The practitioner and client share the power. Mehti has been receiving bodywork from Jameson for more than 3 years. She appreciates Jameson's work because he has successfully treated her chronic low back pain. In her first appointment with Jameson, she was impressed with how attentive he was while listening to her describe the pain she was feeling. Mehti welcomed Jameson's invitation to share with him any knowledge she had about what might have caused her low back pain as well as what she had already tried to remedy it. Jameson also let Mehti know that she was welcome to give him feedback about what she experiences during the treatment and to let him know right away if she needed anything changed such, as the depth of pressure or room temperature. After 3 years, Jameson is still including her in all decisions regarding her treatments, invites her to give him feedback, and immediately incorporates it whenever possible. Jameson's use of open-ended questions demonstrates to Mehti that Jameson is interested in understanding her experience with bodywork sessions so that together they develop the most effective treatment plans to meet her needs.

Jameson is actually telling Mehti that they have a mutual investment in the therapeutic relationship. Jameson demonstrates to Mehti that she has an equal role by inviting her to collaborate in the treatment process. Jameson has a thriving practice because he is able to cultivate a healthy working relationship with his clients. He shares with them the responsibility of setting treatment goals, implementing the goals, and regularly assessing if progress is being made.

There are many other ways power differences manifest in the bodywork profession, including the following:

- The practitioner is always clothed, whereas the client may not be.
- The client sits or lies down, whereas the practitioner is in a physically higher position, leaning over him while standing or kneeling to apply techniques.
- The client can refuse payment if dissatisfied with the treatment.
- The client does not have the therapeutic knowledge of his body that the practitioner does, so he may defer to the practitioner, even when

something the practitioner is doing does not feel comfortable to the client.

- The client assumes the practitioner will be available whenever he wants a treatment, because he is paying for it.
- The manager of a bodywork office does not honor employee requests for time off without lowering the practitioner's seniority status.
- The manager of a bodywork office does not take seriously an employee's concern about an inappropriate client and requires the practitioner to work on the client under threat of losing her job.

Strategies for Working Within Power Differences

Power differences are part of many different interactions people have with each other. In the bodywork profession, they are present in work situations in which there are employers and employees, employees who have varying seniority or skill levels, and male and female power differences. One of the most obvious power differences, though, is between the client and practitioner.

Your attitude toward your clients is a factor that influences the power differential. For example, you may attach a high degree of self-importance to your job based on your education and experience as a bodywork practitioner. As a result, you could dismiss your clients' needs and requests or, worse yet, judge them as insignificant because you know more than clients do. Do not view your knowledge and skills as a means to wield power over clients but rather as a means to connect with them to provide the best possible care.

Likewise, if one of your clients expresses an attitude of inflated self-importance or insists on directing the entire treatment, you do not have to compete with him or her. Your job is to continue to present yourself professionally while working toward a cooperative therapeutic relationship. Keep in mind that clients often come to you suffering from pain, which may influence a client's attitude. When trust, safety, and confidence are communicated to clients through touch and behavior, often (but not always) the power imbalance begins to come into balance.

Client-Practitioner Relationships

In *The Psychology of the Body,* Elliot Greene and Barbara Goodrich-Dunn's research on the psychological impact of the client–therapist relationship is discussed: "The therapeutic relationship is a key to healing and the effectiveness of the therapeutic process. The importance of this observation cannot be overemphasized. Literature on the therapeutic relationship suggests that it is the single most powerful predictor of therapeutic outcome....Clients reported that the quality of their relationship with their therapist was more important in their work than the techniques that were used."[5]

This statement embodies the role that bodywork practitioners often experience. Therapeutic skills are only one feature of the job that clients notice. The primary aspect tends to be the degree to which the client feels a connection with the practitioner through a trusting relationship. This connection is expressed when clients request a regular appointment and keep it without fail, refer family and friends, or convey a sincere interest

Food for Thought
Think of a time in which there was a power difference between you and someone else. Who had the greater power, and who had the lesser power? What did the relationship feel like? What do you think were the benefits and what were the drawbacks to the power difference?

in your well-being. Be mindful and sensitive to these expressions of connection so that you do not inadvertently cross the line between professional and personal boundaries.

Power differences are innate in the service industry because of how the industry is structured. One person provides a service (practitioner) while another receives the service (client). Who has the power in the relationship, though, is a matter of perspective. It could be said that the client is always in the position of power because she is paying for the service, directing how the service is to be provided, and ultimately assuming responsibility for whether the practitioner has a job. Looking at it from the practitioner's perspective, it could be said that the practitioner has the position of power because without him there to provide the service the client would not have her needs met. For example, the practitioner may have a firm policy in place regarding a required time frame for the client to arrive for the service, and if the client is late, the service is reduced, or if the practitioner determines that the client was inappropriate he can terminate the session and still require payment.

These are extreme examples of how policy guidelines that reflect boundaries could be interpreted as power differences. However, if the therapeutic relationship is based only on the policy guidelines, chances are there will not be a sense of warmth and connection between you and the client. In fact, when the focus is on the rules and the procedures of who is responsible for what, the goal of the relationship, which is providing a safe and comfortable environment to facilitate therapeutic change for the client, gets lost. Instead, the intention that both you and the client share in the successful outcome of the therapeutic relationship creates a spirit of collaboration. Working together to make sure that each of you respects and trusts the other, and both know what to expect from each other, diminishes the need for one of you to be in a position of power over the other.

Creating mutual agreements about what you and your client expect as an outcome of the treatment is one strategy that can be implemented to reduce a power dynamic. Ideally, during the pretreatment interview, you and your client share information and agree on a plan that works toward accomplishing the goal of the treatment session. Each of you is responsible for being honest and forthcoming about your expectations and desired outcomes. You should also note that both you and your client have the right to ask for clarification or suggest a change in plans as the treatment progresses. Even with the most thorough interview and assessment skills, it is possible that the agreed-upon treatment plan may need to be altered once the treatment is underway.

Examples of areas of mutual agreement that might be focused on include the following:

- What area of the client's body the practitioner will work on
- How much of the treatment time will be spent on each area
- What areas of the body to avoid (e.g., hair, abdomen)
- What type of lubricant to use
- What method of draping will be used
- Specific techniques that will be used
- Specific techniques that will not be used
- What type of music is appropriate

- The overall length of time the treatment will take
- How and when feedback will be given

Empowering Clients in the Therapeutic Relationship

The term **empower** refers to the process of helping people who do not have power to gain it so that they can improve their personal or professional circumstances. Social scientists believe all individuals have the right, and should be encouraged, to develop to their full potential. In the bodywork profession this means having the ability to grow and develop skills that allow us to achieve our goals of having a thriving professional practice.

From this perspective, the concept of empowerment is the process of helping individuals, families, groups, and communities to increase their personal, interpersonal, socioeconomic, and political strength and to develop influence toward improving their circumstances. Important points to consider in this definition include the following:

- Empowerment is a dynamic process.
- Empowerment involves two people of differing positions of power.
- The one of lesser power is open and willing to receive input from the other.
- The one of greater power passes on knowledge and skills that have been proved to strengthen one's position of power.
- The outcome of this relationship results in increased awareness and competency of the person of lesser power, so that he or she may improve current circumstances.[6]

This definition emphasizes the role of receiving support and guidance from someone who has already achieved a level of success either personally or professionally. It is a positive example of how people who are in positions of power use it to assist others in gaining power. At the same time, the person receiving support is not resentful or suspicious of the one providing the knowledge. There is a mutual understanding that each person has positive intentions for this relationship to succeed.

Being **self-empowered** implies that you have the means within yourselves to overcome doubts and insecurities rather than relying on an external support system. Self-empowerment typically follows a period of receiving support from others until you can manifest this support for yourself. This can occur by working with trusted mentors and supervisors, developing a network of supportive colleagues, taking courses that enhance skills and knowledge, and, most of all, being able to see the progress we are making.

Clients may need our help in becoming self-empowered in the therapeutic relationship. Often they feel powerless regarding their treatments, for any number of reasons. Perhaps the client feels vulnerable during the session and does not want to be perceived as complaining. Perhaps the client has deferred all the power to you because you are the professional (or are on your way to becoming the professional). Therefore, you are the expert who can fix whatever problems the client has. Many clients do not even realize it is within their rights to state their preferences for the treatment.

It is in the area of client preferences that you, as the practitioner, can have the most impact on empowering your client to state her needs. By telling your client during the intake interview that you welcome any feedback she may have during the session, and to mean it, she is more likely to say her preferences. If a need is not being met, she may be more comfortable speaking up because you gave her permission to do so. You may even consider giving her some examples on what she may want to comment. Consider the following examples:

"At any point during the treatment, if you don't feel comfortable, the pressure isn't enough, a stretch isn't comfortable, or anything like that, please let me know. I'm very open to your input because I want to make sure you're getting the treatment you want."

"Don't hesitate to tell me at any point in the session if you need more or less pressure, a particular technique isn't comfortable, or anything else that may get in the way of you enjoying your treatment. I appreciate your feedback so that I can be sure to make adjustments in the moment so that the treatment is meeting your needs."

"Please feel free during the session to let me know how you are feeling about the work. This could include the pressure being too deep or not deep enough, you feeling cold or hot, or a technique not being comfortable for you. Don't worry about hurting my feelings, because I actually prefer it when a client lets me know what isn't working so I still have time to change things in the session, and you are getting the treatment you came in for."

The key points in these examples include the following:

- The client is given permission, and encouraged, to speak up.
- You give examples of what the client may choose to give feedback about.
- You let the client know that you do not take feedback personally so she does not have to worry about being offensive.
- You mention that timing is important so change can happen immediately, thus increasing client satisfaction.
- The client is reminded that the session is about her needs and not yours.

Educating clients on what to expect and what not to expect during the treatment is another way of increasing their comfort level concerning speaking up when their needs or expectations are not being met. One way of thinking of this is that a verbal contract was created between you and your client when you described the treatment plan and the client provided informed consent by agreeing to it. You are fulfilling your half of the contract by giving the client as much information as possible and providing structure and a sense of safety for the client. Optimally, the client will feel this safety and advocate for her needs, fulfilling her half of the contract (Table 6.1).

However you choose to let your clients know they can offer you feedback about their treatment experience, be authentic in your presentation style. Practice some different approaches of what to say ahead of time so that you will not be caught off guard, or so that you will not come off as, for example, apologetic, stern, uninterested, or controlling. Letting your clients know that this is a mutual therapeutic relationship and that their feedback is welcome builds trust and rapport. Clients are less likely to view you as having all the power and all the answers and instead see themselves as being an equal partner in the therapeutic relationship.

Table 6.1	Phrases That Do Not Empower the Client and Phrases That Do Empower the Client

Does Not Empower the Client	Does Empower the Client
Let me tell you what you need in today's session.	Tell me what you need in today's session.
If you don't do the exercises I gave you, your back pain will not go away.	Because the exercises we discussed last week didn't work for you, let's find another way to help decrease your back pain.
If you can't make your appointment on time, I'm going to start charging for the full session even though you aren't here.	Let's talk about your appointment time. Because you have been late the past 2 weeks it seems that we need to look at another day and time. Otherwise, I'm only able to work with the remaining time while charging you for a full session.
Don't worry if you feel some pain with today's treatment. That's what we call a "working sign" that lets me know the technique is being done right. You don't want to be a "wuss," do you?	You may feel some discomfort or even pain during today's treatment. There are times when the pain or discomfort cannot be avoided because we will be working on vulnerable and tight areas. Please do not hesitate to tell me when you start feeling discomfort so that I can make appropriate adjustments.
I do my best work in silence. Try not to talk during the treatment.	You are welcome to give me any feedback during the session to let me know how it is. I will be checking in as well. Otherwise, focus on your breathing while bringing your awareness to your body so that you can get the most out of the treatment.
I just went to a workshop on deep neck massage. You're going to love it!	I just completed training on deep neck massage techniques. I think you would benefit from what I learned. Do you want to hear about them and decide if you would like to try something new?

Once you have given the client permission as well as educated her about giving feedback, you must trust that the client will respond as she needs to. You can role model and give examples of what authentic feedback is; sometimes, however, a client simply chooses not to give feedback. There really is nothing you should do to force the issue. If you do not believe that the client's actual experience is in alignment with what you are sensing intuitively or physically through your work on the client's body, you should check in one more time, but then let it go. Continuing to ask a client for feedback during a session quickly gets annoying and, in itself, becomes a problem. If you know that you have been professional and clear in giving the client information on how to best receive the treatment, then you have done your job, and it is up to the client to decide if she wants to respond or not.

Who has the power if one party is not willing or able to speak up? Could the client be doing this out of lack of clarity concerning her role in the treatment session, or from a deep-seated belief that she should never tell someone else that she does not like what he or she is doing? Some people would rather tolerate pain and discomfort, or simply never return for treatment, than let someone else know that something is not right. You might find it helpful to know that this type of thinking exists, and you are not responsible if a client behaves this way.

■ **CASE PROFILE**

Edward is a student at a massage therapy school. One of his assignments is to receive a massage from a professional in the community and write a paper describing his experience.

Edward schedules a treatment with Dara in her home office. At the time of his appointment Dara conducts a brief intake interview, tells Edward to get on the massage table face down, and leaves the room. As he is undressing Edward realizes he forgot to tell Dara not to work on his feet because he has painful blisters he developed hiking the day before. He decides to leave his socks on, figuring that because Dara is a professional massage therapist she will know not to massage his feet. He lies on the massage table prone, as instructed.

When Dara returns, she announces, "I have a heat pack to help loosen up your back." She briskly proceeds to undrape Edward's entire back and place the pack on his sacrum. Edward jumps slightly, not expecting to feel such intense heat on his low back. Dara begins the massage by removing Edward's socks and massaging both feet at once. Edward does not say anything, even though he is wincing in pain, because he thinks he should have said something in the pretreatment interview. Meanwhile, the hot pack on his sacral area begins to feel very hot. Again, he does not say anything. He has not yet learned in his massage therapy program how to use heat packs, so he assumes this is how it is supposed to feel.

When Dara removes the heat pack, she exclaims, "Gosh, Ed, you should have told me this pack was too hot! I hope you don't get a burn from this. I better not work on this area."

Describe the power differentials in this scenario.

Discuss Dara's behavior and what messages she is sending.

Discuss Edward's behavior and what messages he is sending.

Do you think Dara and Edward will be able to establish a therapeutic relationship? Why or why not?

What would you have said and done differently if you were Dara?

What would you have said and done differently if you were Edward?

Managing Difficult Client Behaviors

No matter how mindful practitioners are in their interactions with clients, there will still be clients who are difficult to satisfy or unpleasant to work with. Although the vast majority of clients are polite, there will be those clients who are demanding, rude, or disrespectful. This distinction is made so that you can note the difference between the client as a person, and the behavior of the client. There are many reasons that a person may behave in such a way, and these reasons are not really the issue. Instead, your job is to manage difficult client behavior so that you are still able to perform effective treatments.

Managing difficult behavior is easier when the focus is on the actions of the person rather than on the person herself. In other words, you cannot expect to change an individual's way of being in a treatment session. However, you can be clear and specific in your communication about what is appropriate behavior in the treatment room. When the client is informed of what behavior is appropriate and what the consequences are if behavior becomes inappropriate, then you have the choice of either continuing or discontinuing the treatment based on the client's ability to remedy the behavior.

What follows are some examples of difficult client behavior, along with brief suggestions of what to say to manage a situation.

Malingering Clients

Malingering clients tend to ask for more work beyond the agreed-upon end of treatment. These are not clients who are simply unaware that the treatment time is coming to a close, but those who are trying to manipulate you into giving a few extra minutes for free. They typically ask for more time to be spent on a particular region or ask you to return to an area that was previously worked. An appropriate response to curb this type of behavior might be the following: "I'm sorry, but our time is up for today's session. Remind me to start with that area the next time you come in." **or** "If you're requesting a longer treatment, I can accommodate your request but I'll have to charge you for the extra time." This response should be used only if you are willing and able to provide the extra time. If you are not, then that would need to be communicated to the client. The emphasis, though, should be that the client does not get a longer treatment for free.

Another ploy a malingering client may use is to imply that you have not done a complete job and need to spend the extra time to satisfy the client. If this is the case, an appropriate response might be the following: "I'm sorry that area is still giving you problems. If you had spoken up sooner I would have been able to return to the area for some more attention. However, our session has come to an end for today. Next time, be sure to let me know as soon as possible if an area does not feel complete."

It is important you respond respectfully to the client, and not be rude. The purpose is to continue to educate the client on the importance of following the agreed-upon time frame.

Excessive Talking

Clients who talk excessively before, during, or after the session can create difficulty on many levels. If the talking occurs during the session, it may be distracting to you, thus causing you to lose focus. Excessive talking could also pull you into the conversation to the point that the session runs over time, or you do not meet the goals of the treatment plan.

When a client talks a great deal before a treatment, then the treatment may start late and may then end late as well. You are then required to decide whether to alter the length of the treatment to accommodate the talking, or try and give the client the full treatment length. If you choose to shorten the treatment length, then the client will certainly notice, and may become angry that she or he has not received the full hands-on time. If you choose to give the client the full treatment length, it can shorten the time you have until your next client is scheduled. This decision may cause a domino effect on the start times of the rest of the day's schedule, and is not fair to the other clients if their treatments start late. You are also not being fair to yourself because you will have less setup time and time to center yourself before the next client. To address this issue, you might say something such as the following as you are guiding the client into the treatment room: "Let's continue this conversation while you're on the table. We don't want to cut short your hands-on time."

A strategy to use on the client who tends to chat after a session, seemingly unaware that you have a schedule to follow, is to quickly find a pause in the conversation, thank the client for coming in, and walk toward the door. The client may recognize this nonverbal cue, and wrap up the conversation and leave. If the door is open and the client is still deep in conversation, then you might need to be more direct. You can offer something such as the following: "Gosh, it seems like today's treatment really energized you! I do have to excuse myself and prepare for my next client. Thank you so much for coming in and I look forward to seeing you next week."

With experience, you will likely be able to spot excessive talkers immediately, and take measures before a pattern is established in which the client assumes that the excessive chatting is acceptable.

Inappropriate Emotional Outbursts

Clients who use the treatment session as an opportunity to have an audience watch them be emotionally distraught, or to treat you rudely by using inappropriate language to express dissatisfaction are exhibiting inappropriate emotional outbursts. An inappropriate emotional outburst might be loud and excessive crying that interferes with other clients' treatments. It might also be the client who chooses to shout at you about how unhappy he is with the treatment he received. It is important that this kind of behavior not be tolerated and that the client be informed of the consequences if it continues. For example, if a client chronically complains that he is not satisfied with the treatments he receives, it would be beneficial for you to sit down with the client, and discuss exactly what his expectations are and whether those expectations are reasonable.

Rude clients are dissatisfied clients. The key is to determine what it is that is not working and attempt to fix it. However, if it is not a matter of being able to make something better for the client, but a personality clash instead, then it may be time to discuss referring the client to another practitioner who would better match his needs. You are not required to tolerate disrespectful and offensive behavior.

It is most important that you remain calm and professional. The client who acts out in a rude and disrespectful manner needs to be informed that such behavior is not permissible and that he will no longer be able to receive treatments if it continues. This conversation must be very direct and not allow for further verbal abuse by the client. Examples of what you might say include the following: "I understand that you are upset. However, it is not acceptable that you speak to me in that manner. If you are not able to lower your voice and discuss your concerns in a courteous manner, I will ask you to leave."

You might also say the following: "I would be happy to discuss your concerns, but not until you lower your voice and show me the professional courtesy that I am offering you."

If the client is not willing to abide by this guideline, then it is within your rights to walk away from the client, or, if you are talking to the client on the phone, tell him that you will be hanging up because he is not changing his tone and demeanor.

There are also clients who have a history of mental illness who may have a psychotic break during a session. If this happens, call 911 and ask for immediate crisis intervention services. This will most likely disrupt the flow and schedule of your entire day. However, these situations must be addressed with appropriate crisis professionals and it would not be appropriate for you to walk away from the client and leave him or her alone before help arrived. In your role as the practitioner you must stay with the client, as long as there is no danger of harm, and ensure the client's behavior affects others in the treatment center as little as possible, until help arrives. If you work in a setting with other practitioners, it may be possible to move clients to another practitioner so that there is no disruption in service.

After such a breakdown, a decision must be made concerning whether this client is able to return for treatments. A doctor's release indicating that the client is able to receive bodywork may be necessary. You must then make a decision about whether you are able to work with the client should he choose to return. If not, then you should refer the client to another practitioner.

Clients Who "Hijack" the Session

"Hijacking" refers to clients who think they have more knowledge and experience than you and do not hesitate to make this known. This client will, for example, interrupt you and question why you are doing a certain technique and not another, or she will disregard your expertise entirely and direct each portion of the treatment.

When you encounter such a client, there are basically three choices that you can make:

1. Fulfill all the requests made by the client.
2. Refuse to accommodate the client and discontinue the treatment.
3. Collaborate with the client to inform him how his behavior is affecting your ability to perform the treatment, and find out why the client is being so demanding in the session.

Each of these choices has its own merit in certain situations. The first choice, fulfilling all the requests, may lead you to feel resentful or take offense toward the client. The reality is that you must be able to decide if what is being asked is indicated for the safety of the client. It is your job to determine

 Food for Thought

Think about a time you had an interaction with someone who was rude or disrespectful to you. Did you talk to this person in a respectful manner about his or her behavior? If so, what was the outcome? If you did not talk to the person, why not? How did you feel about not talking to the person about his or her behavior?

what is appropriate and necessary for a successful treatment outcome. You also have a duty to the client to inform him that the behavior involving managing the treatment is interfering with your ability to work.

Resentment can build if you feel less and less acknowledged and respected for the talents and knowledge you bring to the treatment session. You may even think your skills and knowledge are being dismissed because of the client's need to be in charge. In an extreme situation, if you do not maintain your professional demeanor, you may even feel pushed to an unprofessional display of anger or bitterness toward the client that could have negative consequences for both of you.

The second choice, refusing to make any accommodations at all, is not a viable option as it denies you and the client the opportunity to find a successful working relationship. When you make a unanimous decision such as this, you are acting in the same controlling manner as the client. The practitioner who chooses this response is mirroring the behavior of the client needing to be in charge and not willing to hear other possibilities of what adjustments could be made in the treatment.

The third choice, collaborating with the client, allows mutual exploration of the dynamic between you and the client to determine what is motivating the client to act in this way. The client's behavior is an expression of needing to feel in charge of his environment and well-being in order to experience the treatment. The most fundamental need humans have is to feel safe. What would it take for this client to relinquish control and trust that his needs will be met without the constant directional barrage to the practitioner? To obtain this information you might make the following comment: "I'm noticing that you're making a lot of requests about how you would like me to give this treatment. What can I say or do that would allow you to relax into the session and not feel responsible for giving me directions?"

You might also say the following: "I have to be honest with you. I'm feeling confused and distracted right now because of all the directions you're giving me. What do you need from me to trust that I am fully present and capable of meeting the treatment goals we discussed?"

You are informing the client about what you are experiencing during the treatment, and the client is invited to express which of his needs are not being met. It is helpful when you are specific about what you are experiencing as well as asking for specific feedback from the client. This direct and nonjudgmental way of communicating with the client allows you to find a solution that meets the needs of both you and the client. You can then work without constant interruption and guidance and the client can let go of the need to direct and simply receive.

Strategies for Workplace Settings

Empowerment needs to happen on an organizational level where teamwork is the expectation of a successful business. For example, many bodywork practitioners work in clinics and spa settings where it is important that everyone is committed to creating and maintaining appropriate working relationships. Recall that the primary goal of empowerment is to be

Words of Wisdom

I accept whatever the client says at face value; I don't delve into the client's story or melodrama. This makes it okay for the client to say whatever they want, instead of me getting wrapped up in their drama and not being able to do therapeutic work.

—Barbara Grandstaff, certified Neuromuscular Massage Therapist (St. John Method) since 1986, certified in Yamuna Body Rolling since 2007, and certified in Kinesio Taping since 2008 able to trust your strengths and believe in your potential to make the right decisions. When this happens you will likely feel confident in proceeding with your work.

In the context of workplace settings, empowerment means giving coworkers more latitude to make decisions and allowing them the resources to implement them. In *Leading Self-Directed Work Teams*, Kimball Fisher developed an "empowerment formula," which can be adapted to professional bodywork settings:

$$Empowerment = (A \times R \times I \times A)$$

where

A = authority, R = resources, I = information, and A = accountability

When we have the **A**uthority to act, the **R**esources that we need to do the job, accurate and timely **I**nformation regarding the nature of issue, followed by **A**ccountability, you cannot go wrong.[7]

What is important about this formula is that each of the four variables must be present for empowerment to truly be present. Fisher states, "To feel empowered, people need formal authority and all of the resources (like budget, equipment, time and training) necessary to *do something* with the new authority. They also need timely, accurate information to make good decisions. And they need a personal sense of accountability for the work."[8]

The following is an example of how this formula might work in an organization in which an individual is given tasks that are designed to move the business forward:

Imagine that you are the local manager of a spa franchise. The owner has given you the responsibility of creating a marketing campaign in the community to increase revenue. As you began to work on your task, you realize that you need information about the current financial health of the franchise so you can determine your advertising budget. When you ask your boss for this information, you are told it does not matter and just to proceed with a plan. You put together some designs for print advertisements, contacting several local printing companies to get estimates on their prices. Once this information is gathered and you present it to your boss, you are told that you are not allowed to use a local printing company because all printed materials have to go through the corporate headquarters.

At this point you decide to ask for some guidelines on how your boss wants you to create the new marketing campaign. You share honestly with your boss that you did not feel empowered to make decisions on a local level. You say, "I don't believe I'm given enough information or resources to create a campaign I can believe in, because the corporate headquarters has such tight restrictions on what I can and cannot do." You make it clear that because the franchise is a local business, it needs to support other businesses within the community, not one in a distant state. After thinking it over, your boss tells you to proceed with your ideas. You are given complete authority to make decisions and access to all the resources and information you deem necessary. As a result you feel a personal sense of responsibility for wanting to see your spa franchise succeed.

The principle that all should be treated with respect and fairness should guide the management of power differences in the workplace. This does

Food for Thought

How does the example mirror the client–practitioner relationship?

Take each of the four variables of the empowerment formula (authority, resources, information, and accountability) and define how each one of them is expressed in your professional relationships and in your client–practitioner relationships.

How does having successful client–practitioner relationships predict the success of employee–employer relationships? How does having successful client–practitioner relationships predict the success of relationships among coworkers?

not always happen, of course. There are distinct power differences between employers and employees, and, not necessarily so obvious, there will sometimes be power differences among coworkers.

Employers and Employees

Because employers have the power to hire and fire, there is an implication that the employee has less power in the power difference and should defer to the employer. However, there is increased productivity and loyalty from employees if employers have a management style of collaboration and joint decision making. This does not necessarily mean that the employees have as much power as the employer, but it does mean that their input is valued and respected.

Ideally, employers provide training sessions for employees on how to appropriately offer input to management, along with other training necessary for the workplace setting. However, this will not always be the case. If there are circumstances that you, as an employee, find are hindering your ability to provide effective treatments, work well with other employees, and grow in your skills and responsibilities, it would be worthwhile for you to devise strategies to discuss the issues with your supervisor.

You should keep in mind that communication in the workplace is a two-way street. Employers cannot always expect to be the only one involved in making decisions about the workplace. The following strategies will empower you to talk with employers:

1. Identify what the most important issues are that the employer must hear from you and other employees, perhaps by polling the other employees.
2. Once the issues are identified, you should have very specific reasons why the issues are important.
3. As a team, create solutions for how you and the other employees would like the employer to address the issues. Be realistic about what the employer is actually capable of doing or providing.
4. Arrange to meet with the employer at a time outside of your workday. Come to the meeting prepared and willing to listen.
5. Present the issues in a respectful manner.
6. Schedule a time with the employer to meet again to follow up on the issues discussed.

Consider the following: Karey works at a clinic with 12 other bodywork practitioners. The owner of the clinic provides all managerial support except a receptionist. Answering the phone, scheduling appointments, and greeting clients are duties shared by all of the employees. Over the past 6 months, Karey has noticed that the workload of these duties has increased. A small storefront has been added to sell bodywork products, books, and small gift items. A computer system has been implemented to accommodate the store and to handle the scheduling; clients now have the option of booking appointments online. As a result of these changes, the employees are experiencing a lot of stress trying to figure out the new systems. A feeling of resentment is building among them because they do not think it is fair that they should take on these tasks. Karey can tell that emotions are climbing and that office morale is sinking, so she decides to take action.

Karey asks each of her coworkers if they would like to meet with the owner to tell her about their concerns. Everyone thinks it is a good idea as long as Karey is the one who has the actual meeting with the owner. Karey agrees and proceeds to pass out a survey for all the employees to complete regarding the operational duties, why the new system is causing distress, and what possible solutions they would recommend. Karey compiles the information into a report and sets up a formal meeting with the owner on Karey's day off. At the meeting, Karey explains the purpose of the meeting and presents the report outlining the employee concerns and suggested resolutions. The owner is initially taken aback, because she did not know there is so much unrest among the staff that a report had to be written. Karey assures the owner that she created the report so that she would be well prepared for the meeting. At this point, the owner becomes more open to the information and a productive discussion follows.

The outcome is that the owner would explore the possibility of two part-time receptionists for a total coverage of 6 days a week. After the receptionists are hired, a follow-up meeting is set up. The owner and Karey have both noticed that morale has begun to grow and the staff all seem to be less stressed.

If you were one of the 12 employees, what would you have wanted the owner to know about the situation and why?

If you were the owner, what would have been your reaction to Karey's request for a meeting? What would have been your response to her report?

Coworkers

Unless practitioners are working alone in their business, most will find themselves in an environment that requires them to share workspace, treatment rooms, computers, clients, and so forth. Although this is not true of everyone, many people in Western society tend to compare themselves to those they work with, sometimes to the point of ranking everyone based on age, experience, education, and skill level. The bodywork profession is certainly not immune to this way of thinking.

The practitioner who believes that she has more status than others she works with based on work experience, amount of education, or simply amount of time spent at the workplace could use that perceived status to create a power difference over her coworkers. She may choose to display her perceived power by bragging, which will most likely result in her not having much support from the other practitioners. Perhaps the practitioner's ego will tell her that the lack of support results from the others' jealousy, but in reality people tend to find this behavior to be disrespectful to them and so are not willing to invest any time or effort to connect with this kind of individual.

Other issues you might experience with coworkers can include the following:

• Coworkers who leave the treatment space a mess
• Coworkers who habitually end their treatments late, usurping the next practitioner's time in the treatment space

- Coworkers who take the last of supplies and do not inform anyone else
- Coworkers who form cliques, leading to the exclusion of certain practitioners
- Coworkers who talk to other practitioners in rude and disrespectful tones
- Coworkers who gossip about other coworkers
- Coworkers who gossip about clients
- Coworkers who try to steal clients from other practitioners by downplaying the other practitioners' skills
- Coworkers who engage in loud conversations with their clients, or with other coworkers, right outside the treatment space
- Coworkers who engage in unprofessional and unethical behavior, such as scheduling clients for treatments outside of the treatment space if this is expressly forbidden by the business, keeping gratuities meant for other practitioners, or stealing supplies from the business

Unless there is a leader among the staff, a strong supervisor, or an outside facilitator to confront these dynamics and offer strategies to resolve them, office morale will most likely decline. Practitioners are then more likely to leave to find somewhere else to work, and clientele can suffer. All of these negatively affect the success of the bodywork business. The following are some suggested strategies for you to practice open communication with coworkers:

1. Ask to meet with your coworker outside of work to discuss work-related issues. Choose a neutral meeting place, and one where you will not run the risk of being overheard by other employees. Ask another employee you trust to go with you if you believe you will need support or another perspective on the issue.
2. At the meeting, depersonalize the issue and make it clear to the coworker that it is the behavior he is demonstrating that is the issue.
3. Ask the coworker for feedback on how he views the workplace, the issues brought up, and what he needs to have happen for a more comfortable work environment.
4. Brainstorm together ways to minimize the tension and enhance cooperation. If this is not possible, brainstorm ways to minimize contact with each other or determine and agree on acceptable behaviors that would limit the conflict.
5. Make a commitment to check in with each other every week until it feels that there is a resolution.

■ CASE PROFILE

Gabriel and Leo have been mandated to meet to resolve an ongoing issue between them, or else both will be required to leave the clinic at which they both work. Gabriel, a recent graduate of massage school and the newest employee, has a tendency to laugh and talk a lot during his sessions. Leo, a senior member of the staff, has been practicing shiatsu for 10 years and is very quiet and soft spoken. Leo has grown tired of

Case Study Continued from page 214

asking Gabriel to be quiet. The issue escalated to the breaking point when Leo, out of frustration and egged on by his client, pounded loudly on the wall between the two treatment rooms after Gabriel let out a peal of laughter that could be heard clearly in Leo's treatment room. Gabriel's client complained about the pounding, requiring the clinic to offer the client a complimentary treatment. When Leo's client hears this, she demands a complimentary treatment as well because, as she put it, "That other guy's noise started the whole thing!" At this point the owner of the clinic orders the two men to work it out or leave the clinic because the entire staff has grown tired of their drama.

What do you see as the fundamental issue between Gabriel and Leo?

What role does power or status play in this scenario?

Which one of the practitioners do you relate to? Why?

If you were Gabriel and Leo's boss, how would you have handled this situation?

As a coworker of Gabriel and Leo's, what would you want them to know and why?

Challenges of the Genders

Generally, history shows that one's gender has an impact on what jobs people are drawn to, who gets paid more, and who is discriminated against. For the most part, throughout history, males have had the most power. Just look at the number of men in political, legislative, judicial, and military power; the higher economic status of men over women; and the freedom, for the most part, of working full-time or part-time without worrying about child care. Although women have made great strides in equality during the past 40 years, there are some stereotypes that still stand:

- Women are more nurturing than are men.
- Men are more aggressive; this is respected in the workplace.
- Women who are aggressive are viewed negatively.
- Men are stronger physically and emotionally.
- Women are weaker emotionally and physically.
- Women are safer than men, both emotionally and physically.
- Women are more concerned with their families than are men.
- Men will take on leadership roles and be given leadership roles more often than will women.
- Men deserve to be paid more than women because they work harder than women work.
- When women are at work, their minds are on their families, not on their work.
- Women are more concerned with "soft news," such as fashion and celebrities.
- Men are more concerned with politics, the economy, and world news.

Traditionally, society has also assigned different roles to each of the genders. For instance, men have been thought of more as leaders, problem solvers, and "movers and shakers." Until recently, when the titles CEO, judge, general, doctor, president, and professor were mentioned, most people automatically assumed that men were being talked about. Women have been thought of more as comforters, nurturers, and peacemakers. When talking about nurses, elementary school teachers, nannies, stay-at-home parents, social workers, and office assistants, the assumption was that these were all women.

Of course, thinking has changed quite a bit as more men have moved into jobs traditionally held by women, and more women have moved into jobs traditionally held by men. If, say, a man becomes a nurse, he is no longer referred to as a male nurse, but simply as a nurse. The same is true for women who are doctors; they are no longer called "women doctors."

Impact of Societal Roles in the Bodywork Profession

The bodywork profession has not been immune to the traditional gender roles either. Although there have always been male practitioners, in recent history, more practitioners have been female. This could be because bodywork is considered a nurturing profession, and in the early part of the 20th century, it had a close association with nursing. As times changed, and more men have become interested in the bodywork profession, the idea that it is an occupation mainly for women has changed. In fact, part of the reason the term "massage therapist" was created was because the previous terms for practitioners of massage were "masseuse" for a female practitioner, and "masseur" for a male practitioner. Massage therapist makes no distinction about the practitioner's sex.

Deborah Tannen, a scholar and professor of linguistics at Georgetown University in Washington D.C., focuses her research on the influence gender has on communication styles. In *You Just Don't Understand: Women and Men in Conversation,* she writes: "For women, intimacy is key in a world of connection where individuals negotiate complex networks of friendships, minimize differences, try to reach consensus, and avoid the appearance of superiority, which would highlight differences. In a world of status, independence is key, because a primary means of establishing status is to tell others what to do, and taking orders is a marker of low status. Though all humans need both intimacy and independence, women tend to focus on intimacy and men on independence. These differences can give women and men differing views of the same situation."[9]

Women seek intimacy, connection, and symmetry as a means of communicating with others. Women find value in processing information, seeking to understand and find meaning in their contact with others. A female bodywork practitioner may place great value on the need to create a nurturing safe space for her clients by asking detailed questions in the interview session and allowing her clients to share as much information as they need to feel heard. When she focuses her attention on these practices, she is confident that she is laying the groundwork for a successful client–practitioner relationship. It is possible that this female practitioner tends to have trouble with time management in her sessions because she is so intent on understanding completely what the clients need.

Men value independence, status, and asymmetry in the navigation of their environment. They tend to be focused on the here and now, seeking to get things done in a timely manner so that they can move on to the next thing that needs to be done. This is not to say that men are not paying attention to what they are doing; they just do not feel the need to linger once the job is done or the words are said. A male bodywork practitioner may choose to conduct an intake interview that is brief yet concise, relying on the written information from the intake form rather than take time away from the hands-on portion of the treatment session. The challenge for this practitioner is that he may be perceived as being aloof and lacking the warmth that some clients prefer.

Although everyone has their own unique style of communicating and connecting with others, as a practitioner you might find yourself following these gender tendencies. Neither one is better than the other. Instead, think of these tendencies as ways to understand how people of the opposite sex communicate, thereby giving you the opportunity to prevent or resolve issues that may come up.

Consider the following: Both Lisa and Mark are massage therapists who have clients with low back pain. They have determined that the psoas muscle is the culprit and should be the focus of the massage treatment.

Lisa says to her client: "Your low back pain may be related to your core muscles. Often when they're tight they can cause your back to hurt. I would like to do some deep work through your abdomen that will address this issue, specifically on a muscle called the psoas. The psoas is very deep and can be very tender. Sometimes clients have an emotional release when I work in that area. I'm telling you this so you can be prepared for whatever may happen. There's nothing wrong with having an emotional release. In fact, it's quite normal and a way for your body to tell you there may be something going on you haven't been aware of until now. Because the psoas is very deep, I'll be asking you to do some particular breathing techniques and movements to help me reach it. It might be a good idea for you to go to the bathroom before we start so that you can be comfortable, because I'll be working over the bladder. Again, if you have any questions or concerns please feel free to speak up and let me know. Do you have any questions right now?"

Mark says to his client: "Your low back pain may be related to your core muscles so I'm going to do some deep abdominal work today to help your low back release some of the tension. Do you have any questions? Go ahead and use the bathroom before we get started. I'll meet you back in the treatment room in about 5 minutes. I'll be sure to knock before I come in."

These different approaches touch on the fact that some women practitioners may overanalyze the situation and want to give the client as much information as possible. This is how they feel connected with the client as well as create a therapeutic relationship. If they did not do this, they may think they have not done their job well, and may not feel confident performing techniques.

Conversely, some men practitioners may be all about doing the work without offering any detailed explanation. They know that if anything comes up for the client during the session they can deal with it then. However, they

🍎 Food for Thought

If you are a female practitioner, does Lisa's approach sound like your approach? Why or why not? If you are a male practitioner, does Mark's approach sound like your approach? Why or why not? Overall, how would you describe your approach to clients?

do not see the need to spend a lot of time explaining ahead of time what might happen. They may think that because the client is there to receive a treatment, it is best to get to the hands-on work as soon as possible.

Today, although bodywork is considered a viable profession for both genders, female practitioners still tend to outnumber male practitioners. It is a self-empowering profession for women. Women have taken leadership roles in professional organizations; founding and running spas, wellness centers, and schools; writing bodywork textbooks; and providing continuing education workshops.

Nonetheless, some societal roles continue to affect the bodywork profession. These can be seen in some of the myths about male practitioners, and some of the myths about female practitioners.

Myths About Female and Male Practitioners

Myths are generally created out of fear, a lack of information, a narrow-minded perspective, or grandiosity placed on ordinary achievements or events. All professions are subject to myths that the public believes to be true, including the bodywork profession. Consider the following myths:

- Male practitioners will sexualize the bodywork treatment. Although there have been isolated cases, and male practitioners seem to be shown this way in all forms of entertainment media, it certainly is not true of most male practitioners. Men in the bodywork profession, though, need to be keenly aware of this myth, and make sure that anything they say or do cannot be misconstrued as either sexual innuendo or as being outright sexual. They need to keep in mind that if a client already has a concern that this may happen, it would not take more than, say, an ill-placed hand on the client's hip to send a client to the manager to complain.
- Male practitioners are the only ones who can provide deep pressure during techniques. This myth may have resulted because men generally have a larger body size then women; therefore, the thinking is that men are stronger. However, women learn the same bodywork techniques, and if they learn proper body mechanics they are just as capable of applying appropriate deep pressure.
- Male practitioners will be "all business" and not care about the emotional aspects of bodywork. This myth does not take into account that men are just as capable of emotional connections as women when they are appropriate and necessary for the therapeutic relationship.
- People are more afraid of male practitioners. This myth implies that because men are generally stronger than women, they will hurt their clients or, worse, want to be sexual with clients or even predatory. This myth does not take into account that men learn the same bodywork techniques as women and so know how to perform effective treatments without hurting clients. Also, all men, of course, are not looking for ways to be abusive to others. Many have worked hard to assist survivors of abuse in healing, some of whom did not think that they could work with a male practitioner.
- Female practitioners are available for sex. This myth dates back to the era when massage parlors were in existence and the women who

worked in them were prostitutes. It is also reinforced by how the popular media portray most female massage therapists. Today's female bodywork practitioner is a proud professional with expertise in facilitating the healing process.

- It is more difficult for male practitioners to build a clientele than it is for female practitioners. Actually, there is some truth to this, mainly because of the mistaken notion that some have that male practitioners will hurt clients or are sexual predators. Sometimes clients simply prefer a female practitioner. However, the practitioner's gender is not the sole factor involved in building a clientele.
- In a bodywork business, the male practitioner is the boss and the female practitioner is his employee. As with the myth that male practitioners are better at business than are female practitioners, this myth is easily proved wrong by the number of successful female bodywork business owners in any given community. The opportunity to be the employer and the opportunity to be the employee are equal in the bodywork profession.
- Male practitioners make better business owners and supervisors than do female practitioners. This myth is false because the ability to be an effective supervisor is not based in gender, but is based in having the skills to manage a budget, hire and manage staff, find investors for the business, and market and network effectively.

Challenges Between the Genders

The bodywork profession is enriched because of the diversity that exists among its practitioners. Diversity not only means people of different ethnicities, ages, countries of origin, age, and skill level, it means gender as well. Although there are many challenges in the bodywork professions, one of the major reasons for its successes is the ability of practitioners to cooperate and work together to promote the industry. Given that, there can still be challenges that gender may contribute to the profession.

Much has been talked about in terms of the communication styles of men and women. It has been proved that men and women do, indeed, communicate differently, sometimes to the point at which they have a difficult time understanding each other. Women tend to be relational and value the process of conversation with colleagues. Although men value conversation, they tend to focus more on ideas than on relationships, and do not seem to have the same need as women do to talk things over with others. Male practitioners, then, may view female practitioners as talking with each other a lot, but not really saying much, which they can find tedious. Female practitioners, then, may view male practitioners as unfeeling and unconcerned about anything except that which the male practitioner finds interesting.

Communications studies professor Julia T. Woods uses the term "speech communities" to describe a group of people who share norms about communication. She says that "a speech community exists when people share understandings about goals of communication, strategies for enacting those goals, and ways of interpreting communication. This is an important definition for our discussion of gender and communication because it emphasizes the importance of both parties having similar methods of communication as well as expectations for the outcome. If we have been socialized to think that women are always seeking relationships and like to talk about feelings but that men never do those things, then we run the risk of seeing our communication styles as black and white when in fact our world is full of shades of gray."[10]

One challenge arises from the way that practitioners choose to resolve conflict with one another. In general, men tend to resolve conflict by coming up with solutions that involve specific steps. The sooner the conflict is resolved, the better it is, so that everyone can move on. Women, conversely, tend to want to discuss what happened, and may need to do so more than once, and work together to create a solution. Male practitioners, then, may view female practitioners as needing to talk about a particular issue over and over again, and think that it is pointless to do so once it has been solved. Female practitioners, then, may view male practitioners as being in a hurry to accomplish something and not caring about what others think.

Awareness is the first step needed to ensure that these challenges do not cause conflict or strife between coworkers. A successful practice will hold regular staff meetings to give the practitioners an opportunity to discuss what is and is not working. It is also an opportunity for coworkers to make requests of one another in terms of what would be helpful to increase cooperation.

Chapter Summary

Power differences occur in many professions, and bodywork is no exception. Practitioners need to use their power in a way that earns client trust and creates therapeutic relationships to have a long and successful career. A power difference occurs when, in a relationship, one party has greater control, or power, over the other. In the bodywork profession, you are perceived by clients as having greater power in the therapeutic relationship because you are the expert, and clients think you must know what you are doing. To reduce the power difference between you and your client, you can create mutual agreements about what you and your client expect as an outcome of the treatment. You can empower your client by setting treatment parameters, soliciting feedback, and educating clients on what to expect during the treatment. Learning to work with clients who are difficult and unpleasant also requires understanding the power difference.

Practitioners who work in a setting with other practitioners are likely to experience power differences between employers and employees and among coworkers. With employers and employees, it is important to remember that communication is a two-way street and to use strategies that will empower you to talk with your employer should an issue arise. The same is true of coworkers. Finally, practitioners must learn to deal effectively with issues and myths of gender in the bodywork profession, both with clients and other coworkers.

Food for Thought

Think about interactions you have had with people of the same sex, and people of the opposite sex. What were some of the challenges you experienced while communicating with them? What were some of the successes you had? Why did you have these challenges, and why did you have these successes?

Review Questions

Multiple Choice

1. The person who has the means to overcome doubts and insecurities without relying on an external support system is said to be:

a. High in status

b. Self-empowered

c. In authority

d. Having a gender challenge

2. The practitioner who remains clothed while the client is not is an example of:

a. Empowerment

b. Status

c. Power differences

d. Malingering

3. Power from our formal place within an organization or group is power from:

a. Expertise

b. Relationships

c. Status

d. Position

4. A way to reduce a power dynamic between you and a client is to:

a. Speak about how highly skilled you are

b. Create a mutual agreement about the structure of the treatment session

c. Tell the client what type of music you will be using during the treatment

d. Discourage feedback

5. If a client has an inappropriate emotional outburst, the most important thing to do is to:

a. Remain calm and professional

b. Raise your voice to be heard over him

c. Call the police immediately

d. Say nothing about the incident

6. The client who insists on directing the practitioner's every move during the treatment can be described as the client who:

a. Hijacks the session

b. Has emotional outbursts

c. Is malingering

d. Talks excessively

7. A common myth about male practitioners is that they:

a. Are worse at business than women

b. Can provide more emotional support to their clients than women

c. Make better supervisors than women

d. Make more people afraid than women do

Fill in the Blank

1. Power has much to do with how we _____ ourselves.

2. _____ refers to the process of helping people who do not have power to gain it.

3. Our level of skill and knowledge is referred as _____ .

4. If a client has a psychotic break during a session, you should call 911 and get immediate _____ .

5. The empowerment formula is Authority × Resources × Information × _____ .

6. An effective strategy for an employee to address issues with his employer is to identify the most important issues the employer must hear by _____ the other employees.

7. When women communicate, they tend to be _____ and value the process of conversation with colleagues.

Short Answer

1. Give at least three examples of behaviors that make clients perceive you, as a bodywork practitioner, as a person of power.

2. List five ways power differences can occur in the bodywork profession.

3. List at least five phrases that do not empower the client. Rephrase each of these in a way that will empower the client.

4. Describe at least three ways practitioners can manage malingering clients, clients who talk excessively, inappropriate outbursts from clients, and clients who hijack the session.

5. Explain the six steps that will empower you to talk with an employer if an issue arises.

6. Describe at least five issues you might experience with a coworker and what you might do to resolve each one.

7. List at least six myths about male and female practitioners, and explain why they are not true.

Activities

1. Choose two of the following scenarios. Either by yourself or with another practitioner, discuss the issues involved, and decide how you would address them with the client.

- A client who has a pattern of showing up 10 to 15 minutes late for appointments and expects to receive the full-body, 1-hour session
- A client who delays leaving the office by 10 or 15 minutes by writing out the check for payment, then engages you in a story before handing you the check
- A well-paying, regular client who develops the pattern of calling at the last minute for an appointment, and offers you more money when you say you are not available
- A client who makes frequent comments comparing your work to another practitioner in an unflattering fashion
- A client who tells you stories about another practitioner that the client thinks is funny, but raises your concerns about the practitioner's ethics, use of boundaries, and ability to follow the policies and procedures of the clinic

2. Choose three of the following scenarios. Either by yourself or with another practitioner, discuss the issues involved, and decide how you would address them with your coworker.

- You share a treatment room with a coworker who never ends her treatments in enough time for you to prepare for your client and start your session on time.
- You are employed at a destination resort and are scheduled to perform a treatment on a famous celebrity. After the interview, you leave the room to gather supplies for the treatment. When you return you are informed that another practitioner stepped in to do the treatment because he admires the celebrity.
- You are part of a cooperative clinic setting. All practitioners are responsible for documenting each treatment immediately after completing the treatment. You notice one coworker always leaves her documentation to do later, and often does not complete it at all.
- A coworker confides in you that twice a week he has friends call to make an appointment for his last session of the day under a false name and phone number with the intention of not keeping the appointment so your coworker can leave early.
- You suddenly have the opportunity to attend a 2-day workshop that starts tomorrow, which is the last day of your weekly shift. The management has told all practitioners that they must give 3 days' notice if they want to be released from a shift or they will not be able to get the time off. You call in sick to attend the workshop. When you arrive, the person taking registration is your manager.
- You work in a clinical setting in which teamwork is emphasized for the successful completion of daily tasks. One employee makes it very clear that she is not a team player and does not plan to become one. She does not participate in employee meetings but is the first to complain about a new procedure or chooses not to follow it because she does not agree with it. The employee also monopolizes conversations in the break room and has the habit of telling off-color and inappropriate jokes. Over time, the dynamic in the office has become stressful and uncomfortable.
- You are a female working with two other practitioners, one of whom is male, in a cooperative setting. One day this coworker announces to you and the other practitioner that he has created a marketing plan and has taken out an ad in the newspaper. He asks you to contribute one-third of the price of the ad.

3. Describe your perspective on the role of gender in the bodywork profession. Consider it as a practitioner, and then as a client.

4. Call bodywork businesses in your community to find out how many are owned by men and how many are owned by women. Interview several of the male owners and several of the female owners to find out their challenges and their successes, and what has contributed to the success of their businesses and what has not.

Guidance for Journaling

 Some key areas to think about while journaling for this chapter include the following:

- Your sources of power
- How you feel about your personal, relational, expertise, position, and status power
- What power differences you have experienced in your life and how you have felt about them
- What strategies you are likely to use when working within power differences between yourself and your clients, as an employer or employee, and with your coworkers
- Roles society has assigned to each of the genders and how these roles affect you personally
- Roles society has assigned to each of the genders and how these roles affect you as a bodywork profession
- Myths about male and female practitioners and whether these apply to you
- Challenges each of the genders faces in the bodywork profession
- How you will meet the challenges as a male or female bodywork practitioner
- The challenges between the genders in the bodywork profession
- How you meet challenges between the genders as a bodywork practitioner

---

References

1. Harvard Business School: *Power, Influence and Persuasion: Sell Your Ideas and Make Things Happen.* Boston, Harvard Business Publishing, 2005, p xi.
2. Tubbs, S.L., and Moss, S.: *Human Communication: Principles and Contexts,* ed. 10. Columbus, OH, McGraw-Hill, 2006, p 298.
3. Ibid.
4. Harvard Business School, *Power, Influence and Persuasion,* p 16.
5. Greene, E., and Goodrich-Dunn, B.: *The Psychology of the Body.* Baltimore, MD, Lippincott Williams &Wilkins, 2004, p 17.
6. Zastrow, C.: *Introduction to Social Work and Social Welfare.* Stamford, CT, Brooks/Cole Cengage Learning, 2004, p 59.
7. Fisher, K.: *Leading Self-Directed Work Teams.* New York, McGraw-Hill, 1999, p 14.
8. Ibid., p 16.
9. Tannen, D.: *You Just Don't Understand: Women and Men in Conversation.* New York, HarperCollins, 2001, p 26.
10. Wood, J.T.: *Gendered Lives: Communication, Gender, and Culture,* ed. 8. Boston, Wadsworth Cengage Learning, 2009, p 125.

Ethical and Legal Parameters of Practice

LEARNING OBJECTIVES

After studying this chapter, you will be able to:

1. Explain what a scope of practice is.

2. Explain the ethical and legal parameters involved in scope of practice.

3. Explain how scope of practice affects client retention and how to know when to refer clients.

4. Define "confidentiality," and explain its role in documenting treatments.

5. Explain what HIPAA is and how it affects the bodywork profession.

6. Delineate the different types of licenses that bodywork practitioners need.

7. Explain the importance of ethical accounting and tax payment and why insurance is necessary.

8. Define and describe the components of informed consent.

CHAPTER OUTLINE

KEY TERMS

Business privilege license: required by municipalities for individuals or businesses that sell products

Certification: a process in which a person has completed a formalized program of study, and has passed one or more tests demonstrating competency in the area of study

Competency: the ability to perform a specific task, action, or function successfully

Consensus: general agreement, or the judgment arrived at by most of those concerned

Diagnosis: to assign a name or label (such as disease, disorder, or condition) to a certain group of signs or symptoms. Diagnosing falls only within the scope of practice of medical physicians.

HIPAA: The Health Insurance Portability and Accountability Act; a law enacted in 1996 to protect the privacy of people's health-care records

Informed consent: the process by which clients have been fully informed about what to expect during the bodywork treatment

Occupational license: a license needed by people who provide services, such as attorneys, chiropractors, and bodywork practitioners

---

Dylan is a successful self-employed practitioner and massage therapy instructor. He specializes in rehabilitative care and injury management of soft tissue and sees about 15 clients a week. In addition, he teaches 10 hours a week at the local massage school. Because of his busy schedule, Dylan has little time for keeping up with the paperwork involved in running his business. To help keep his paper work to a minimum, he does not accept third-party insurance payments. Instead, Dylan's clients pay him directly after each treatment and then they submit receipts to their insurance companies for reimbursement.

Dylan began working with Mae 2 months ago after she suffered severe whiplash in a car accident. One day Mae leaves an angry message on Dylan's cell phone. She says that, thanks to him, her insurance company will not reimburse her for payments that she has made to Dylan for the massages she received from him. She wants all of her documents from him tomorrow or she will report him to the Better Business Bureau; she has already filed a complaint with the state licensing board. When Dylan calls her back to find out what is going on, Mae says the insurance company denied her request for reimbursement because Dylan does not have a current massage therapy license.

Dylan is stunned. He had no idea this could happen. He had received a notice to renew his license several months ago and has been meaning to do so. It is now 2 weeks past the deadline but Dylan assumed that because he had been licensed for several years without interruption, he would be given a grace period in which to renew his license. Dylan also realizes that he has another problem. Mae's treatment documentation is not up to date. In fact, of the eight treatments he has given Mae, only the first one is completely charted. Dylan also kept meaning to update his files but he has not yet found the time to do so.

At first glance, the ethical and legal parameters of a bodywork practice may seem fairly straightforward. As a bodywork student, you learn information and techniques you will be using as a professional practitioner; therefore, logically, it would seem that these determine the limits within which you will work. Also, many regions of the country have licensure requirements that delineate what education bodywork practitioners must have, what practitioners are legally able to do in their practice, and the consequences for not staying within the law.

In real life, and in real practice, however, events do not always unfold in such a straightforward manner, as is shown by what Dylan experiences. During your bodywork program, you may learn methods of stretching that you can show your clients to assist them in developing or maintaining flexibility. However, if you set up your practice in a region in which the law says that educating clients about stretching can be done only by physical therapists, you may be in violation of the law. Furthermore, ignorance of the law is considered inexcusable by legal authorities; if you proceed without researching the law ahead of time, you will still be held accountable.

Aside from the legal considerations, practitioners must consider the ethics of the issue, as well. Using the example of educating clients about stretching, if you believe that showing clients how to perform their own stretches will help them increase their health and wellness, you have an ethical dilemma. Should you still show the stretches to clients even though it is against the law? Should you not show the stretches to clients, thereby risking clients losing out on a beneficial complement to bodywork? Should you refer the clients to physical therapists to learn the stretches? What if you do not know any physical therapists to which to refer clients? The clients will then have to take the time and effort to find one to work with. What if the clients cannot afford both physical therapy and bodywork? Then you are risking a potential loss of income if they choose physical therapy over your treatments.

Practicing bodywork, then, means more than being able to perform techniques skillfully and to communicate with clients effectively. This chapter covers the definition of "scope of practice"; the legal and ethical responsibilities that practitioners have to stay within their scopes of practice; and the roles of education, competency, and self-accountability in staying within scope of practice. The impact of scope of practice on client retention, and how practitioners will know when to refer clients are also discussed.

Confidentiality of client information is absolutely essential in the bodywork profession. How and why confidentiality should be kept is discussed, along with ethical documentation procedures. Also included is an overview of the Health Insurance Portability and Accountability Act (HIPAA) and why bodywork practitioners need to understand it and follow its guidelines.

Other legal parameters of practice covered in this chapter include why practitioners need to understand the different types of licenses required to practice legally, what the difference between licensing and certification is, and the importance of ethical accounting and tax payment procedures as well as the importance of carrying insurance.

Informed consent, touched on briefly in previous chapters, is one of the foundations of the therapeutic relationship. It is absolutely necessary for providing safe and effective treatments. Therefore, a discussion of the factors involved in informed consent, including appropriate disclosure on the part of clients and practitioners, rounds out the chapter.

What Is Scope of Practice?

Recall from Chapter 5 that scope of practice is a set of guidelines that clarifies exactly what professionals can and cannot do based on laws, completion of a course of education or training, and competency of skill and techniques. To define it further, it is a term used by state and/or local licensing boards for various professions that defines the procedures, actions, and processes that are permitted for the licensed individual. Correspondingly, laws, licensing bodies, and regulations describe specific requirements for education, training, and competency.

In this way, the professions are able to establish their own standards, direct their own practices, determine who is qualified to practice, and determine what services can be provided to whom, where, and under what conditions. Scope of practice may also list specific methods (e.g., facials or ultrasound treatments) that practitioners may not offer because a separate license is required. Each profession has legal limits to what the members of the profession can do, say, or perform. This is so the members of professions do not encroach on the scope of practice of other professionals.

Ideally, scopes of practice are established by **consensus** of the members of each profession along with legislators, such as city or state councils. "Consensus" means general agreement, or the judgment arrived at by most of those concerned. As many representatives from the profession as possible should take part in the process. Because bodywork encompasses many different modalities, it is important to hear from many practitioners of different bodywork modalities, such as craniosacral therapists, Rolfers, shiatsu practitioners, reflexologists, and so forth. Defining what practitioners can and cannot do as professionals should not be determined by a select few people. The process should include discussion and active participation by many members of the profession to reach an outcome that satisfies the majority of the people involved.

Having a standard level of competency in performing the techniques of the profession is an important hallmark of the scope of practice. When members of the profession come together to pool their ideas, resources, and measurements of competency, it allows realistic and practical expectations for the members of the profession to accomplish.

As discussed in Chapter 5, often the term "scope of practice" is used interchangeably with the term "standards of practice"; however, it is important to differentiate between the two terms, even though they seem to be similar. Recall from Chapter 5 that standards of practice are specific rules and procedures for professional conduct and quality of care that are to be followed by all members of a profession. Standards of practice describe appropriate and expected conduct of the members of a profession and reflect the most commonly held values of the profession. They describe the professional conduct expected of members to preserve and enhance their professional reputation as well as the general reputation of the bodywork profession. Furthermore, standards of practice seek to protect the general public. They are tools to assist practitioners in making ethical decisions while practicing bodywork so that they stay within their scope of practice.

Although standards of practice are foundational for the development and delivery of the profession's educational programs, membership organizations, and testing for certification credentials, scope of practice is foundational for the regional legal determination of who has the right to practice and who does not. Another way to think of these two concepts is that standards of practice apply to the profession as a whole, whereas scopes of practice are defined by laws that apply to each individual municipality, whether it be a town, city, county, or state.

Laws defining scope of practice affect all practitioners in the region, and punishment for infractions may range from civil penalties such as fines or loss of credentials to criminal penalties. Legal factors have to be changed collectively by many individuals through an often lengthy process. Thus, it is important that people who actually participate in the profession take responsibility for identifying specific issues that need to be addressed in laws governing bodywork. The more that members of the profession become involved in this process, the more useful and practical the outcome will be. In other words, it helps to have people who actually do the work be the ones to decide what limits and boundaries should be set and why. Taking responsibility and ownership of this process gives the members of the profession more authority to establish the standards necessary for the profession to thrive as well as have a hand in directing where the profession will go in the future.

Examples of Scope of Practice

The intention of scope of practice is to give practitioners, clients, potential clients, insurance companies, and mass media clarity about the actual work done in the profession. It is designed to protect both practitioners and clients, and to prevent as much misunderstanding as possible about the profession. For example, if the practitioner is not able to work on a client because a condition the client is presenting with is considered out of the practitioner's scope of practice, then the practitioner is ethically bound to refer the client to an appropriate resource. By doing so, the client is protected from potentially being harmed by an unskilled practitioner, and the practitioner is protected from acting unethically by performing a treatment that may harm the client.

In her book *Massage Therapy Principles and Practice,* Susan Salvo defines "scope of practice" as the profession's working parameters. These parameters are a result of identifying the legal definition of massage and articulating what professional boundaries and limitations the bodywork practitioner must follow with clients. Salvo states, "As massage therapists we have a license to touch. Scope of practice defines what services that massage therapists can and cannot provide. Being aware of our limits of competency and being clear of our scope of practice ensures us the objectivity to refer a client elsewhere when the need arises."[1]

Competency is defined objectively by passing required examinations such as a state licensing examination or a national certification examination. There is also a subjective component in which only practitioners can determine for themselves their levels of competency. If you are a practitioner who is learning new techniques, it is important that you practice them to gain competency. However you must not represent yourself as competent until you have demonstrated that you have reached a personal level of knowledge and skills to the point that you are ready to share them as a professional.

Exhibiting yourself as being competent requires ethical self-assessment. You need to be honest about your qualifications and level of proficiency. You have to take personal responsibility to make sure you are accurately representing yourself to your clients. If you are unsure whether you are ready to offer new skills and techniques to paying clients, you may find it worthwhile to seek support from a trusted advanced practitioner. He or she can assist you in this process by receiving a treatment from you and giving you feedback and suggestions.

Because scope of practice is involved in legalities, where, when, and how professionals can practice can be quite complicated, and can vary greatly throughout geographic regions of the country. Currently, because the United States has not standardized the scope of practice for bodywork, the scope of practice varies from state to state or even city to city. It is your responsibility to be aware of what is required for you to practice in your locality.

As an example, the following are summaries of scope of practice for massage therapy in three regions of the United States. Note, however, that state laws can change over time; consult each state's Web site, as provided, for up-to-date information.

Licensed Massage Therapist, State of Arizona

Note: This section is reprinted with permission from the Arizona State Board of Massage Therapy's Web site: http://www/ massagetherapy.az.gov/rules.asp

A massage therapist means a person who is licensed to perform massage therapy, which means the manual application of compression, stretch, vibration, or mobilization using the forearms, elbows, knees, or feet or handheld mechanical or electrical devices of the organs and tissues beneath the dermis, including the components of the musculoskeletal system, peripheral vessels of the circulatory system, and fascia, when applied primarily to parts of the body other than the hands, feet, and head. It also includes any combination of range of motion, directed, assisted, or passive movements of the joints, and hydrotherapy, including the therapeutic applications of water, heat, cold, wraps, essential oils, skin brushing, salt glows, and similar applications of products to the skin. These techniques are undertaken to increase wellness, relaxation, stress reduction, pain relief, and postural improvement or provide general or specific therapeutic benefits. The practice of massage therapy does not include the diagnosis of illness or disease, medical procedures, naturopathic manipulative medicine, osteopathic manipulative medicine, chiropractic adjustive procedures, homeopathic neuromuscular integration, electrical stimulation, ultrasound, prescription of medicines, or the use of modalities for which a license to practice medicine, chiropractic, nursing, occupational therapy, athletic training, physical therapy, acupuncture, or podiatry is required by law.

Applicants need to have successfully completed a course of study of massage therapy or bodywork therapy consisting of a minimum of five hundred classroom hours of supervised instruction at a board recognized school in this state that is accredited by an agency recognized by the secretary of the United States Department of Education, or successfully completed a course of study of massage therapy or bodywork therapy consisting of a minimum of five hundred classroom hours of supervised instruction at a school in this state that is licensed by the state board of private postsecondary education or at a school outside of this state that is recognized by the board, and successfully passed an examination administered by a national board accredited by the certifying agency that has been approved by the national commission on competency assurance and that is in good standing with that agency or have successfully passed an examination that is administered or approved by the board.[2]

Licensed Massage Therapist, State of New York

Note: This section is reprinted with permission from the Office of the Professions of the New York State Education Department's Web site: http://www.op.nysed.gov/mtlic.htm

The practice of the profession of massage therapy is defined as engaging in applying a scientific system of activity to the muscular structure of the human body by means of stroking, kneading, tapping and vibrating with the hands or vibrators for the purpose of improving muscle tone and circulation. Any use of the title "massage therapist" or "masseuse," "masseur," or any derivation of the title, within New York State, requires licensure as a massage therapist.

Educational requirements include completing high school or its equivalent and graduating from a school or institute of massage therapy with a program registered by the New York State Education Department as licensure qualifying, or its substantial equivalent in both subject matter or extent of training, provided that the program in such school or institute consists of classroom instruction with a total of not less than 1000 hours in specific subjects satisfactory to the Department. Complete coursework needs to include anatomy, physiology, neurology, myology or kinesiology, pathology, hygiene, first aid, CPR, infection control procedures, the chemical ingredients of products that are used and their effects, as well as the theory, technique and practice of both oriental and western massage/bodywork therapy. Within the 1000 hours of education, students need to have had to complete a minimum of 150 hours of practice on a person. Also required is passing the New York State Massage Therapy Examination, which is given twice a year, once in January and once in August.[3]

Licensed Massage Therapist, State of Missouri

Note: This section is reprinted with permission from the Missouri Secretary of State's Web site: http://www.sos.mo.gov/adrules/csr/ current/20csr/20c2197-2.pdf

Requirements include completing massage therapy studies consisting of at least 500 clock hours of supervised instruction in a Coordinating Board of

Higher Education (CBHE) certified school, Missouri Department of Elementary and Secondary Education (DESE) approved vocational program or school, or school, college, university, or other institution of higher learning in the United States accredited by a regional accrediting commission recognized by the United States Department of Education or an equivalent approving body for out-of-state applicants.

The massage therapy studies need to include at least 300 clock hours dedicated to massage theory and practice techniques, 100 clock hours dedicated to the study of anatomy and physiology, 50 clock hours dedicated to business practice, professional ethics, hygiene and massage law in the state of Missouri, 50 clock hours dedicated to ancillary therapies that can include but not be limited to cardiopulmonary resuscitation (CPR) and first aid. Additionally, passing a national certification exam such as the National Certification Examination for Therapeutic Massage and Bodywork (NCETMB), or passing the Massage and Bodywork Licensing Examination (MBLEx) is required.[4]

Researching Scope of Practice

Part of the responsibility of being a professional practitioner is knowing exactly what your legal scope of practice is. Because the administrators and instructors in most educational programs are well aware of the laws that govern their profession and their schools, and most are diligent about giving this information to their students, you should have a fairly good idea of your scope of practice by the time you graduate from your educational program.

However, there can still be some confusion when graduates apply for licensure, especially if they are choosing to practice in a region other than where their bodywork program is located. If professional practitioners decide to move from one region to another, the laws governing their practice in their new location may be quite different from those in their old location.

There are several resources you can use to research what your scope of practice is in the area in which you practice or plan to practice. You may contact the licensing agencies directly. To find state licensing agencies, you may need to consult telephone directories or conduct an online search. To find state legislative information online, type in www., the two-letter state abbreviation, then .gov. For example, to find state legislative information for Oregon, type in www.or.gov; for North Dakota, type in www.nd.gov; and for Mississippi, type in www.ms.gov. Once at the state Web site, type in a keyword such as "massage therapy" or "Healing Touch" in the search box. Local licensing agencies may or may not have the information online, and so your only option may be to use telephone directories to find the appropriate contact information.

You may also contact bodywork program administrators and instructors. Practitioners new to an area may want to consider contacting local schools for information. Yet another resource is membership organizations. For example, Associated Bodywork and Massage Professionals (ABMP; http://www.abmp.com) and the American Massage Therapy Association (AMTA; http://www.amtamassage.org) provide legislation information relevant to the bodywork profession. The AMTA also has state chapters with boards of directors who may be contacted for information.

If you are planning to move to another location to practice your profession, it is important that you do some homework to be sure you know what you will need to do to begin working as soon as possible. Figure 7.1 is a worksheet designed to make the process easier for you.

Staying Within Scope of Practice

When a new profession is established, there must be a starting point at which the scope of practice is defined by the individuals in the profession

---

• Where do you want to work?_____

• Who regulates the professional bodywork you are going to do in this area?

_____ State _____ City _____ County _____ There is no regulation (if there is no regulation then you do not need to fill out the rest of this form)

• Contact information for the regulating body:

Telephone: _____ Website: _____

Mailing address: _____

• What are the regulations for the professional bodywork you are going to do in this area?

_____ State license _____ Certification _____ None

• How many educational hours are needed to qualify to work in this area?_____

• Is there a licensing or certification exam required? _____No _____Yes

• If a licensing or certification exam is required, what type is it? Check all that apply and list the organization's contact information to find out how to register for the exam.

_____ State   Contact information:_____

_____ NCBTMB   Contact information:_____

_____ MBLEx   Contact information:_____

_____ NCCAOM   Contact information:_____

• How much will it cost to become licensed/certified?_____

• How long does the license/certification last?_____

• What are the requirements to renew the license/certification? _____

_____

• How many hours of continuing education are required to renew the license/certification? _____

• Are there any additional requirements? Check all that apply.

_____ None

_____ First Aid certification

_____ CPR certification

_____ Background check:

_____Fee of $_____ paid by applicant

_____Fee paid by regulating body

_____ Local requirements apply

_____ Accredited school only

_____ Physical exam

_____ Health certificate

_____ TB test

_____ Proof of no contagious disease

_____ Jurisprudence exam (some areas use this to cover the legal parameters of the profession in their area)

_____ Other: _____

_____

_____

Figure 7.1 Relocation worksheet.

who are familiar with the work because they are the ones performing the work. These individuals know the issues affecting the profession as well as what circumstances need to be monitored or not allowed. In the bodywork profession, this hands-on knowledge and experience gave early practitioners the capability of articulating what behaviors represent the profession with honesty, integrity, and fair treatment of both the client and the practitioner.

Eventually, all the ideas surrounding these behaviors were pared down to a concise record that identified the limits and boundaries of bodywork practices. The key word is "practices," as it highlights specific actions and behaviors. These behaviors and actions then must be monitored so that practitioners are held accountable for following the established parameters of the scope of practice.

One factor that will determine your scope of practice is the education you receive. Your education provides you with an understanding of the human body and how it responds to bodywork. You must also be able to know when a bodywork treatment is contraindicated. Knowing when not to treat a client is just as important as knowing the latest techniques. You must always represent yourself within the level of expertise based on your body of knowledge and ability.

Your scope of practice will change each time you increase your training as a professional. You can embrace this dynamic aspect of the profession by regularly conducting a self-inquiry to assess whether you are happy with your approach to your career. If you want to make changes, you can look for classes that interest you and are taught by qualified teachers, then budget to pay for continuing education classes.

As previously discussed, local and state laws also determine your scope of practice. These legal guidelines are in place to regulate the profession to ensure that practitioners are providing safe treatments, and are proficient and qualified to provide the service.

Legal Responsibility to Stay Within Scope of Practice

Practitioners have, of course, a legal responsibility to stay within their scope of practice. There are three ways that state, county, and local governments regulate the scope of massage therapy practice: licensure, certification, and registration.

Licensure is the process of receiving a license from a governing body that allows you to conduct a professional bodywork practice. Licensure will require you to have completed a specific level of educational training or attained a certain level of experience in addition to the successful completion of some type of practical evaluation and a written examination. Licensure also gives title protection, meaning that only those who have met the criteria for the license can give themselves a specific title. For example, if you are licensed as a massage therapist you can legally call yourself a massaged therapist. Others in your community who do not have a license to practice massage therapy but call themselves massage therapists can be prosecuted under the law.

Certification is another process to demonstrate your credentials in the profession. This is typically voluntary, as it is offered by a nongovernmental agency or organization as a means to identify practitioners with advanced knowledge and skills. It involves an evaluation process, such as an examination, to determine the proficiency of the candidate. One example is the certification given by the National Board for Therapeutic Massage and Bodywork. Passing the National Certification Exam for Therapeutic Massage (NCETM) earns the credential Nationally Certified in Therapeutic Massage (NCTM); passing the National Certification Exam for Therapeutic Massage and Bodywork (NCETMB) earns the credential Nationally Certified in Therapeutic Massage and Bodywork (NCTMB). These credentials can then be used only by the practitioners who have passed these examinations.

Registration is yet another process that is employed by a professional organization to keep track of practitioners in a database. Some states may require that professional bodywork practitioners have a certificate of registration in that state to practice legally. This system is designed to give the governing body a method to keep track of its registered practitioners.[5]

All of these legal regulations are in the best interest of the client. Consumer protection is an important feature of certification or licensure; consumers are given an avenue by which the bodywork profession can investigate and follow up on any grievances and enforce disciplinary action if necessary. Disciplinary action can result in the practitioner defending his or her actions before a board of practitioners. The end result may be a reprimand, suspension, criminal penalty, or revocation of the license if the offense warrants it.

Ideally, scopes of practice are written clearly within the law so that there can be no misunderstanding, but this is not always the case. For example, the state of Arizona massage therapy law states, "A massage therapist means a person who is licensed to perform massage therapy, which means the manual application of compression, stretch, vibration or mobilization using the forearms, elbows, knees or feet or handheld mechanical or electrical devices of the organs and tissues beneath the dermis, including the components of the musculoskeletal system, peripheral vessels of the circulatory system and fascia, when applied primarily to parts of the body other than the hands, feet and head."

The law also states, "Persons and activities not required to be licensed include:

- When the customer is fully clothed, the practice of movement educators, such as dance therapists or teachers, yoga teachers, personal trainers, martial arts instructors and movement repatterning practitioners.
- When the customer is fully clothed, the practice of techniques that are specifically intended to affect the human energy field."

Although it may seem that shiatsu practitioners are exempt from being licensed as massage therapists because their clients (called "customers" by law) are fully clothed and their "techniques are specifically intended to affect the human energy field," the techniques also include manual application of compression, stretch, vibration, or mobilization using the forearms, elbows, knees, or feet of the organs and tissues beneath the dermis, including the components of the musculoskeletal system, peripheral vessels of the circulatory system, and fascia. Shiatsu practitioners are also not specifically mentioned as being exempt anywhere in the law.

Food for Thought
What would you do if you were a shiatsu practitioner in Arizona? Why would you choose to do this?

This has led to considerable confusion, with some shiatsu practitioners being told by members of the licensing board that they do, indeed, need to be licensed as massage therapists in order to practice, some being told that they do not, and some being told that although the law is unclear, if they are caught practicing without the massage therapy license they could be penalized.

Unfortunately, scenarios such as this one in Arizona are not unique. Practitioners everywhere struggle with laws that are written unclearly or perhaps even unfairly. The only solution seems to be for practitioners to come together and demand changes to the law, a time-consuming and costly process.

Consider the following: Wes, a massage therapist, has a client named Ella who has come to him off and on for the past year to treat her low back pain. During a recent massage session interview, Ella discloses that she has been diagnosed by her doctor as having a herniated disc between L1 and L2, and that she was given a referral to see a physical therapist for six visits. Her insurance will cover the 60% of the physical therapy appointment. Ella does not want to go to physical therapy because she prefers massage therapy. She tells Wes that she went to the physical therapist one time and all he did was hook her up to some machines. She plans to ignore the referral and continue to see Wes because she likes his work. She does not want to spend a lot of money on a physical therapist who will barely touch her.

Wes, however, is greatly concerned about Ella's diagnosis; this is the first he has heard about it. He explains that treating a herniated disc is out of his scope of practice. Although there are some techniques that might be helpful to relax the muscles around the area of the herniated disc, he needs a release form from Ella's doctor stating that it is safe for Wes to give her treatments. He asks her to sign a release of information form that will allow him to consult with her primary care physician, the orthopedic doctor, and the physical therapist. Having access to all of Ella's information will help Wes make the right decisions about her care. Wes says he believes that physical therapy is the best option for Ella right now and massage may be able to complement those sessions but he needs clearance from her health-care providers first.

What do you suppose could have happened if Wes agreed to work with Ella without her the doctor's permission? What if Wes made this choice and injured Ella's back? What do you think the legal and ethical consequences could be?

Diagnosis Versus Assessment

Bodywork practitioners learn information about medical conditions for two main reasons. First, practitioners must know what a condition is when a client presents with it. The purpose of learning about diseases and conditions is not so that practitioners can tell clients they potentially have a disease when they describe certain symptoms that may be characteristic of particular diseases or disorders. Instead if a client has, for example, rheumatoid arthritis, practitioners need to know enough about the disease to make safe technique decisions while performing bodywork.

Second, practitioners must be clear about what to do when a client presents with signs and symptoms that indicate a medical condition beyond the scope of what practitioners can safely work with or are qualified to treat.

In Western medicine, a **diagnosis** is the assignment of a name or label (such as disease, disorder, or condition) to a certain group of signs or symptoms. Diagnosing falls only within the scope of practice of medical physicians. The process involves performing some type of assessment (evaluation), sometimes referred to as medical tests, and based on the findings, assigning a name or a label to a person's problem. When assigning a name or label to something the person is experiencing and stating to the person what disease, disorder, or condition he or she has, then that is considered diagnosing.

In his book *Orthopedic Massage, Theory and Technique*, Whitney Lowe, director of the Orthopedic Massage Education & Research Institute, defines assessment as an evaluation process that allows a practitioner to explore a client's condition. Lowe asserts that a medical diagnosis is a statement that identifies a disease, illness, or a condition made by a licensed medical professional. Bodywork practitioners should never tell clients they have a specific condition.[6]

The assessment skills that bodywork practitioners learn are methods for gathering information to make informed decisions about if and how treatments should proceed. Because assessment is really information gathering, practitioners cannot apply any kind of treatment without performing some level of assessment. The assessment can be visual, such as noticing that one of the client's shoulders is higher than the other or seeing how far to the left the client can comfortably turn the head, or palpatory, such as feeling where muscle tissue is tight or feeling restriction in movement of a joint when performing a passive range-of-motion technique on the client.

The purpose is to gather information about the client to determine if and how the bodywork treatment should proceed. It also gives the practitioner and the client an opportunity to collaborate in developing a treatment plan while establishing trust and rapport. However, should the practitioner use the information gained through assessment to tell the client that he or she has a particular condition, then the practitioner is diagnosing. Practitioners should be mindful of making sure that any information from assessments they give clients, document in client files, or discuss with other practitioners, is based on observed facts, not diagnoses. Whatever the outcome of the assessment, it is essential that the practitioner communicate the information in a descriptive manner rather than make an absolute statement naming the condition, which would be diagnosing.

For example, if the practitioner assesses that the client has a lateral curve of the spine, with tight, shortened erector spinae on one side of the spine, and tight, elongated erector spinae on the other side, the practitioner can state this factual information to the client and still be within bodywork scope of practice. If, however, the practitioner says to the client, "You have scoliosis," then the practitioner is diagnosing. What follows are some more examples of assessments versus diagnoses.

Assessment: Based on what you've told me and my palpation findings, you have tender points along your low back, your upper shoulders, and the base of your neck and on your knees.

Diagnosis: You have fibromyalgia. I know because you have all the classic tender points of fibromyalgia.

Assessment: During the interview you said you've been feeling some tingling sensations down your arm and into your fingertips.

You also mentioned that you sit at a computer for hours at a time, 5 days a week. When I massaged your anterior neck muscles they felt very tight. I also noticed that your shoulders are rounded, giving you a bit of a "caved in" posture. Both of these conditions can interfere with the nerves that runs down your arm and into your fingers.

Diagnosis: Whenever there is a tingling or numbness in the fingers like you have it's carpal tunnel syndrome. Lots of people who work at computers get that.

Ethical Responsibility to Stay Within Scope of Practice

Even though every health and service profession has techniques and understandings that may be unique, many professions may actually share common knowledge and methodology. Because of this shared information, the parameters defining a profession's scope of practice are not always clear, and overlap can occur.

It is important that practitioners be consistent with what they state legally as the parameters of their scope of practice as well as how they conduct themselves on a daily basis. Staying within the scope of practice, regardless of what a client may request or what a practitioner may think she can "get away with because no one else is watching," is the sign of an ethical practitioner. This practitioner knows that it does not matter if anyone else knows what she did; she herself will know. Therefore, she practices accordingly to maintain her integrity as well as the integrity of the profession.

Consider the following: Patrick is teaching a workshop on the first day of a 5-day national massage therapy convention. The workshop is about specific techniques for treating pain caused by tight low back and gluteal muscles. There are 50 participants in the workshop, one of whom Patrick invites to be the demonstration body while he is teaching the techniques. Because of time limitations Patrick does not conduct a pretreatment interview with the volunteer. He also starts demonstrating the techniques without spending much time warming up the client's tissues. Forty-five minutes later, the volunteer is experiencing severe pain in the area where Patrick has worked. The pain is so severe that the volunteer has to leave the convention, losing $500 in registration fees.

Did Patrick behave ethically toward the workshop volunteer? What would you have done differently if you were Patrick? What would you have done differently if you were the volunteer?

As a professional bodywork practitioner you must be willing and able to evaluate your acquired body of knowledge and skills realistically to determine the parameters of ethical practice within your scope of practice. Ethical professionals understand the limits of their technical skills and scopes of practice. To assist you in determining how to be ethically responsible and stay within your scope of practice, there are three main factors you should keep in mind: your education, competency, and self-accountability.

Education

Laws, licensing bodies, and regulations describe specific requirements for education, training, and competency for scope of practice for many professions.

Often, there is common information and training used in the profession's education process to meet these requirements. This is certainly true of medical, nursing, chiropractic, physical therapy, and acupuncture schools. Their basic training programs are fairly consistent across the country in terms of what they teach the students.

Bodywork training programs, however, are quite diverse. The result, at this time, is reflected in the disparity among local laws governing bodywork. There is no national standard that says how much and what type of training are adequate. Practitioners need to realize that while laws serve as guides for accepted knowledge and practice, bodywork practitioners regulated by the same laws may have significant differences in what and how they can practice based on their education and unique knowledge base.

Therefore, as an ethical practitioner you must be mindful about the extent of your training, regardless of what you are lawfully permitted to do. For example, if the licensing law allows you to provide your clients with information on basic nutrition, such as the recommended daily intake of water and what percentage of the diet should be carbohydrates, proteins, and fats, but you have no educational background in nutrition, then you would be out of your scope of practice if you offered this type of information to clients.

These issues apply not only to entry-level bodywork education but to continuing education as well. Continuing education is designed for you to gain and improve your hands-on skills and knowledge. By doing so, you are meeting one aspect of professionalism—the commitment to gain more training and expertise so that you can be of better service to your clients. Continuing education is so important that many laws have a continuing education requirement for license renewal.

Some of these laws are specific about how many continuing education hours are required, the maximum number of hours that can be taken through online courses, and the types of courses that qualify for license renewal. Coupled with the fact that continuing education courses are just as or more diverse than basic bodywork programs, and you may have difficulty choosing the courses that are right for you.

To assist you, the following include some of the factors you should keep in mind when choosing continuing education courses:

- How many hours of continuing education are required by the laws governing your practice? How many can be completed online, and how many need to be acquired through physically attending seminars?
- Do the laws governing your practice have stipulations about courses? For example, a massage therapy law may state that only courses in which hands-on techniques are taught qualify, and that the course involves techniques performed on humans. This means that a course in energy work, such as Reiki or Healing Touch, or a course on animal massage would not count toward license renewal.
- What types of courses are you interested in taking?
- Who is the course instructor? What credentials and experience does the presenter have? Will you be getting good value for your money?
- Has the course been approved by an agency recognized by the bodywork regulatory bodies in your location? For example, some laws

require that continuing education courses be taken through schools accredited by their state education departments or presenters, either individuals or organizations, which are NCBTMB-approved providers.

- What is your continuing education budget? If there are courses you would like to take but do not have the money for, setting up a budget so that you can save for the courses is an option.
- Where are the courses located?
- How much do the courses cost?
- What are the other costs associated with taking the courses? Will there be travel, hotel, and food costs to budget for?
- When must the courses be completed? It is better to plan ahead so that you are not in the position of having to take, for example, 20 continuing education hours in a 2-week period.
- Are you able to take the time off to take the courses? If you are an employee, you will most likely have to request time off from your supervisor. If you are in private practice, you will need to schedule time off to take the courses, and you will need to keep in mind that you will lose income while attending the courses.

Online courses and reading articles in bodywork journals and then answering questions online for credit are also becoming more and more popular. They can be less costly than attending a live seminar, and can be completed at your convenience. When choosing these methods of earning continuing education credit, you should also evaluate the course or article to make sure that it is given by a credible source, that what you learn will be useful to you, and that you are getting good value for your money. You should also keep in mind that many licensing, credentialing, and professional organizations place a limit on the number of continuing education hours you can earn through these methods.

Competency

In most regions, the laws governing bodywork state that competency is presumed once the required number of hours of entry-level formal education have been completed. Practitioners may also be required to pass a written examination and possibly a practical examination to become licensed.

For you to provide service to clients ethically, **competency,** the ability to perform a specific task, action, or function successfully, is of critical importance, perhaps more so than education. Even after meeting all legal and educational requirements, ethical practitioners self-evaluate their training, experience, and confidence level before offering professional treatments to clients. It is the responsibility of bodywork students to practice the skills they learn in class until they are competent in them before performing them as professionals on clients.

According to Gerald Corey, Marianne Schneider Corey, and Patrick Callanan in their book *Issues and Ethics in the Helping Professions,* competency is gained by receiving training and developing skills to treat clients effectively in a specific area of practice. It is the practitioner's responsibility to make sure that he is getting the most out of his training program as well as seeking support if he finds that he is lacking a particular skill. Peer supervision groups can assist him in discerning if he is lacking in competency or if he is simply unaware that a particular skill needs more development.[7]

Some practitioners who have worked in the profession for a length of time have taken at least one continuing education course and then failed to practice the skills they learned until they were competent, resulting in a loss of those skills. Similarly, practitioners might be competent in certain skills at one point in their careers and then, after a period in which they did not perform those skills, they lost that competency. Serving clients with rusty skills or using techniques that the practitioner has not been trained in is ethically problematic.

You also need to be mindful of the credentials with which you are presenting yourself. Ethical practitioners are those who study new modalities in depth before offering them to their clients. For example, taking a 14-hour shiatsu workshop does not qualify someone to be a shiatsu practitioner, nor does watching a 2-hour video on reflexology make someone a qualified reflexologist. Practitioners need to have significant mastery of a particular modality, not just a passing familiarity.

Certificates of completion for continuing education courses are sometimes confused with **certification.** As discussed in the section "Legal Responsibility to Stay Within Scope of Practice," certification means that a person has completed a formalized program of study, and has passed one or more tests demonstrating competency in the area of study. The tests can be written, verbal, or practical, or any of a combination of the three. Certificates of completion, sometimes called certificates of achievement, mean that a person has attended and participated in a course, but that there were no tests of competency. Practitioners also cannot ethically and, in many areas, legally present themselves as being certified in a modality unless they have gone through the certification process. Figure 7.2 presents an example of certificate of certification, and Figure 7.3 presents an example of a certificate of completion.

Self-Accountability

Don't bother just to be better than your contemporaries or predecessors. Try to be better than yourself.

—William Faulkner

Self-accountability is the most decisive factor that keeps practitioners functioning within their scopes of practice. Practitioners are answerable and responsible for what they say and do, even when there is no external authority present. Governing laws, education, training, and competency all influence practitioners' ability to stay within their scope of practice, but only by obeying the laws, carrying out what they have learned and been trained to do, and performing their work competently, even if no one is providing oversight, all define what it means to be ethical practitioners.

Self-accountability is the cornerstone of and sustains personal and professional ethics. It keeps you functioning within the parameters of your scope of practice. In short, self-accountability enforces scope of practice. Examples of behaviors that demonstrate accountability include the following:

- Keep all your licenses, credentials, and certifications current.
- Maintain liability insurance (discussed in the section "Other Legal Parameters of Practice")

Food for Thought

A shiatsu practitioner who works in a spa setting is told by her supervisor to give massages to clients even though the shiatsu practitioner has had no training in massage therapy. What do you think the shiatsu practitioner should do? Why do you think the shiatsu practitioner should do this?

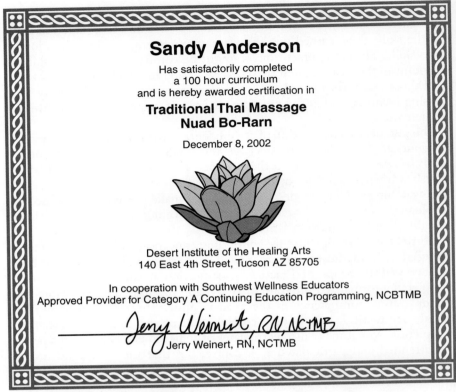

Sandy Anderson

Has satisfactorily completed
a 100 hour curriculum
and is hereby awarded certification in

**Traditional Thai Massage
Nuad Bo-Rarn**

December 8, 2002

Desert Institute of the Healing Arts
140 East 4th Street, Tucson AZ 85705

In cooperation with Southwest Wellness Educators
Approved Provider for Category A Continuing Education Programming, NCBTMB

Jerry Weinert, RN, NCTMB

Figure 7.2 Certificate of certification.

- Take the required number of continuing education credits.
- Maintain CPR certification.
- Recognize when you are suffering from burnout and seek support to renew and rejuvenate yourself so that your clients can continue to benefit from your work.
- Realize that if the needs of a client are beyond your personal scope of practice, it is your responsibility to refer the client to a practitioner who can help him or her.

Figure 7.4 presents a visual representation of the way that education, competency, and self-accountability fit together when you are determining how to be ethically responsible and stay within your scope of practice.

Scope of Practice and Client Retention

There is a direct correlation between staying within scope of practice and client retention rate. The more specific you are about the policies of your practice, and the techniques you perform, the safer clients are likely to feel with you, and the more likely they will be to return for treatment. Trust develops because clients always know what to expect from you.

Transparency in your words and actions is essential. There should be congruency between what you say and what you do. This congruency is evident when you are comfortable, at all times, with others knowing what you are

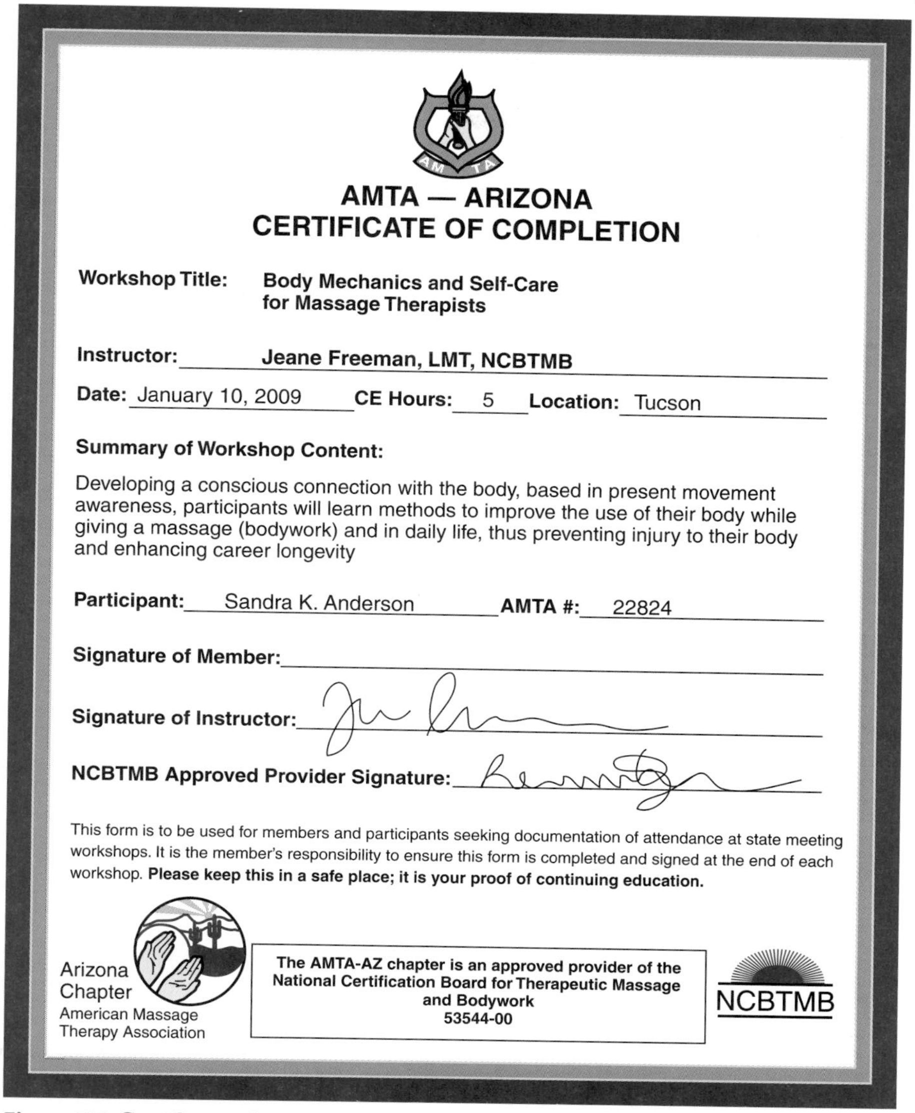

AMTA — ARIZONA
CERTIFICATE OF COMPLETION

Workshop Title: Body Mechanics and Self-Care
for Massage Therapists

Instructor: Jeane Freeman, LMT, NCBTMB

Date: January 10, 2009   **CE Hours:** 5   **Location:** Tucson

Summary of Workshop Content:

Developing a conscious connection with the body, based in present movement awareness, participants will learn methods to improve the use of their body while giving a massage (bodywork) and in daily life, thus preventing injury to their body and enhancing career longevity

Participant: Sandra K. Anderson   **AMTA #:** 22824

Signature of Member:

Signature of Instructor:

NCBTMB Approved Provider Signature:

This form is to be used for members and participants seeking documentation of attendance at state meeting workshops. It is the member's responsibility to ensure this form is completed and signed at the end of each workshop. **Please keep this in a safe place; it is your proof of continuing education.**

Arizona
Chapter
American Massage
Therapy Association

The AMTA-AZ chapter is an approved provider of the
National Certification Board for Therapeutic Massage
and Bodywork
53544-00

NCBTMB

Figure 7.3 Certificate of completion.

doing in your work, and in being willing to share your work. You are not covert about client interactions, business practices, or personal boundaries. When you are aware and deeply understand the importance of being consistent in your words and actions, you are demonstrating self-accountability and ethical behavior.

Knowing When to Refer Clients

"It is essential for professionals to know from the outset the boundaries of their own competence and to refer clients to other professionals when working with them is beyond their professional training or when personal factors

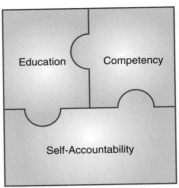

Figure 7.4 Education, competency, and self-accountability fit together in ethical responsibility of staying within scope of practice.

would interfere with a productive working relationship," state Gerald Corey, Marianne Schneider Corey, and Patrick Callanan in *Issues and Ethics in the Helping Professions.*[8] Knowing when you have reached your ability to help your client is a self-accountability trait that is essential for all practitioners to develop. By staying within scope of practice and referring clients when necessary, you are showing clients that you have their best interests in mind.

The length of the professional relationship you will have with the same client is determined by the following factors:

- The quality of the therapeutic relationship.
- Whether there is notable progress in meeting the stated goals of the treatments.
- Client satisfaction with your work and the therapeutic relationship.
- Your satisfaction with the therapeutic relationship.

The first step in knowing when to refer a client to another practitioner or resource is being able to assess the progress in the treatment plan. If progress is not being made, is it because there is an uneasy fit between you and the client? Are there transference or countertransferance issues present that interfere with achieving the goal of the treatment plan? Or is the reverse true— are the treatment goals successfully achieved, and there is nothing more that you can do for the client?

Another good measurement you can use to decide if it is time to refer a client elsewhere is for you to notice how present you are with the client during the treatments. Have the treatments become so routine that you are bored and therefore not paying attention to the details of the client's condition? Has the client developed a pattern of complaining about the work not being satisfactory, yet is unwilling or unable to give you reasons? Would the conditions the client has be better treated by another practitioner or resource? Taking some time to ponder these reflective questions may help you decide the best course of action.

Any one of these, or a combination of these and other factors, is an indicator that it is time for the therapeutic relationship with your client to end. In current culture, the thinking is that "the customer is always right," so it may be difficult for you to convince clients that their needs may be better served by another practitioner. Conversely, it may be difficult for you to recognize when you need to make a referral to another practitioner or resource.

Ethically, you should discuss with the client what the issues are, and why it may be time for the client to consider terminating treatments from you and seeing another practitioner or resource. Listening to what the client has to say demonstrates that you understand that there are two people in the therapeutic relationship and both have a say about what happens.

The conversation can be difficult if the client is unaware that something is amiss in the therapeutic relationship, or if the client does not wish to see someone else because he simply likes your work. Clients, of course, have the right to refuse to accept a referral. You then need to decide for yourself if you can continue working with the client, or if it is time to set a really strong boundary and insist that the client move on.

The art of making referrals is based in the communication skills you use to inform the client. Consider the following:

Effective Referral Statement

Katie, I know when you first started seeing me for treatment of your hamstring pull, we had discussed the probability of four treatments being enough to facilitate repair of this tissue. Next week is our fourth session and I don't think we progressed the way we should have by now. I'd like to refer you to a colleague of mine who has had great success working with this type of injury. Would you be willing to meet with her so you can have a second opinion of what may be going on with your leg?

This statement and query allow for a dialogue between the client and the practitioner to decide what the best course of action is. The practitioner is stating facts and emphasizing that he wants what is best for the client, yet he is inviting the client's participation in the decision.

Ineffective Referral Statement

Katie, I'm really frustrated that your hamstring pull has not improved more by now. I don't know what's going on and I don't have the time to figure it out. I'm going to set you up with my buddy Al who can work that area out. After next week's session you can start seeing him. I've already called him and he has lots of openings.

This statement does not honor the client's experience or allow her to have any input into the decision. In fact, the practitioner is making it clear that the decision is all about his own needs, that he has already made the choice not to work with her, and is telling her he is passing her off to another practitioner. As a result of the practitioner's dismissive message, the client may decide not to continue treatment. This could be harmful for the client, as it may interrupt the healing process of her hamstring pull.

Referral Resources

As an ethical practitioner, you understand your scope of practice, the limits of your training and knowledge, your personal and professional limitations, your areas of weakness, and your blind spots. Accordingly, you need to develop a network of professionals whose work you know to be of the highest quality to refer clients to when necessary. Ideally, you will cultivate ongoing professional relationships with these resources and communicate with them directly. This list of reliable resources should be readily accessible. Clients and colleagues can act as resources for the development of this network.

Table 7.1 provides a tool designed to assist you in developing your own referral list.

■ CASE PROFILE

Before becoming a professional massage therapist, Judy worked at a natural foods grocery store as the manager of the supplements and vitamins department. Judy taught herself about how to use herbs, essential oils, nutrition, and meditation for maintaining a healthy and emotionally sound body. Judy is particularly proud of the fact that she has not been sick in over 10 years because of a personal regime she follows to stay healthy.

During her stint in bodywork school, Judy is very willing to share her knowledge of alternative methods of healing with her classmates and instructors. She is very critical of the diet that the majority of her classmates follows, and also frequently gives advice on what nutritional plans people should follow. She often tells people on campus what she thinks they are suffering from and how they could find a remedy for it at a health food store. There are also times Judy brings teas and tinctures to school for various people who she thinks will benefit from their use.

At one point, Judy talks with Azad, a student who is diabetic and needs insulin. Judy is convinced that, given the research she has done on diabetes, Azad can stop taking insulin and manage his condition with a change in diet, and by taking certain dietary supplements that affect blood sugar levels. Azad is very excited to hear Judy's plan for him because he finds his insulin pump expensive and inconvenient to use, and he wants to stop taking insulin.

What is Judy's intent with Azad?

Describe Judy's behavior in terms of scope of practice.

If you were one of Judy's instructors and overheard her talking to Azad, what would you do?

Confidentiality

Chapter 5 discusses confidentiality in detail. However, it is worth revisiting the topic here because confidentiality is an essential component of ethical and legal parameters of practice. Recall from Chapter 5 that "confidentiality" means ensuring that information is accessible only to those authorized to have access. In the bodywork profession, it means being entrusted with clients' personal and private matters, and treating these matters as privileged. Clients have the right to expect that communications will be kept within the bounds of the professional relationship.

Confidentiality applies to every client, regardless of the client's age, status (e.g., social, financial, health), or relationship of the client to the practitioner

Table 7.1	List of Conditions and Appropriate Referrals
Condition	**Referral**
Poor circulation in the extremities that does not improve with TX	Vascular physician
Cluster headaches	Craniosacral therapist
Severe migraine headaches that impair the client's daily activities for days at a time	Neurologist Craniosacral therapist
Emotional despair	Mental health professional (e.g., counselor; psychotherapist*)
Injury rehabilitation from a work-related accident or car accident	Orthopedic physician Neuromuscular physician Physical therapist
Injury rehabilitation from a sports injury	Neuromuscular physician Orthopedic physician Sports massage therapist
Stiff and painful joints	Orthopedic physician Rheumatologist
Digestive disorders	Gastroenterologist
Constipation issues	Shiatsu practitioner, Chi Nei Tsang practitioner
Sexual assault survivor	Crisis counselor specializing in sexual assault

*The difference between a counselor and a psychotherapist is determined by the level or type of education the individual received. Psychotherapists tend to have an advanced degree, such as a doctorate degree in psychology. A counselor is typically a practitioner with a master's degree.

or another client. It is important for you to inform clients before the first treatment session that confidentiality is maintained at all times.

Violating a client's privacy by breaking confidentiality is a serious breach in ethics and your code of conduct. Sometimes the consequences may be minimal, such as the loss of the client's trust, although the client may still see you for treatments because the client likes your work. However, it is highly likely that the client no longer trusts you. The consequences can also, of course, be much more severe; you may lose the client, or you may even be arrested or sued for serious infractions. However, if you are conscious of boundaries, do not discuss clients outside of the treatment room, and are regularly supervised by a trusted mentor, breaking confidentiality is less likely.

Confidentiality also relates to Web sites and electronic communications that you may have with your clients. In addition to having a statement of confidentiality on your intake form or a sign posted in your office, consider posting a statement on your Web site.

The following is an example of a Web site privacy policy: "Protecting your privacy is important to us. We collect no personal information about you unless you choose to provide that information to us. When you do provide personal information, such as an e-mail address, we keep that information confidential. Our Web site does not identify visitors. Anonymous tracking information is collected to analyze how many times our site is visited. The only time the Web site acquires information from you is when you use the contact form or sign up for our newsletter. We will not disclose, give, sell, or transfer any personal information about our visitors or clients unless it is required by law. We reserve the right to update this privacy policy statement without notice. Please review it periodically for updates. If you have any questions regarding our privacy policy, please contact us."

Documentation

Recall from Chapter 2 that documentation refers to the process of writing down notes, or charting, each therapeutic session you have with clients. It should be a systematic method of organizing the information for decision making. As Diana L. Thompson puts it so well in her book *Hands Heal,* we chart because we care about the safety of our clients and we want to provide the best service possible.[9]

Thorough and accurate documentation is important because it is a record of specified treatment goals, tracks the techniques performed during the treatment, provides the history of treatment progress the client has achieved, gives information on how the treatment plan may need to be changed to meet the needs of clients, and is a brief yet concise history of treatment plans that can be shared with other practitioners who may also be working with the same client. It also demonstrates to other health-care providers your abilities to maintain client records in a professional manner.

In certain cases, you are legally bound to provide accurate information about the work being done with the client. The legal system has the right to subpoena your client lists or even client records. In addition, many state licensing boards are requiring that treatments be documented, and the documentation can be used in peer reviews and concerns about licensing as well as legal proceedings.

If you do business with insurance carriers, you need to keep treatment notes since most insurance companies require subjective, objective, assessment, and plan (SOAP) notes before reimbursing the client. In this case, remember to keep detailed notes of those client treatment sessions and submit them promptly when asked. Insurance companies are also particular about how SOAP charts are written and what abbreviations are used.

Documentation benefits both you and the client in many ways.

Client Benefits:
• It builds trust between you and the client.
• The client has a historical record of all treatment plans, goals, and outcomes.
• Written documentation promotes safety and accuracy.
• The client has documented proof of progress.
• Quality assurance and value are demonstrated by tracking positive outcomes.
• It encourages the client to participate in the therapeutic process.

Practitioner Benefits:
• It demonstrates professionalism.
• There is financial security, as clients recognize positive outcome of the treatments.

- There is legal assurance that insurance companies will reimburse practitioners because there is a record to show proof of treatment.
- If there is a malpractice case, documents will show what work was done.
- It enhances the professional image and credibility of the practitioner and the profession.
- It assists in communication with a health-care team.
- It provides a historical record of all treatments.
- It provides safety of care because of access of client information.
- It outlines which treatment plans are effective and which ones are not effective so that the practitioner can be efficient in the care of the client.
- It demonstrates clear boundaries to differentiate the client and the practitioner's experience.

The best time to document is immediately after the treatment session. Documenting days, weeks, months, or even years later is risky, and even unethical, because it is difficult to remember a particular treatment session after several, or many, other sessions have blurred the details.

Consider the following: Campbell does not keep detailed charts of his work with clients at the massage therapy clinic at which he works. He assumes that because he sees all of his clients on a regular basis, he can remember what specific needs each one has without writing down all the details. When Campbell is involved in a minor car accident one day, Gary is called in to cover Campbell's shift until Campbell is able to return to work. Gary has a difficult time preparing for each client, as the client charts do not contain any specific information about any needs and treatments the clients have been receiving. The first client does not receive a full treatment, because Gary uses an oil that causes her to break out in an allergic rash. Her reaction is so severe that she goes into anaphylactic shock and paramedics need to be called. Gary feels really terrible about this but manages to pull himself together for his next client. This client becomes really annoyed because he does not like his feet touched and the first thing Gary does is to attempt to work on his feet. After loudly complaining to the clinic manager, this client is given a complimentary coupon for his next treatment. These situations could have been avoided if Campbell had documented essential information in the clients' charts. Because he did not, one client had a life-threatening experience (and will likely never return to the clinic), the clinic lost money because of the need to give out a complimentary coupon, and Gary had what was probably the worst day of his life as a massage therapist.

Health Insurance Portability and Accountability Act

Prior to the computer and electronic age of information, patient health-care information was written or typed onto paper documents and stored in one area, usually file cabinets within physicians' offices. If information was needed by, say, an insurance company, the patient's records were photocopied, and the paper copies were mailed out. Patients rarely had direct access to their files.

With the increasing use of computers, e-mail, the Internet, and electronic claims submission, medical records and other private information began to

Words of Wisdom

Good documentation can help with client retention. Clients will return because you paid attention during the consultation and documented the therapies you performed and those you discussed for their next visit. Remembering details to ask at their next visit shows them that their health is important to you. Everything the client mentions during the consultation can help with the design of the proper modality to help them achieve their goal. For example, I watch for physical gestures when going over the client profile sheets with the client. He might write down his chief concern is his right shoulder, but while discussing it, he may be pointing to his left shoulder. Questions of an injury or conditions help determine the best modality to use for them. The proper choice in massage and add-ons will customize their treatment plan, and encourage them to rebook.

—Kathleen Smith,
  Licensed Massage Therapist
  since 1976, Certified
  Neuromuscular Therapist,
  and Spa Director

be transmitted through these means. Without adequate laws and protection in place, people lost jobs, bank loans, and life insurance policies because their medical records and other private information were too easily accessed. Many times the information was incorrect, and people did not know it until a major problem arose. Although some states had laws governing these aspects of client privacy, there was no national system in place.

The Health Insurance Portability and Accountability Act **(HIPAA)** is a law that was enacted in 1996 to protect the privacy of people's health-care records. In general, HIPAA requires health-care providers to inform patients (clients) about their right to privacy and how their personal information can be used. Providers must implement procedures to keep patient records private, and train employees to comply. In fact, in an office or clinic, there must be a designated person who is responsible for seeing that privacy policies are followed.

The three main purposes of HIPAA are the following:

- Protect and enhance the rights of consumers by providing them access to their health information, having mistakes in their records corrected, controlling the inappropriate use of that information, and knowing who has accessed their records. Patient (client) records must be kept secured and away from anyone who does not need to see them. For example, physical records should be kept in locked file cabinets, preferably in separate, limited access records rooms. Passwords should be required for access to computerized client files. Patients (clients) must give written consent for use and disclosure of information for treatment, payment, and health-care operations.
- Improve the quality of health care in the United States by restoring trust in the health-care system among consumers, health-care professionals, and the organizations and individuals committed to the delivery of care. Most disclosure of patients' health information is restricted to the minimum needed for researchers, other health-care providers, and other professionals, and there are criminal and civil sanctions for improper use or disclosure.
- Improve the efficiency and effectiveness of health-care delivery by creating a national method for health privacy protection that builds on efforts by states, health systems, organizations, and individuals.[10]

Practitioners who use business software and store their client files on computers need to be especially careful to follow HIPAA regulations. Even if bodywork practitioners keep all their client information as paper documents, they must be mindful of HIPAA regulations. If practitioners need to send any client information by fax, e-mail, or in any other electronic way, then HIPAA regulations apply. Many practitioners bill insurance companies or health-care plans for client treatments. These businesses submit information electronically, even if practitioners give them paper documents. Any information that is or will be transmitted through any electronic method needs to be handled according to HIPAA requirements, even if the information was originally on paper.

HIPAA is administered by the U.S. Department of Health and Human Services (HHS), and enforcement and complaints are handled by the HHS

Office of Civil Rights (OCR). Information about HIPAA can be found on the HHS Web site, http://www.hhs.gov/ocr/hipaa

Other Legal Parameters of Practice

Other legal parameters of practice include knowing what different types of licenses exist, knowing which licenses are needed by which practitioners, having a clear understanding of informed consent and why it is important to obtain it from clients before the treatment starts, knowing what legally appropriate disclosure is and its importance in the bodywork profession, and understanding the importance of proper accounting and tax paying procedures, as well as the importance of liability insurance for practitioners.

The Different Types of Licenses

Ethical practitioners comply with all legal requirements that pertain to them. This shows respect for their clients, the profession, and the community in which they live. It also reflects a level of integrity. Four levels of government make laws that affect practitioners: federal; state; county; and city and town, or local, municipalities. As a practitioner, you need to make sure you understand what laws are in place and at which level you are governed.

In the bodywork profession, the federal government imposes taxes, and authorizes the accreditation of schools. The state, county, and local governments are also involved in levying taxes as well as issuing licenses and permits. Licenses and permits are one of the ways governments raise money. They are also set in place to protect the health and safety of the public.

People who provide services, such as attorneys, chiropractors, and bodywork practitioners, are usually required to have an **occupational license.** Some regions require that practitioners present evidence of completing state or locally approved entry-level bodywork programs and perhaps passing a licensing examination before they can apply for their occupational licenses; some regions do not. In those areas of the country that require bodywork practitioners be licensed by the state, the locality in which the practitioner works may require that practitioners obtain an occupational license as well.

Business privilege licenses are those required by municipalities for individuals or businesses that sell products. This type of license provides a method for the products sold to have taxes levied on them. If you sell products, even on a small scale, you will most likely be required to obtain a business privilege license in addition to your occupational and/or state practitioner's license.

Practitioners who own their own businesses are subject to other legal requirements as well. Depending on the region in which the private practice is located, there can be state and municipal zoning, licensing, and sanitation laws to adhere to. These laws and regulations will vary by locality. Regulations are not necessarily always clear and sometimes it is difficult to wade through the legalese of statutes and zoning codes.

Start with your municipal licensing office to find what your laws and regulations are for your area. Check your local telephone directory for its location and contact information. Internet research is also a possibility, because most local, regional, and state licensing and regulating bodies have their laws and regulations available online. Working with legal counsel might also be a proactive step in ensuring that the private practice or treatment center meets all requirements.

You also need to be aware that following all the legal steps necessary to start and maintain your private practice can be time consuming. Remodeling or expanding a physical site may require building permits. There will also be inspections of the construction, and inspections to ensure the facility meets zoning codes and health and sanitation standards. There can be inspections for the structure, electrical wiring, plumbing, and any equipment. Sometimes one city or county representative can make the entire inspection; most often, each inspection needs to be done by a different person.

Depending on the municipality's workload, these inspections may take a long time to schedule and carry out. You need not only to plan for costs and time required to build and install equipment, but for time for inspections as well. Many business owners have been surprised that their time frames for expansion have had to be greatly expanded.

Because of all the work and expense necessary to open a private practice, some practitioners may choose to ignore the legalities and start a business without obtaining the proper permits and licenses. This is not only unethical, it can be legally risky as well. At the very least, they may have to pay fines and close down the business until they have met all the legal requirements for their business. At most, they can lose their license to practice and perhaps even be arrested.

If you want to open a private practice, careful research and preparation need to be carried out first. It is much better to spend the time and effort necessary to determine what local and state regulations exist regarding the bodywork office than to invest time and money only to discover that you have not met certain legal requirements or, worse yet, that the treatments are not allowed by law in the location you have chosen.

Accounting, Taxes, and Insurance

Professional practitioners are responsible for abiding by state and federal guidelines to report income as well as pay taxes on the income. Accurate accounting is an ethical consideration because it demonstrates that you are not trying to "beat the system" by not recording all sources of income.

Practitioners are often conflicted about whether to record cash income. Federal and state tax guidelines are inflexible on this point, but some practitioners choose to withhold reporting cash payments for personal reasons, or to exaggerate their business expenses to reduce the amount of taxes they have to pay. Practitioners who sell products in states that collect sales tax may be tempted not to collect and remit sales tax. Ethically, of course, practitioners must keep accurate records and work with a trusted accountant to find legitimate ways to reduce tax liabilities. According to Cherie Sohnen-Moe, in her book *Business Mastery,* "An ethical practitioner keeps precise records, declares all income received, refrains from inflating expenses and accurately files governmental reports."[11]

Another way some practitioners may choose to cut costs is not to maintain adequate business and liability insurance coverage, even though it is required in some localities. This is short sighted on the part of practitioners. In the short term it may be a money-saving strategy. However, if something were to happen, such as a client being injured on the practitioner's property or by a technique performed by the practitioner, without proper coverage, the practitioner could be out a considerable amount of money.

Informed Consent

Informed consent has been mentioned throughout this text. Because it is crucial to the safe performance of bodywork, informed consent is explored in more depth here. **Informed consent** refers to the process by which clients have been fully informed about what to expect during the bodywork treatment. The primary purpose of informed consent is to increase the chances that the client will become involved, educated, and a willing participant in his or her treatment.[12]

Informed consent is part of client empowerment, and serves as protection for the client. The key to this process is that practitioners provide clients with all of the information they need to make a fully educated decision about accepting the terms of the treatment, whether they want a particular therapist to work with them, and whether the professional structure, including client rules and regulations, is acceptable to them. It reflects the ethical principle of client participation and self-determination in a client-centered approach.

Informed consent benefits and protects clients because it does the following:

* Gives the client the opportunity to ask questions about the treatment.
* Promotes complete understanding of the policies and procedures of the treatment.
* Clarifies expectations for the client about what will happen and what will not happen.
* Names the benefits of the treatment as well as the contraindications of the treatment.
* Empowers the client to make choices during the treatment.
* Permits the client the option to refuse treatment or stop the treatment at any time.
* Validates the therapist credentials and expertise.[13]

Informed consent can be given verbally, or, better, clients can sign a written agreement giving consent for the treatment to be performed. The written consent can be kept in the client's file. Aspects of informed consent include that you, as the practitioner, do the following:

* Define what the treatment plan will be, for example, describing the techniques that you will use, and the reasons for them.
* Inform the client what to expect as a result of the treatment plan. This should include benefits the client may experience, such as loosening of tight muscles, as well as risks of the treatment, such as feeling sore over the course of a few days.
* Discuss alternatives to the proposed treatment plan.

The consent given is not considered valid unless clients understand the information given. Ethically speaking, clients need to be well informed. This means using clear language that is understandable to clients, and not using scientific terms for anatomy and physiology or bodywork lingo unless clients have indicated they have a good working knowledge of these.

For example, saying to the client, "To find out whether I need to focus on the muscles on the right or left side of your neck, I'm going to test the range of motion in your cervical vertebrae by having you rotate your head ipsilaterally and contralaterally" may be perfectly clear to you, but may leave the client totally confused. It is much better to inform the client in a manner that he or she may find more understandable: "To find out whether I need to focus on the muscles on the right or left side, let's see how much movement you have in your neck. First, I'll have you turn your head to the right to see how far it goes; then I'll ask you to turn your head to the left to see how far it goes."

Informed consent concludes with acknowledgment from clients that they either agree to the treatment plan or refuse the treatment plan. You should inform clients that they have the right to refuse treatment at any point during the session, without stating a reason, even if they have already given written consent. You need to hear the client say yes or no to the treatment or see that they have agreed to it by signing the informed consent statement. Some practitioners have an informed consent statement on the intake form for the client to sign. Figure 7.5 presents an example of an informed consent statement on an intake form.

However, even though this states that the client is willing to receive a treatment, it does not list specifics of the treatment plan. Once the intake interview is complete and the treatment plan is discussed, you need to ask whether the client agrees to the treatment plan before beginning the treatment, and to remind the client that he or she has the right to tell you to stop the techniques you are performing, or stop the entire treatment at any time.

Even after they are given this information, some clients still do not think they can verbally say no to you. Therefore, you should be alert to nonverbal signals from the client. Should this occur, you should immediately stop what you are doing and ask the client if it is permissible to proceed with the technique. If the client says no, then do not proceed with the technique. The client may want to end the treatment completely at that point, in which case, you are ethically bound to respect the client's wishes.

Informed consent between you and your clients provides the framework of an ethical and safe experience for both of you. When informed consent is conducted properly, it enhances the level of trust between the client and you, especially as it allows the client to withdraw consent if he or she finds that actual experience is not acceptable.

The following are examples of verbal informed consent:

Nick is working on Penny, who is receiving a massage for the first time. After doing some assessments, he determines that Penny would benefit from some myofascial release in her upper trapezius.

Ineffective Informed Consent

Nick: I'm going to do some myo work on your shoulders. It will help loosen things up. When I ask, let me know if you are feeling pain. Even if it hurts, I'll keep going because that's the only way you'll benefit from this. When I'm done, you should feel a lot better.

Therapeutic Massage by Patricia Holland, LMT, MC
520-555-7517
Client Intake Form

Date: _____

Name: _____

Address: _____

Occupation: _____

Email: _____

Phone: home: _____ cell: _____

Emergency contact: _____ Phone: _____

Date of birth: _____

What is your goal for today's treatment?

Please circle all that apply:

Have you received a therapeutic massage before?   Yes   No

Do you wear contacts?   Yes   No

Are you pregnant?   Yes   No

What is your preference for pressure?   Mild   Moderate   Firm

Do you currently have – or have you had in the last 2 years – any problems or discomfort in the following areas?
Please circle all that apply.

Back/spine issues	Arthritis	Athlete's foot/fungus	Legs/feet
Digestive issues	Sinus	Arms	Hands
Skin issues	Neck	Shoulders	Varicose veins
Joint issues	Hearing	Headaches	Respiratory/lungs
Insomnia	Sciatica	Diabetes	Cancer
Cardiovascular/heart issues		Numbness/tingling	Limited range of motion
High blood pressure		Low blood pressure	Vision issues

Describe any of the previous conditions, or any other conditions that may affect your ability to receive a therapeutic massage today.

List any hobbies, sports exercise or other activities that you do regularly.

List any surgeries, accidents or injuries you have had in the last 2 years with dates.

List any medications you are taking including self-prescribed.

List any medical treatment or bodywork that you are currently receiving.

Name of Primary Care Physician: _____ Phone: _____

Do I have your permission to contact your physician should the need arise? ___Yes ___No

I, _____, understand that the therapeutic massage provided by Patricia Holland, LMT, MC is intended to enhance relaxation, decrease muscle tension, increase circulation and range of motion. I further understand that the nonsexual, therapeutic massage treatment provided by Patricia is not a substitute for medical treatments or prescribed medications. I have been informed by Patricia of the benefits of the treatment plan we discussed, I have been invited to provide feedback at any time during the session and I may ask for the session to stop at any time if necessary. Lastly, I understand and agree that I am required to provide a 24 hour notice of cancellation or I will be charged for my appointment. This agreement is for the duration of our professional therapeutic relationship.

_____   _____
Client Name   Date

Figure 7.5 Example of an informed consent statement on an intake form.

As the treatment gets under way, Penny expresses discomfort. Nick does not say anything. When she speaks up again, Nick sighs and says, "That's a good sign that I'm getting the work done." Penny does not say anything for the rest of the treatment. The next day she calls to tell Nick that there are bruises along the top of her shoulders and that she cannot lift her arms above her head. She cancels her next appointment, and it is a very long time before she is brave enough to try massage again.

Effective Informed Consent

Nick: Given our discussion of the pain you're feeling in your shoulders and the results of the assessments we did, I'd like to recommend that we do some myofascial release on your shoulder area. This technique involves very slow movement across that area while I slowly sink my fingers into the tissue to engage and stretch the tissue.

At this point Nick asks Penny for her arm and, with her permission, does a sample myofascial stroke so that she has a sense of what he means by engaging the tissue and to give her a sense of what the depth of pressure may feel like.

Nick: The benefit of this work is to help lengthen the fascia that has shortened around your muscles, which is causing the discomfort you're feeling. The technique will increase blood flow to the area as well. What you should feel is a slight burning sensation and a "hurts so good" type of pain. If the pain isn't tolerable, let me know immediately and I'll stop. If this work doesn't sound appealing to you, I could place a moist heat pack on your shoulders to help soften the tissues, then do other massage techniques instead. Do you have any questions? Would you like to try the myofascial release technique? Yes? Great. Remember, at any point you can tell me to stop if you do not want me to continue.

Shortly after the treatment begins, Penny expresses discomfort. Nick immediately stops what he is doing and asks if the work is too intense for her. Penny says yes. Nick then asks if she would like the hot moist pack and other massage techniques instead. When she says yes, he redrapes her back, gets the heat pack, places it on her and proceeds to perform the rest of the massage without incorporating the myofascial technique. Afterward, Penny thanks him for the treatment and schedules another for the following week. After three more appointments, she is ready to try the myofascial technique again.

Disclosure

Disclosure is important for clients to give informed consent. Recall from Chapter 1 that disclosure is revealing information. A certain amount of disclosure is essential in the client–practitioner relationship. In the case of informed consent, disclosure refers to the responsibility of clients as well as practitioners to provide accurate and complete information about the treatment. Clients are responsible for informing you of all facts necessary for the formation of the therapeutic relationship so that you can design and perform

Food for Thought
Think of a situation in which you were not fully informed about what would be happening to you. How did you feel? What do you wish had been explained to you? Would you have agreed to proceed if you had had full information? Why or why not?

treatments specific to their needs. In addition, if clients do not provide full disclosure about previous health conditions, then you cannot be held liable should the treatment aggravate a preexisting condition the client has.

Clients are expected to disclose all health-related information during an initial intake and interview. But how many times have you been performing a treatment and come across a scar, sign, or symptom that could be due to a condition that the client did not write down on the intake form or reveal during the pretreatment interview? Clients sometimes forget certain aspects about their health or not realize that something they have experienced is relevant to the treatment they are about to receive. For example, while working on a client you discover he has a scar that he tells you resulted from open heart surgery. He did not check off the section on the intake form that asks if he has any heart problems, nor did he mention anything about it in the pretreatment interview. Because the surgery prevented the heart attack he had been about to have, he does not think he has heart problems any longer and did not think that you would need to know about the surgery.

Clients may also speak up with information about their health during the treatment because they suddenly remember it as you are working in a particular area. For example, you may find out about the car accident that a client was involved in 2 months ago while you are addressing trigger points in his neck muscles.

Situations such as these are opportunities for you to educate the client about how health information, even if they think it is trivial or irrelevant, is useful for you to know to tailor the treatment to his or her needs, or to identify contraindications so that you will not harm the client. Also, often clients can begin to see the connection with symptoms they may have had for years with previous injuries, accidents, or illnesses.

Sometimes clients do not feel comfortable revealing their health history. It may take some of them a while to feel that they can trust you; establishing rapport, therefore, is an essential skill. Perhaps the intake form does not have enough space for thorough answers, or the pretreatment interview may not include enough time for clients to give complete information. These shortcomings can be remedied by ensuring there is enough room on the intake form, and giving clients plenty of time to fill it out. Also, be sure not to rush through the pretreatment interview. Allow the clients enough time to express themselves clearly.

You should note that, no matter how skillfully you communicate with your clients, some will still choose to keep certain information private. You are then not responsible for the treatment outcome based on this choice. Having a signed informed consent form is essential in this case because, by signing it, the client states that he or she is in agreement with the treatment plan that you have developed based on the information you have been given.

In turn, your responsibility concerning disclosure involves providing complete and accurate information about your skills as well as your ability to provide treatments. Appropriate professional disclosure includes describing your training and experience with the intent of instilling confidence in your clients. Disclosure on your part must be only that which will be helpful to the client. If there is consistency between what you say you can do and what you can actually do, then you are acting ethically and working inside your scope of practice.

Chapter Summary

"Scope of practice" is a term used by state and/or local licensing boards for various professions that defines the procedures, actions, and processes that are permitted for the licensed individual. Correspondingly, laws, licensing bodies, and regulations describe specific requirements for education, training, and competency. Practitioners are responsible for finding the scope of practice that applies to them in the region in which they practice. The ethical side of staying within scopes of practice involves the practitioner's education, competency, and self-accountability.

Confidentiality of client information applies to every client. Documentation is the process of writing down notes, or charting, each therapeutic session practitioners have with clients. HIPAA is a law that was enacted to protect the privacy of people's health-care records. Practitioners need to ensure they follow HIPAA regulations.

Occupational licenses are required for practitioners to practice in most regions of the country; business privilege licenses are usually required if practitioners sell products. Practitioners need to be mindful of ethical accounting and tax payment procedures, as well as the importance of carrying insurance. Informed consent is the foundation of the therapeutic relationship and directs the treatment plan. Practitioners need to be aware that consent given is not considered valid unless clients understand the information given.

Review Questions

Multiple Choice

1. The term for general agreement is:

   a. Scope of practice

   b. Consensus

   c. Standards of practice

   d. Competency

2. The ability to perform a specific task, action, or function successfully is called:

   a. Education

   b. Self-accountability

   c. Certification

   d. Competency

3. If a client has a pattern of complaining about the work not being satisfactory, yet is unwilling or unable to give specific feedback about why, it may be time for the practitioner to:

   a. Stop seeing the client immediately

   b. Continue treatments but say nothing to the client

   c. Refer the client to another practitioner

   d. Ignore the client's remarks

4. Which of the following is a consideration when choosing a continuing education course?

a. How much it costs

b. Where it is located

c. Who the presenter is

d. All of the above

5. Which of the following helps practitioners enforce scope of practice the most?

a. Self-accountability

b. Education

c. Competency

d. Certification

6. HIPAA applies to practitioners who:

a. Submit client records to insurance company.

b. Keep client records in computer files

c. Transfer client files by fax, e-mail, or other electronic methods

d. All of the above

7. Providing accurate and complete information on the part of both the client and the practitioner is known as:

a. Informed consent

b. Client retention

c. Disclosure

d. Documentation

Fill in the Blank

1. _____ is a term used by state and/or local licensing boards for various professions that defines the procedures, actions, and processes that are permitted for the licensed individual.

2. The term for the process of doing an evaluation is _____ , whereas the term meaning assigning a name or label to a certain group of signs or symptoms is _____ .

3. Completing a formalized program of study and passing one or more tests demonstrating competency in the area of study is the definition of _____ .

4. The term for ensuring that information is accessible only to those authorized to have access is _____ .

5. _____ refers to the process of writing down notes, or charting, each therapeutic session that practitioners have with clients.

6. The law enacted in 1996 to protect the privacy of people's health-care records is _____ .

7. Practitioners who sell products are likely to need a _____ license.

Short Answer

1. Explain the differences and similarities between scope of practice and standards of practice.

2. Describe three ways that practitioners can research what their scope of practice is in the area in which they practice or plan to practice.

3. Explain why ethical professionals choose to network with other professionals for the best possible outcome for the client.

4. Describe the role that scope of practice plays in client retention.

5. Explain what informed consent is, including at least three factors involved in it.

6. What are the three main purposes of HIPAA?

7. Explain the difference between an occupational license and a business privilege license.

Activities

1. Choose a region of the country in which you would like to practice bodywork. Conduct an online search to find the laws and regulations in that state or locality that governs the type of bodywork you want to practice. Did you find any of the laws or regulations surprising? If so, how were they surprising?

2. List some conditions that you think would blur the line between offering a diagnosis to a client and offering information gained as the result of conducting an assessment with the client.

3. Give three examples of diagnoses, and three examples of assessments. Rewrite your three examples of diagnoses as giving the client information you found through assessment instead of as diagnoses.

4. Describe what competency as a professional bodywork practitioner means to you. Be as specific as possible about what traits, characteristics, or skills you would want others to use when describing you as a competent professional bodywork practitioner.

5. Explain what self-accountability means to you. List the ways you hold yourself accountable as a student, professional bodywork practitioner, friend, and an employee.

Guidance for Journaling

 Some key areas to think about while journaling for this chapter include the following:

- The scopes of practice for various professions, and how the scopes of practice for the bodywork profession impact you
- What the standards of practice are for various bodywork modalities, and what your own personal standards of practice are
- What your legal responsibility is to stay within scope of practice
- What your ethical responsibility is to stay within scope of practice
- How diagnosing versus assessing affects you as a bodywork practitioner
- How education, competency, and self-accountability can assist you in your ethical responsibility to stay within scope of practice
- What you would look for when choosing continuing education courses
- Why and how staying within scope of practice can help your client retention
- When you will know it is time to refer a client
- The importance of confidentiality and its role in documenting your treatments
- How HIPAA affects you as a bodywork practitioner
- The types of licenses you need as a professional bodywork practitioner
- Why it is important to be ethical in your accounting and tax payments, and why carrying insurance is necessary
- How informed consent is necessary for bodywork, and how it will help you strengthen your therapeutic relationships with clients

References

1. Salvo, S.G.: *Massage Therapy Principles and Practice,* ed. 3. St. Louis, MO, Saunders Elsevier, 2007, pp 23–24.
2. Arizona State Board of Massage Therapy (2010). Retrieved 8 July 2010 from www.massagtherapy.az.gov: http://massagetherapy.az.gov/rules.asp
3. Office of the Professions, New York State Education Department (2009). Retrieved 8 July 2010 from www.op.nysed.gov: http://www.op.nysed.gov/prof/mt/
4. Missouri Secretary of State Robin Carnahan (2010). Retrieved 8 July 2010 from http://www.sos.mo.gov/adrules/moreg/previous/2004/v29n1/v29n1b.pdf
5. Braun, M.B., and Simonson S.: *Introduction to Massage Therapy,* ed. 2. Philadelphia, Lippincott Williams & Wilkins, 2008, p 32.
6. Lowe, W.: *Orthopedic Massage, Theory and Technique*, ed. 2. St. Louis, MO, Mosby Elsevier, 2009, p 6.
7. Corey, G., Corey, M.S., and Callanan, P.: *Issues and Ethics in the Helping Professions*, ed. 7. Stamford, CT, Brooks/Cole Cengage Learning, 2007, p 314.
8. Ibid.
9. Thompson, D.L.: *Hands Heal,* ed. 3. Philadelphia, Lippincott Williams & Wilkins, 2006, p 74.
10. U.S. Department of Health & Human Services (2010). Retrieved 8 July 2010 from http://www.hhs.gov/ocr/privacy/hipaa/understanding/index.html
11. Sohnen-Moe, C.: *Business Mastery,* ed. 4. Tucson, AZ, Sohnen-Moe Associates, 2008, p 87.
12. Corey, Corey, and Callanan, *Issues and Ethics in the Helping Professions,* p 156.
13. Braun and Simonson, *Introduction to Massage Therapy,* p 45.

Boundaries, Transference, Countertransference, and Dual Relationships

LEARNING OBJECTIVES

After studying this chapter, you will be able to:

1. Discuss the importance of boundaries in the bodywork profession.
2. Explain how to develop and maintain personal and professional boundaries.
3. Explain the importance of establishing boundaries for self-care, and the role of self-care in terms of responsibility to clients.
4. Define "transference" and "countertransference," and identify strategies to manage them.
5. Define "dual relationships" and "multiple relationships" and explain how these can occur in the bodywork profession.
6. Explain the risks and benefits of dual and multiple relationships.
7. Delineate appropriate parameters for successfully navigating dual and multiple relationships, and identify dual roles that practitioners should avoid.
8. Explain strategies for managing dual and multiple relationships, including how to make appropriate choices, when to ask for help, and when and how to end them.
9. Clarify dual and multiple relationships with family, friends, and coworkers, including likely issues they will encounter and solutions for these issues.

CHAPTER OUTLINE

KEY TERMS

Boundary: a limit set to inform others where one's personal space ends and public space begins

Countertransference: a defense strategy that bodywork practitioners employ when they have unresolved issues from their past, have perceptions about someone from their personal history, or have feelings from their past and are transferring these feelings and thoughts onto a client

Dual relationship: a relationship in which a professional assumes a second role with a client, becoming friend, employer, teacher, business associate, or family member

Emotional baggage: latent, unresolved issues; misguided anger; unrealistic expectations

Emotional environment: the atmosphere or energetic sense of the therapeutic relationship

Healthy insulation barrier: a boundary structure that is permeable enough to allow experience to penetrate the inner self but solid enough to protect it from being overcome by internal impulses and external demands

Multiple relationship: a relationship in which people have more than two different roles with each other

Overlapping relationship: a relationship in which two people can shift back and forth between dual or multiple roles, depending on the situation and the factors involved

Positive transference: a situation in which the client projects positive feelings or good qualities onto the practitioner

Role blending: a situation in which roles and responsibilities in dual or multiple relationships are combined

Self-care: the ability of practitioners to ensure a healthy emotional state, a sound physical state, and the awareness of how self-care affects the practitioners' work

Sequential relationship: a relationship in which one set of roles completely ends before the beginning of a new set of roles

Transference: a situation in which a client who has unresolved issues in his past is projecting, or transferring, these issues onto the practitioner

---

You are an avid hiker. You have decorated your treatment center with photographs you have taken from your many hikes. It is common for your clients to comment on them and ask about where the photos were taken and about hiking in the areas you like to go. One client, Eddie, is particularly curious and has been asking you to be his guide on a particular trail he has always wanted to hike but has been afraid to go on alone. You agree and set a date for the hike.

Shortly after you start the hike, Eddie starts to complain about how hot it is and that his knee is hurting, and implies that he wants to schedule a massage after the hike because he is straining his body. He has quickly run out of water because he did not bring enough and now he is asking for some of yours. When he mentions, for the fourth time, that he would like to schedule a massage after the hike, you tell him that you are not available. He gets upset with you and demands to know why not. He then starts to blame you for taking him on a hike that is too strenuous for him and then being unwilling to work on him afterward. When you say that you have a number of referrals that Eddie could call instead he refuses, stating that you are the only one he trusts to work on him.

Eddie does not notice a rut in the trail, which causes him to injure his knee severely. He now gets very angry and starts yelling at you for taking him on such a dangerous trail. When you finally make it back to Eddie's car, he tells you that he expects to get as many treatments as it takes from you, free of charge, to heal his injury. Eddie's last words before leaving are, "If it weren't for you I wouldn't have even been on this trail in the first place!" You are so shocked you do not know what to say. You also have no idea how you managed to end up in this situation.

Creating and maintaining boundaries are important to the success of bodywork practitioners. Boundaries are necessary to maintain a sense of self, to define personal space, and to provide protection for both the client and the practitioner. Boundaries help to clarify the practitioner's and the client's roles in the therapeutic relationship, and determine who is responsible for what, the expectations of the client and the practitioners, and the limitations of the therapeutic relationship. The purpose of boundaries is to create a sense of safety and security as well as a predictable relationship for both clients and practitioners.

Not only are boundaries necessary for practitioners to be able to make clear and informed decisions about their professional and personal lives, they can also help to prevent burnout. This chapter discusses how to set boundaries around issues such as finances, religion and spirituality, and sexuality in bodywork practices. Personal boundaries for practitioners are explored as well as the distinction of professional boundaries from personal boundaries. Boundaries around practitioner self-care are also crucial to a successful bodywork practice. Such boundaries help practitioners stay fit and healthy physically and emotionally so that they can provide effective treatments. Suggested ways to develop a self-care plan are covered, as well as strategies to use to communicate self-care needs to employers.

In addition, sometimes clients and practitioners are not able to keep their personal feelings separate from the therapeutic relationship. Clients who subconsciously project their feelings about other people in their lives onto the practitioner are transferring them. Practitioners who subconsciously have the same feelings toward a client as they do toward other people in their lives are exhibiting countertransference. Both situations can interfere with, harm, or even irretrievably damage the therapeutic relationship.

The topics of transference and countertransference and how they may interfere with the therapeutic relationship are presented in this chapter. Also included are ways to recognize when this is happening and how to manage the issues of transference and countertransference effectively.

In the bodywork profession, dual or multiple relationships often occur because bodywork practitioners choose to extend a connection with the client beyond the treatment room. This is especially true for practitioners and clients who have similar interests and values. Sometimes practitioners may have two or more roles at the same time or sequentially with a client, relative, or friend of the client; other practitioners; other health-care providers; and employers and supervisors.

Having dual and multiple relationships with family, friends, and coworkers is inevitable. To help you navigate dual and multiple relationships successfully, this chapter defines these concepts, covers their benefits and risks, and provides suggestions for defining appropriate parameters. Emphasis is placed on dual roles you should *never* enter into. Strategies for managing dual and multiple relationships are presented, including how to make appropriate choices, the factors involved in successful relationships, and when and how you should ask for help. Sometimes a dual or multiple relationship becomes unmanageable or not useful and therefore should be ended. Methods to help you determine when and how to do this are presented.

Importance of Boundaries in the Bodywork Profession

A **boundary** is a limit set to inform others where one's personal space ends and public space begins. Another way to think of a boundary is as a limit set by an individual that informs others what behaviors are acceptable in her presence, what topics of conversations are appropriate, and to what extent she is able and willing to provide support to others. When boundaries are set, they provide a sense of safety and security for the person to move forward in the world.

Boundaries exist in many forms and are essential to our well-being and functioning in our family, school, society, and profession. When you set a boundary you are declaring who you are, who you are not, what you are willing to do, and what you will not do. In essence, boundaries create a sense of safety and security by defining roles, responsibilities, expectations, and limits. This clarity of purpose engenders trust, which, as discussed throughout this text, is a necessary component of a successful therapeutic relationship.

In the bodywork profession you need to be connected to your clients on one level to establish a positive therapeutic relationship. At the same time you need to be separated enough from your client to avoid becoming enmeshed in the emotional or personal aspects of the client's life. It is possible to navigate these borders when we are clear of what our intent is for the relationship. It is a balancing act that begins with an awareness of your ability to identify your boundaries and the boundaries of others. The next step is recognizing that you have the right to choose when you allow another person to share your personal space, as well as recognizing that others have the right to choose when you will share their personal space.

In the bodywork profession, boundaries are set by practitioners to define appropriate behavior. These boundaries can include those for physical, financial, and emotional well-being. For example, a practitioner may set one of her physical boundaries by defining how many treatments she will perform in a day to ensure quality work with clients and to protect her physical well-being. Another physical boundary is using draping with a massage therapy client to inform the client that he will be safe and the practitioner will respect his body during the session.

A financial boundary can be affected if the practitioner keeps changing the price of his treatments to accommodate clients' needs rather than establishing a set rate. If the practitioner is not valuing his work by setting a fee and expecting clients to meet the fee, then clients are driving the decision about what they will pay for the massage. The practitioner's power is diminished and the client's power is increased in this particular aspect of the practitioner's business, and it can affect the practitioner's ability to succeed and be respected for his work.

Boundaries are essential for healthy relationships to exist, both personally and professionally. If you are not clear about your boundaries or you choose to ignore the proper use of boundaries you are essentially saying that you do not care about the safety and the protection of your client. This lack of respect for the client is also a lack of respect for yourself and for the bodywork profession. Many boundary violations or abuses occur because bodywork practitioners do not take boundaries seriously and think they can handle on their own whatever situation may crop up. It is risky to think and behave this way. It takes only one complaint to bring a successful career to an end.

Types of Boundaries

There are many different types of boundaries people can set for themselves. There are physical boundaries, such as people determining for themselves how their bodies will be touched and by whom. There are mental and emotional boundaries, such as how much time and attention people will give to others. Emotional boundaries are important so that people do not continually give time and attention to others until they have nothing left for themselves.

Boundaries can also be set to define the limits of finances, religion and spirituality, and sexuality. For example, someone can decide how much his skills and experience are worth and choose to set a minimal acceptable salary. Another example is lending others money. Some people choose never to lend money; others do so, depending on certain circumstances; yet others lend money to anyone. Each of these situations involves boundary setting on different levels.

What follows are explanations of various boundaries in the bodywork profession and some assessment questions to help you identify what each boundary means.

- **Physical boundaries.** These enclose the actual space in which practitioners and clients feel safe.
  - **Your treatment office.** Is the office in a low-crime area? Is the entryway clean and accessible for all clients? Is there good lighting so that clients who have evening appointments feel safe? Is the office clean and clutter free? Is the decor appropriate? Are there any offensive odors in the air? Is the background music in the lobby congruent with the setting?
  - **Your treatment room.** Are the decor, the lighting, and the choice of music appropriate? Is the room clutter free? Are there blinds on the windows to ensure privacy? If you share a treatment room with another practitioner, do you communicate expectations and needs about how the treatment room is kept?
  - **Draping (for modalities involving unclothed clients).** Is it professional at all times? Are the linens thick enough that you cannot see through them? Are the linens clean and comfortable? Do you communicate to your clients the intent of the draping and ask for feedback to be sure the clients feel secure?
  - **Personal space.** How much distance do you prefer between you and others when you are in conversation? What is your preference for noise or conversation in a community workspace such as a break room?
- **Social boundaries.** These determine our comfort in connecting with others. What is your comfort level when:
  - Meeting new clients?
  - Meeting new coworkers?
  - Networking with other bodywork practitioners?
  - Networking to build your practice?
  - Coping with conflict with others?
  - Receiving and giving authentic feedback to others?
- What is your ability to say no when asked to do something you would prefer not to do for a colleague or a client? Are you able to assert your opinions and ideas at staff meetings? Are you able to distinguish between your professional self and your personal self when you are at work?
- **Emotional boundaries.** These define one's capacity for empathy, compassion, and mutuality.
  - Are you able to offer support to your clients or coworkers without taking on their issues? Are you judgmental if your clients do not make the progress you think they should make in their treatments? Do you have difficulty understanding the choices your clients make about their health and well-being? Do you have a tendency to work harder than your clients do in helping them rehabilitate from an injury? How emotionally invested do you become when a client shares a sad or painful story?

- **Psychological boundaries.** These determine how people reconcile that deep longing for intimacy with the need for autonomy, or how people reconcile the need for being with others with the need to be alone.
  - If you are in private practice do you find yourself feeling isolated from peers and substitute your clients for intimate friends? Are you reserved by nature and feel challenged by the task of creating the therapeutic relationship with your clients? Are you a "people person" and consider all your clients to be friends and share your personal life with them openly because to withhold such information would seem rude?
- **Ethical boundaries.** These determine the lines drawn between the moral and the immoral, the acceptable and the unacceptable.
  - What client behaviors and issues do you not tolerate at all? What behaviors and issues do you not tolerate from colleagues? What behaviors and issues do you believe are opportunities for educating clients? Do you maintain confidentiality at all times? Do you take the code of ethics for the bodywork profession to heart and follow it closely? Are your fees consistent for all clients regardless of their income? Do you work within your scope of practice at all times?
- **Professional boundaries.** These distinguish not only what behavior is appropriate with clients and colleagues but also the difference between who you are and what you do.
  - Do you maintain a professional demeanor at all times with your clients and colleagues? Do you limit the amount of personal information you share with clients at all times? Are there some clients with whom you feel comfortable sharing your personal information? If so, why? When you are not working do you feel obligated to uphold professional standards when in public? If you see a client in public do you approach him or her first to say hello or do you let the client initiate a greeting? When away from your office are you able to "turn off" the bodywork practitioner mind and just relax, or do you find yourself always networking, assessing postures, and marketing?
- **Financial boundaries.** These determine our relationship with money and our ability to value our work as well as effectively communicate the value to others.
  - Do you set a fee for your services that is competitive within your community or do you set your fee lower because you assume clients will not pay you the going rate? Do you have an established fee structure that assures equity for all clients at all times? Are you mindful of your income and expenses? Are your bills paid on time? Do you allow clients to owe you for more than one session at a time?[1]

Three especially important boundaries for bodywork practitioners are discussed in greater detail below: religious and spiritual boundaries, sexual boundaries, and dating boundaries.

Religious and Spiritual Boundaries

Religious and spiritual boundaries refer to the limits set by individuals to determine what input they will receive from others as well as what information they will impart to others about faith-based issues. Because of the highly personal and potentially volatile nature of discussions surrounding religion and spirituality, practitioners must approach these boundaries with sensitivity. Generally, practitioners are advised to avoid such discussions altogether, or run the risk of being drawn into conversations that do not benefit the therapeutic relationship, particularly if the practitioner is not in agreement with the client.

Some clients may use the treatment session to try to convert you to their way of believing. Should this happen, a professional response is to be respectful of the client while at the same time letting the client know the conversation is not appropriate. One example of an appropriate response to a client might be the following: "It sounds like you live a life of deep faith and I respect how comfortable you are at sharing your beliefs. However, I prefer that we not discuss these issues during the session."

Another appropriate response might be the following: "I want you to know that I deeply respect how important your life of faith is to you. I want you to know that those issues are very private for me, and I am not comfortable [and/or willing] talking about them during your treatment. I would prefer that we focus our attention on your body and how it is responding to the treatment."

Sometimes there is no easy way to prevent the client from talking about something that is important to her. However, the therapeutic relationship can be placed in jeopardy by pretending that a topic is not interfering with the treatment. The more direct and specific, in a respectful manner, you are with your clients, the more authentic you can be in your interactions with them.

Sexual Boundaries

Sexual boundaries are set limits that determine what is appropriate and safe in terms of behavior and comments on the part of both the practitioner and the client. Being direct and clear about sexual boundaries creates a safe and appropriate environment for the client as well as for the practitioner.

All practitioners know that it is unethical to have a sexual relationship with a client. However, sexual boundaries are not just about the act of sex, but also about the use of language in a session that is sexual in nature. For example, the client may tell a joke or make a comment about the practitioner's touch that has a sexual overtone. This is not appropriate and if left unaddressed, the client will assume that the practitioner condones this type of behavior.

Practitioners must also maintain boundaries and not engage in conversation that has sexual innuendo or sexual overtones. Sexual harassment charges could be brought up against the practitioner if the client perceived the impact of the comment to be harmful, regardless of the practitioner's intention. Also, a person's sexual orientation is not an appropriate topic of discussion during a session because it is highly personal and because it does not play a role in the treatment outcome.

There is always the possibility that a client may ask a practitioner about his sexual orientation because the client is curious or needs to know in order to feel comfortable with the practitioner. However, the practitioner is under no obligation to disclose any information. The practitioner should never ask clients about their sexual orientation either, because this has absolutely no bearing on the treatment.

Practitioners can maintain sexual boundaries in a session by saying, for example, "Sexuality is a very private matter to me and I choose not to discuss it with any of my clients. It is important to me to create a professional and therapeutic environment at all times."

Dating Boundaries

As stated previously, sexual contact with a client is forbidden. However, there are times when a practitioner and a client determine that there is a mutual desire to explore the possibility of a romantic relationship outside of the professional relationship. When this is the case, *the professional relationship must be terminated immediately.*

The following are some of the factors involved when a practitioner and a former client are considering dating:

- The nature of the professional relationship. This includes the number and frequency of sessions, types of issues dealt with in treatments, and intensity of issues dealt with in treatments. Generally, the greater the number of issues that are dealt with during treatment sessions, the greater becomes the potential for problems when forming a relationship outside the therapeutic relationship.
- Emotional maturity and stability of the former client. To what degree is the former client able to relate to the former practitioner as an equal? Does the former client have any emotional conflicts that would interfere with making a successful transition to a different type of relationship? Is the client trying to meet unsatisfied social needs or resolve personal problems by forming this relationship?
- Emotional maturity and stability of the practitioner. To what degree is the practitioner able to relate to the former client as an equal? Is the practitioner trying to meet unsatisfied social needs or resolve personal problems by forming this relationship? Does the practitioner have sufficient emotional and professional support such as mentoring or supervising?[2]

These factors provide the practitioner with a framework in which to consider whether terminating the professional relationship and dating the client would be a wise or emotionally safe decision. Because of the power differential in the therapeutic relationship or the possibility of transference issues (discussed in the section "Transference and Countertransference"), it is possible that the client has the practitioner on a pedestal and may not see him or her for who he or she truly is. A healthy connection is based on mutual respect and mutual contribution to the relationship.

Boundaries in Bodywork Schools

The physical environment of school offers many educational opportunities as well as avenues for personal development. Most boundary lessons are learned through experience. Spending months or possibly a year or more with the same people will give you many opportunities to practice setting, maintaining, and communicating about boundaries. There may also be a supportive environment present in the form of faculty, staff, and administrators who are willing to work with you to provide feedback on handling specific boundary issues that may arise.

 Food for Thought
Think about boundaries you have surrounding your finances, religion, spirituality, and sexuality. Have you spoken about your boundaries to another person? If so, how did you feel? How did the other person respond? Do you think your boundaries were respected? Why or why not?

Because bodywork schools are typically nontraditional educational settings, there are some unique challenges concerning boundaries. Generally, in bodywork schools, students take most or all of their classes together throughout the entire program. In a university setting or a more traditional vocational setting, students mix and mingle in a variety of classes throughout their time at school. They may not get the chance to get to know one another very well. They are also not required to disrobe, lie under a sheet on a massage table (for modalities involving unclothed clients), and be touched on a daily basis by fellow classmates.

This is one reason boundaries are unique in a bodywork school as opposed to other educational institutions—the intimacy and trust students need to have as they learn hands-on techniques by practicing on each other. Intimacy and trust also play a huge role if instructors demonstrate techniques on students, and as instructors correct the techniques students are performing on each other.

This distinctive learning environment found in bodywork schools requires an astute awareness of personal and professional boundaries for both students and instructors. They need to be able to identify boundaries, communicate their boundaries to others, recognize when a boundary has been crossed, manage the outcome when the boundary crossing has been acknowledged, and know when to make a boundary more flexible or less permeable.

Appropriate professional boundaries need to be modeled at all times by bodywork school instructors, staff, and administration. Students of any age are very impressionable and are quick to judge an instructor's teaching style and sense of humor. They certainly notice if there is not equity in the teacher's attention toward all students. Therefore, teachers of bodywork students have the responsibility of being deliberate and mindful in their thoughts, words, and deeds when instructing a class.

Students at bodywork schools must also be mindful of boundaries implicit in an educational setting. Some students may be older than the instructor, causing the students not to respect the instructor's knowledge and experience. Another common challenge in the classroom is what to do when students disagree with the instructor. When students exhibit disrespectful behavior or talk back to an instructor, a boundary has been crossed in the classroom. If appropriate boundaries are set that honor and respect the power differential that is innate in a learning environment, then the student and the teacher can work together to overcome these differences.

The standard form of training in bodywork school is to learn a modality by receiving the modality as well as by performing the modality. Therefore, the classroom is a place to practice maintaining appropriate boundaries and modeling professional behavior at all times. How you treat one another as fellow students and as practice clients is an indicator of your ability to develop successful therapeutic relationships as a licensed professional.

Role That Boundaries Play in Successful Bodywork Practices

In successful bodywork practices, practitioners set and maintain healthy boundaries so that clients feel a sense of safety and well-being. For example, by defining the parameters of the treatment space and treatment session, clients are informed about what to expect in terms of the length of the session, their treatment plan, a clean and professional treatment space, and the practitioner's skill level and competence. Clients will want to return to practitioners who set such boundaries and standards because there are no surprises and the clients feel well taken care of.

One area of appropriate boundary setting involves having conversations with clients. During conversations you should remain professional, be non-judgmental, and use language that does not invite advances. In turn, the client should be in control concerning the amount of talking that will occur during the treatment. For example, consider the following guidelines:

- Let the client take the lead in how much talking occurs during the treatment.
- Meet hot topics such as religion and politics with professional courtesy and not participate in debates about them.
- Do not invite the client to participate in an outside business venture such as, for example, selling beauty products or nutritional supplements.
- Do not engage in sexual innuendo or direct sexual comments; if the client should do so, let the client know these are not appropriate.

Other appropriate boundaries practitioners can consider to prevent burnout, increase the chances for career success, and ensure career longevity include the following:

- Limit the number of clients seen in a day or a week to avoid repetitive stress injuries, and physical and emotional exhaustion.
- Recognize that you are not responsible for "fixing" the client, solving client personal problems, or being responsible for more than 50% of the therapeutic relationship.
- Protect your privacy by not oversharing about your personal life; oversharing can possibly lead to disclosure remorse, feeling vulnerable to the client, or feeling uncomfortable seeing the client again.
- Pay attention to the needs of the client and respond appropriately and within your scope of practice.
- Inform clients when they have crossed a boundary, and do so by educating them on what is appropriate, and not scolding or shaming them.
- Know when to back off in a conversation when it appears that either you or the client is becoming too invested in being "right."
- Acknowledge that your ability to provide effective treatments is directly related to the honesty of the information the client shares about his health history and preferences. This involves understanding that if the client does not disclose at the time of treatment that he does not like something you are doing, you are able to let it go and not see yourself as incompetent.
- Make the session about the client at all times, and do so with respect.
- Provide a safe, clean, and pleasant atmosphere in which the client is to receive the treatment.
- Be on time for each and every appointment; if you are running late, call as soon as you can to inform the client of your estimated time of arrival.

- Reschedule appointments as soon as possible when the need to cancel arises, and apologize to the client.
- Follow up on all phone calls within a 24-hour time period to demonstrate your dependability.
- Maintain your health; cancel appointments if you are sick so that you do not compromise the health of your clients.
- Take responsibility for missing an appointment because of forgetfulness; reschedule as soon as possible and give the client the treatment free of charge.
- Be consistent with each treatment so the client knows what to expect in terms of treatment structure, time frame, quality of skills, and treatment charge.

It takes time, effort, and practice to set and maintain limits, and, of course, no one does it perfectly all the time, or with every client. Sometimes the best lessons about setting boundaries are those learned from making mistakes. However, as long as you are open to, and willing to respond to, the feedback from a client or colleague when a violation happens, you will become more skillful over time as you continue to refine your skills at setting, maintaining, and communicating your boundaries.

Personal Boundaries

To develop and maintain professional boundaries, practitioners need to understand what their personal boundaries are. A personal boundary is one that you determine is a nonnegotiable limit that must be established in order to feel safe and in control of your surroundings. When you set a personal boundary, you are making that clear to another person.

Often personal boundaries are discovered when people recognize that they were not comfortable with how an interaction occurred with someone else, or how they were spoken to by another. When people feel out of control, afraid, or even angry about an interaction with another, it usually stems from the fact that their stated preferences were not honored or that their feelings were dismissed. Chances are when you feel bad about yourself or about a behavior or a comment, a personal boundary has been crossed. Sometimes the ability to recognize personal boundaries starts when you feel overwhelmed and confused, or you do not feel good about yourself or your family and friends. It may not be until difficult emotional responses occur for you to ask, "What is this about? Why am I feeling this way?"

It can be difficult to define personal boundaries if we are unfamiliar with the concept of setting limits that will enable us to feel good about who we are, and about how we are interacting with others. For some, the process may involve receiving recognition from others for opinions and thoughts they have shared. Once this recognition is felt, they may offer more of their ideas without the fear of being dismissed or humiliated. Others may require privacy before they feel comfortable enough to open up about what makes them comfortable and uncomfortable. Once the right to privacy is respected, they may feel free to disclose more about their boundaries. Still others may have the need to be in control of as much as possible, and may need to set many boundaries.

A starting point for you to recognize your personal boundaries is to brainstorm, create a written inventory on all the areas in your life in which you want to feel safe, secured, respected, and heard. Be sure to include your family, friends, and bodywork practice. For example, you can ask yourself the following questions:

- Do I want to have a phone call before someone shows up at my home for a visit?
- Do I want my friends to ask how I am rather than to assume I'm fine and therefore always available to meet their needs?
- Do I want my significant other to notice I have had a long week and pamper me, or do I prefer to ask directly for pampering each week?
- Am I comfortable discussing my relationship with others or do I consider it off limits?
- What are my belief systems about religion and spirituality? What am I comfortable sharing about my belief systems?
- Do I need time to myself each Sunday night to become centered and organized for the week?
- Do I want to instigate phone contact with my brother, or should I ask him to call me sometimes too?
- Do I want to socialize on a weekly basis with the people I also work with?
- What is the number of treatments I can do in a day and still have quality energy left for the last client?
- Do I need to receive a bodywork session every week, twice a month, or once a month? What fits into my schedule and my finances?
- Do I want to trade with other practitioners to save money on receiving treatments, or do I want to pay for them so that I do not have to schedule an additional treatment each time?
- Do I want to see clients as early as 8:00 in the morning and as late as 8:00 in the evening? What time of day does my energy peak and then drop?

From these self-reflective questions, you can then develop your set of personal boundaries. Whatever they are, you have a right to them, and have the right to inform others of your boundaries as situations arise. The following are examples of what you might say:

- Please don't just drop by my house for a visit; I need you to call first.
- Could you please not wear perfume when we're going to spend time together? I'm allergic to most scents.
- I'm uncomfortable being touched unless I know the person well. Could you please not hug me?
- Please refrain from using foul language.
- I choose not to discuss my personal finances as it's no one's business but my own.
- Please don't call me after 10 p.m. or before 8 a.m.
- I prefer that you not smoke cigarettes in my presence.
- I'm not comfortable with racist jokes or derogatory comments about other people.
- Please don't discuss religion or politics during supper.

Words of Wisdom

I believe that in recognizing and respecting our boundaries we affirm ourselves, our rights in all our relationships and the rights of others. When we fail to defend ourselves, when we fail to stand up for ourselves under attack, we lose some treasured part of ourselves—our integrity, belief in ourselves, the real "I" at the core of the self, and each time this is a little death. And when we fail to respect the rights of others, we inflict losses, large and small, that may shake the core of lives of all we touch.

—ANNE COPE
    WALLACE, author of
    *Setting Psychological
    Boundaries: A Handbook for
    Women*[3]

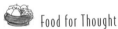

Food for Thought

Off the top of your head, list 10 of your personal boundaries. Why do you think these boundaries came to mind first for you?

- I prefer not to socialize with my coworkers.
- I prefer not to let others borrow my car.
- I choose not to answer questions about my personal life during a bodywork treatment.
- I choose not to give or receive a bodywork treatment if I'm not feeling well.

When stating a personal boundary it is not necessary for you to explain why you are setting it unless you feel compelled to do so. If others press you for reasons why, that itself can be considered crossing a boundary, and you are under no obligation to give answers. If, of course, you would like to give reasons, it should be because it is your choice to do so.

When one or more of your boundaries has been crossed by another person, it is important that you inform who did the crossing what happened and why it was not acceptable. It is also possible that you can cross your own boundaries in an attempt to be accepted by others or to be noticed. If that is the case, it would be beneficial for you to talk with a trusted friend or mentor about why this happened and what you hoped to be accomplished by it. You can then evaluate if crossing the boundary was useful and healthy for you. If not, you can decide what you need to do to not cross the boundary in the future.

How to Develop and Maintain Professional Boundaries

Recognizing personal boundaries is essential to the health and well-being of practitioners because they have so much contact with others. Practitioners should also recognize that their personal needs should be met outside of their bodywork practice. It is unhealthy, and possibly dangerous, to try and have clients meet these needs. This can be a common challenge among bodywork practitioners because of the intimate nature of the bodywork. Because of this, practitioners, in addition to personal boundaries, need to be able to develop, set, and maintain professional boundaries.

Professional boundaries involve your being able to manage client requests, needs, and demands in a manner that does not give the client too much, or too little, power or control in the therapeutic relationship. Professional boundaries also enable you to model for the client appropriate ways to ask for needs to be met. For example, if a client is perpetually late, you have the responsibility to inform the client tactfully how his lateness affects your schedule for the rest of the day.

Without personal boundaries you may end up making yourself available to anyone at all times. Over time, you will have no reserves left for yourself. If this is your history with personal boundaries, you will most likely have the same issues with setting professional boundaries, possibly leading to burnout and a shortened career as a bodywork professional. Therefore, it is helpful for you to develop a list of professional boundaries, much in the same way you can develop a list of personal boundaries.

You can start by spending some time thinking about what it is you want your clients to experience from the treatment sessions, what you want to experience from the sessions, and the best ways to have these expectations met. From there, you can determine what your professional boundaries will be.

An important aspect of developing professional boundaries is to be clear about what is appropriate and what is not. Some areas in which you would benefit from setting clear boundaries with clients are the following:

- Stating procedures for making and canceling appointments
- Sticking to the agreed-upon duration of the treatment (e.g., not allowing the client to persuade you to work longer than the agreed-upon time frame if you are unable or unwilling to do so)
- Determining what techniques will be used in the treatment plan
- Paying for services
- Receiving phone calls after hours
- Clarifying it is a nonsexual therapeutic treatment and refusing anyone who asks for a sexual treatment
- Stating that you do not diagnose conditions
- Refusing to work outside of your scope of practice

Rigid and Flexible Boundaries

It is also helpful for you to be aware of the areas in which you can be flexible and those in which you cannot. A rigid boundary is one that practitioners are unwilling to modify, no matter what, as shown in Figure 8.1A. Although it is essential to have certain rigid boundaries, such as no sexual contact with clients, if boundaries about all aspects of the practitioner's practice are completely rigid, they may run the risk of appearing cold and unfeeling to their clients. This makes it difficult for them to have rapport with clients, and decreases the chances of forming a therapeutic relationship with them.

The opposite of a rigid boundary is one that has so much flexibility in it that there may as well be no boundary at all, as shown in Figure 8.1B. For example, some practitioners can never say no to clients, even though saying yes will require them to make all kinds of changes in their schedules or lives. Then there are those practitioners who have no sense of their own needs because they are always focused on others. These practitioners run the risk of burnout and a shortened bodywork career. Burnout is, in fact, typically described as a sense of having nothing left to give, no ability to care, and a deep sense of despair that things will never change.

It is possible to create a balance between absolutely rigid and absolutely flexible boundaries, as shown in Figure 8.1C. When there is balance in your boundary setting you can experience a sense of satisfaction in being true to yourself. Psychiatrist Louis Ormond called this type of boundary a **healthy insulation barrier.** It is a boundary structure that is permeable enough to allow experience to penetrate the inner self but solid enough to protect it from being overcome by internal impulses and external demands or overwhelmed by toxic stimuli such as critical or negative judgments, ideas, and views, our own as well as those of other people.[4] Having healthy insulation barriers allows you to see a situation for what it is and not doubt what you are feeling or feel bad about the outcome.

Depending on the situation, it is key to have certain boundaries that are flexible. This involves emotional awareness and self-reflection about what you are unwilling to compromise on and why, and about what you are willing to be flexible on and why. Saying, "I don't know; let me get back to you" to those who are asking something of you is a way not to commit to anything

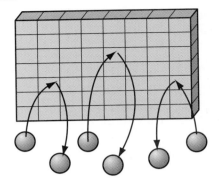

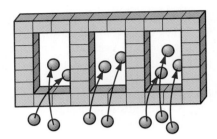

Nothing gets through the boundary – no new ideas, no different ways of looking at things, no changes to accommodate others' needs. The practitioner is unwilling to, or does not know how to, create any
A   flexibility, which would be shown by removing bricks.

Everyone else's needs and requests get through, which can be to the detriment of the practitioner's well-being. The practitioner is unwilling, or does not
B   know how to, set more bricks in place.

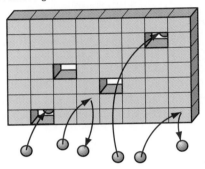

The practitioner chooses what can come through the boundary and has flexibility in meeting others' needs. The practitioner can move the bricks around,
C   adding more or taking some out as she likes.

Figure 8.1 Rigid vs. flexible boundaries. (A) A rigid boundary. (B) A boundary that is so flexible it might as well not be a boundary. (C) A balance between rigid and flexible boundaries.

until you have time to check in with yourself. You can ask yourself whether what you are being asked to do is reasonable, something you really want to do with no strings attached, and is in keeping with your principles.

If you feel resentment, fear, or anger at being asked, then you could explore the source of these feelings. Have you been asked to do this many times before and did not want to do it? Is it because you are afraid of what may happen if you say yes? Do you think no one should ask anything of you, ever? All of these can determine where the balance between rigid and flexible boundaries is for you.

As you gain more experience setting boundaries, you will most likely know when it is appropriate to stay firm and when to lighten up. For example, there is a client who has a perfect record of making his appointments on time. One time he forgets a treatment and does not call. You might decide that it is appropriate not to charge him the full cancellation fee as this was his first offense. By waiving this fee, this one time, you are acknowledging that mistakes happen, but because he has been such a consistent client he will not be charged. Another example of being flexible with a professional boundary would be to allow a client to reschedule an appointment to a different day as long as it is not a hardship for you. Any decision to make exceptions to a boundary must be made with clarity. Otherwise, resentments can build up, which may make your interactions with the client difficult.

In a professional setting it is very tempting to be either hypervigilant and expect colleagues to meet your standards on all operational and client-related issues, or laid back, having no expectations of structure. Some people prefer to go with the flow and not make problems for anyone. These are risky extremes because, on the one hand, you could be considered the high-maintenance, difficult colleague if you enforce your thoughts, ideas, and feelings on others. People tend to act this way to get their need to be in control met and to feel safe in their environment. On the other hand, you could become the go-to colleague whom everyone calls on when they need something done that no one else wants to do, such as covering a shift, giving up the prime treatment room when it is your turn to have it just because someone else wanted it, and working all holidays.

These extremes can happen if you think you are too valuable (They should do things MY way; their way isn't good enough) or not valuable enough (I should do things THEIR way; my way isn't good enough) to be part of a professional team. Either way, you are denying your opportunity to share your talents as equals. Finding the correct balance of professional boundaries is a process that takes time. The key is to stay aware and flexible so that you can adapt accordingly in a healthy and professional manner.

Communicating About Boundaries

Developing appropriate methods of communication about your boundaries is important. Often, practitioners may not want to speak up to a client who has crossed a boundary because they do not want to seem rude or disrespectful. This is a valid concern. However, if you value your time and efforts, then you must relay those values to your clients. Being mutually invested in the therapeutic relationship will benefit both of you, as you will have a shared interest in a successful outcome, which can only come about if both you and your client feel respected.

Communicating about boundaries can be done with a respectful tone of voice, and in a nonjudgmental manner. If you are clear about your intention behind why you have set a particular boundary, and how the client has crossed that boundary, then you have done the appropriate groundwork for communicating your concerns to the client.

The following is an example of such a conversation:

"John, I wanted to take some time before you leave the office today to discuss a concern I have about our treatment sessions. I've noticed that during the past 2 weeks you have been very verbal and descriptive about your new relationship. I'm very happy that you have found someone you are happy with, and it sounds like things are going very well for you. But I'm uncomfortable with the amount of detail you have been sharing with me about your sexual activities. What I would like is for you to keep those intimate details private and share more general details. Again, I want to be clear that I'm happy for you and your relationship and grateful that you feel that you can trust me with such detail. However, it's uncomfortable for me to hear."

This conversation allows the practitioner to assure the client that she is supportive of the new relationship, but that she does not want to be included in the specific, intimate aspects. It also includes nonjudgmental language as well as the acknowledgment that the client trusts the practitioner. This type of honest sharing is modeling for the client that the practitioner in return trusts the client to hear and understand the request that is being made.

Policies and Procedures Document (boundary framework)

A useful method for clearly communicating professional boundaries is for practitioners to design a policies and procedures document. This gives your business structure as well as defines for clients what is expected of them. It also makes it easier for you to maintain professional boundaries. For example, if there is a no-show fee for last-minute cancellations that clients are made aware of before their first session, then you do have to go through the uncomfortable steps of asking for payment or informing clients that payment is due should the client cancel with less than 24 hours' notice. You may still have to remind clients, but because it was part of the initial bodywork agreement, it makes it easier for you to discuss it.

Exceptions, of course, can be made for clients who have emergencies, showing some flexibility with that boundary. But because it was clearly stated in a policies and procedures document, the client has been fully informed and it is up to your discretion if you want to maintain that boundary or not. If you grant the client an exception, then the client knows it is an *exception* to a boundary you have set; communication about the issue is clear.

If there are clients who continually break the last-minute cancellation boundary, then you can choose to make the clients accountable by charging them for the missed sessions. This should come as no surprise to the clients, because it is clearly spelled out in your policies and procedures document.

When considering what type of information to include in your policies and procedures document you can start by looking at the types of business boundaries there are in the bodywork profession. These include the following:

- **Time Frame of Session**
  - What is the length of your sessions—30, 60, 90, or 120 minutes?
  - When is the beginning of the treatment—when the client arrives? When the pretreatment interview begins? When you begin performing the hands-on portion of the treatment?
  - Does the length of the treatment session include time for the client to undress, dress, pay, and give you feedback?
  - When a client is late, will you feel obligated to give him or her a full session even though you may have somewhere else to be?
  - Will you allow sessions to run overtime? If so, how far over? Under what circumstances?
- **Fee and Payment Structure**
  - What fees will you charge?
  - Do you think you are charging what your services are worth?
  - What are you basing the worth of your service on?

- Will you allow a client to owe you money? If so, under what circumstances?
- What do you think about having a sliding fee scale in which you charge people according to their ability to pay?
- Are you willing to make payment plans? Take credit cards? Accept checks? Barter? Will you offer package deals? Discounts?
- Do you want to sell products?
- When do you want to be paid—at the beginning of the session, at the end of the session, or monthly?
- **Communication With Client**
  - How do you want to communicate—by cell phone? Texting? E-mail? Through a social networking site?
  - Will you place limits on when and how often clients can contact you? What would those limits be?
  - Will you limit the subject matter of the content of the call from your clients?
  - How will you handle the initial phone call? Is it brief, then followed by an e-mail? Will you have an initial conversation over the phone to screen the caller (to make sure he or she is appropriate for your office)? What basic information do you want new clients to know before coming to see you for the first time? Will you discuss your cancellation policy?
  - Will you charge for consulting with your client? If so, what type of information exchange qualifies as a consultation? How long must the call be to be considered a consultation? How will you determine a fee for the consultation?
  - How will you handle dissatisfied clients? Can you listen to them calmly and without interrupting? Can you accept that the client's experience is his or her experience and is not something that you can change or correct? Will you ever refund a client's fee or offer a complimentary treatment for the future? If so, under what circumstances?
- **Setting Appointments**
  - Do you have regular appointment times available each week?
  - How far in advance do you want to schedule clients?
  - How quickly would you be willing to perform an unexpected appointment?
  - If you are going out of town, how much notice will you give clients?
  - Will you establish days off? What will cause you to make an exception and come in on one of your days off?
  - Will you encourage clients to have standing appointment times so that there is a continuity in scheduling?

Cancellation Policy

- Do you charge for a missed appointment? If so, how much? Full price? Half price?
- Do you require advance notice for cancellation? If so, how far ahead?
- How do you prefer the client contact you if he or she is going to miss an appointment—by text? Phone? E-mail?
- What is your policy if you miss an appointment or are late to an appointment?[5]

 Food for Thought

Have you read policies and procedures documents for other businesses? If so, what did you think of them? What do you think of the businesses that had policies and procedures documents? Do you think your business could benefit from such a document? If so, how?

Establishing Boundaries of Self-Care

Self-care refers to the ability of practitioners to ensure a healthy emotional state, a sound physical state, and the awareness of how self-care affects the practitioners' work. Self-care deals with maintaining a strong and fit physical body, a body that is capable of providing bodywork services in ways that do not cause pain or injury to the practitioner or to the client. In addition, by taking good care of their bodies, practitioners are less likely to become ill, and, therefore, less likely to take time off from work. By setting a boundary for self-care, practitioners can be more available for treatments, and perform better treatments.

If you are not paying attention to the physical nature of the bodywork profession, then you are running the risk of having a short-lived career. This work is demanding on your body. You need to use proper body mechanics, not just while you are working but in all the activities you do, from those of daily living to the types of recreation and sports you participate in. Regular exercise, eating a diet rich in nutrients, receiving regular bodywork yourself, and getting enough sleep to be well rested and energized are other aspects of self-care. In addition to ensuring your best health and strength, clients tend to feel more at ease with practitioners who are modeling health and well-being.

Sometimes practitioners decide to provide treatments on clients who are ill, or to provide treatments if they themselves are ill. Both of these instances are cases of violating boundaries of self-care. They are running the risk of making the clients' conditions worse, spreading disease to other clients or practitioners, and becoming ill themselves.

Emotional self-care is also important. If people decide to become a bodywork practitioner because it seems like an easy job or it would allow them to work out some issues from their past, then this must be addressed as well. Practitioners cannot ethically use the profession, or their clients, as a means to work out unresolved emotional issues. In addition to the ethical concerns, this method does not stand up to the day-to-day demands of being a professional bodywork practitioner. By working on their personal emotional issues, it interferes with the practitioners' ability to connect with their clients and to be present with them, preventing a therapeutic relationship.

Emotionally healthy practitioners are aware if they need professional counseling services and they follow up immediately. If the practitioner is taking medication to help manage any emotional conditions, the practitioner needs to maintain personal and professional boundaries that involve following doctors' orders so they do not risk harming clients.

Certain practitioners who have histories of mental illness may find themselves attracted to the bodywork profession because of its "touchy-feely" aspects. This may be all right as long as the mental illness is under control, and there is no chance that clients will be affected. If, however, these practitioners notice that they are not feeling quite right, or if they are given feedback by supervisors and colleagues about their behavior, then it is important they work with their health-care provider to clarify what is happening to them, and to get appropriate treatment. Again, this is both a personal and professional boundary about self-care that these practitioners need to set for themselves and adhere to.

Developing a Plan for Self-Care

You can develop a plan for self-care by yourself, or with the assistance of a professional who has knowledge and experience in the self-care arena, for example certified personal trainers, nutritional counselors and registered dieticians, psychologists, counselors who specialize in mental and emotional health, and experienced practitioners who have remained healthy and injury free throughout their careers.

No matter how you decide to develop a self-care plan, there are several core concepts that your plan should include:

- Specific goals that you want to accomplish
- An exercise routine—swimming three times a week, walking daily for 30 minutes, stretching each morning and evening.
- A nutrition plan—eating healthy, nutritionally balanced meals each day, drinking eight glasses of water a day.
- A social plan—contacting three friends each week by phone, going out one evening a week with a friend or partner to socialize.
- Alone time—spending 30 minutes a day in quiet reflection, meditation, journaling, soaking in a hot tub or bath, playing with animals, gardening.
- Stretching at work—stretching before and after each session to ensure continued flexibility.
- Proper medical attention—checking in with a health-care provider if dealing with physical, mental, or emotional issues; taking care of medical issues immediately.

Figure 8.2 shows the practitioner's day filled with self-care and the practitioner's day not filled with self-care.

Because everyone is different, self-care plans should be individualized for each practitioner. The purpose is for you to be conscious of the need to create and maintain balance in life. Because some work best in community, it may be helpful for those practitioners to ask friends and family to support them in their efforts to take care of themselves.

Signs of Needing Self-Care

Even with a plan for self-care, sometimes people allow themselves to become overworked and physically, emotionally, and mentally drained. This can also happen when life demands outside bodywork practices increase, or if there are new or unexpected stresses. Ideally, you would always be able to recognize when this is happening. However, the reality is that often people get so caught up in what they need to get done they may not realize that their lives are out of balance and that they are risking burnout, placing bodywork careers at risk.

The following are signs of needing self-care. Use this list as a self-assessment tool to see if there are changes you need to make in your personal and professional life:

- Wake up dreading the day.
- Finding no pleasure or enjoyment in your work.
- Finding yourself grimly doing things just to get them done.

A Day in the Life of a Bodywork Practitioner with Good Self Care Boundaries	
5:30 AM	Alarm goes off
6:00 AM	Swim laps at the gym
7:30 AM	Beakfast of oatmeal, toast and orange juice
	Meditates (15 minutes)
	Checks email
8:30 AM	Arrives at treatment office
	Sets up treatment room
	Stretches for 10 minutes to warm up
9:00 AM	Appointment with Jose (90 minutes)
10:45 AM	Sets up for next client
	Stretches for 3 minutes
11:00 AM	Appointment with Cal (60 minutes)
12:15 PM	Sets up for next client
12:30 PM	Networking Luncheon at the Holiday Inn (60 minutes)
1:50 PM	Stretches for 3 minutes
2:00 PM	Appointment with Willie (60 minutes)
3:15 PM	Has an apple for a mid-afternoon snack
	Stretches for 3 minutes
3:30 PM	Appointment with Fran (60 minutes)
5:30 PM	Cleans up treatment space
	Checks messages and return calls
7:00 PM	Dinner at a friend's house
9:30 PM	Returns home
	Checks email and reviews schedule for tomorrow
10:30 PM	Goes to bed

A Day in the Life of a Bodywork Practitioner with Less than Optimal Self Care Boundaries	
8:00 PM	Alarm goes off
	Hops in the shower
	Has a cup of coffee on the way to the treatment office
8:30 PM	Appointment with Ken (60 minutes)
9:40 PM	Eats a donut for some quick energy
	Sets up for next client
9:45 PM	Appointment with Sayeem (60 minutes)
10:50 PM	Sets up for next client while checking phone messages
11:00 PM	Appointment with Kathy (90 minutes)
12:40 PM	Sets up for next client
	Notices that there are 5 phone messages but does not have time to listen to them
12:50 PM	Gets fast food lunch and eats in the car on the way to the University
1:00 PM	Attends lecture on Complementary Care Class at the University (60 minutes)
2:30 PM	Appointment with Neville (30 minutes)
3:40 PM	Sets up for next client
	Notices that there are now 8 phone messages but does not have time to listen to them
3:45 PM	Appointment with Carleen (60 minutes)
4:55 PM	Sets up for next client
5:00 PM	Appointment with Ana Maria (90 minutes)
6:45 PM	Eats a candy bar for energy while cleaning up treatment space
	Does not have time to check messages and email or return phone calls so decides to do that first thing in the morning
7:00 PM	Home appointment with Jim and Lydia (2.5 hours)
10:00 PM	Meets friends for a late dinner and drinks at a local bar
2:00 AM	Goes to bed

Figure 8.2 Examples of the practitioner's day filled with self-care and the practitioner's day not filled with self-care.

- Feeling like you are dragging yourself through the day.
- Having difficulty focusing.
- Feeling chronically tired.
- Feeling resentful and angry.
- Not remembering why you are doing the work that you are doing.
- Losing a sense of connection to the values that made you want to do bodywork in the first place.
- Feeling depressed.
- Engaging in addictive or compulsive behavior, in other words, constantly looking to a substance or addictive activity for relief from the tedium and/or agony that work or day-to-day life has become.
- Racing thoughts.
- An internal aggressive emotional climate characterized with negative inner talk directed at yourself or outwardly at others.
- Feeling as if there is no time to pause, rest, or slow down, even when something potentially important is at stake.

- Feeling critical of, superior to, or impatient with others.
- Having difficulty listening to others or hearing them out.
- Lashing out at others.
- Finding yourself interacting with others in confrontational and/or sloppy ways that do not seem clear or right.
- Feeling an increased need and/or desire to control the behavior of others.
- Having a decreased willingness or ability to accept feedback about yourself or your work.

Strategies for Nourishing Yourself

If you think you have signs of needing self-care, then it is time to reevaluate your self-care plan. Is it meeting your needs? Is it time to modify it, or even create a new one? Are you honestly following the best that you can? In addition, consider implementing new strategies that can help you nourish yourself.

Get enough sleep. It is not normal to feel tired during the day, even if your days are busy. Experiment to find out how many hours of sleep leave you feeling rested and replenished. If you are having difficulty believing that sleep matters, look into some of the studies that have recently been done into how a deficit of sleep affects mental functioning, weight gain, and the body's ability to fight off disease.

Eat in a manner that gives you energy rather than robbing you of it. Notice what foods and food habits distract you or deplete your energy. Notice what foods and food habits give you energy and leave you feeling healthy, satisfied, and energized. There is much information in the public domain about what constitutes good nutrition, and there is much information about the different food plans that various people and groups have embraced as a path to good health. Use that information, as well as your doctor's recommendations, as a starting place for conducting your own research into what manner of eating is right for you. A good place to start is the U.S. Department of Agriculture's Web site for healthy eating, http://www.choosemyplate.gov

Set aside a day in which you expect nothing of yourself, a day in which the only thing that you ask of yourself is to listen to yourself and do only that which you really want to do. Also set aside a certain amount of time each day, even if it is only 20 minutes, to engage in some activity (or inactivity) that nourishes, relaxes, or energizes you. Experiment with various types of exercise, meditation, creative endeavors, and hobbies until you find those that are the best fit for you. If you cannot find time in your day for this, try getting up earlier in the morning.

Read regularly those writers whose thoughts motivate you, inspire you, or remind you of who you want to be. Develop relationships with people whose words and actions encourage and support you in living by those key values that evoke passion and that encourage a healthy relationship to work. Discuss dilemmas as well as troubling emotions and issues with people who you can trust to listen attentively and to respond in a way that supports you in becoming the person that you want to be.

Make your work your own and enhance your experience of it by reflecting on it during your downtime. Frequently ask yourself what values you want to give expression to. Ask yourself what values you feel passionately about. Write down what comes to mind. Once you have opened this door, keep listening and writing down what comes to you.

Think about how you can infuse your work with those values. Plan what you will do differently. Mentally practice doing your work in a way that implements those values; that is, during quiet times imagine yourself doing your work in a way that is informed by the values that fire you up. Ask yourself what tends to get in the way of doing your work in such a way that it is an expression of that which you value. Make a plan for and imagine yourself sidestepping those obstacles. Cultivate an appreciation of the work itself. See it as its own end rather than simply as the means to an end. Give yourself permission to slow down and direct your full attention to the process of doing the work.

Observe your body's rhythms, work patterns, and habits and, wherever possible, build your workday around what you discover or know to be true about yourself. When do you have the greatest amount of energy and enthusiasm? When do your energy and spirits flag? What approach to work encourages or empowers you? For example, when some people feel resentful about or overwhelmed by the task in front of them, it helps them to break it down into tiny steps. Some people find it helpful to do the most difficult task of the day first thing. Others need to ease into work by starting with the easiest tasks first. Consider how you feel about breaks. Do you benefit from frequent short breaks or breaks that take place less frequently but last longer?

Make regular time for self-care. Afterward, observe how much energy and enthusiasm you have for your work. How do you feel about your work now as opposed to how you felt about it before taking a break? Do you find that the quality of your work improves, stays the same, or suffers in the aftermath of self-care? Does anything about the way you interact with others change? Observe and compare the results you get when you neglect and when you partake of self-care as to get a sense of which best helps you to be the person and worker that you want to be.

Communicating Self-Care at Work

Practitioners will develop an awareness over time that they can do only so much each day at work before their bodies start to "talk back." Paying attention to this awareness and making adjustments can be difficult if practitioners are financially limited and need to work too much just to make ends meet. If this is the case, it could be beneficial for them to reframe the line of thinking that they must take every job that comes their way because they do not know when the next one will come to limiting the number of treatments they do per week to ensure that they will have a long and prosperous career.

It is easy to operate from a place of fear and limitations when people can see only what is right in front of them—rent is due, the cat needs to go to the vet, the car needs repair. However, if this thinking can be reframed to trusting that needs will be met without having to overwork and potentially harming our bodies, then we are valuing our self-care. This will not necessarily be an easy thought process to embrace, particularly if there are school loans to pay back, and a family to support. But you are encouraged to consider this as a means to honor your health and wellness.

Food for Thought

What do you do for self-care now? How do you think these self-care activities benefit you? Are there ways you would like to improve your self-care? What are they?

If you are employed in someone else's business, it is not always possible to set your own schedule in terms of how much you will work. If this is the case, then it would be wise for you to learn how to communicate with your supervisor about what is needed to maintain self-care. This does not mean demanding to perform only a certain number of treatments. Instead, it can mean discussing scheduling at the clinic, and how it affects you. If the supervisor has a valued employee speak to him about the toll the schedule is taking on her ability to be pain free, it is likely he will be willing to listen.

It is possible to negotiate with an employer or supervisor a schedule that is healthy if you have a good work performance history and are presenting your case respectfully. If the workplace cannot accommodate your requests, then you may want to find out if there is a way to split your schedule up so that you have some down time at some point. The bottom line is that the bodywork business owner should not ignore the fact that to be successful, he needs happy and healthy employees. Presenting the business owner or supervisor with a formal and professional request to look at this issue might help you gain what you need.

If the owner or supervisor does not want to listen and tells you, "Deal with it," you may need to consider if this is the best working environment for you. You should keep in mind that it is not professional to leave in the middle of a shift or to denigrate the management at such a time. Other practitioners in the workplace may not be having the same experience as you. Maintaining morale in the workplace is important.

Transference and Countertransference

Through the use of appropriate boundaries, the practitioner sets the **emotional environment,** the atmosphere or energetic sense of the therapeutic relationship, of the treatment session. In other words, it is the sense the client has about the practitioner, and it determines whether she will continue with the session or, on completion of the session, book another appointment with the practitioner. In fact, the emotional environment of a session can even be set or felt during initial contact between the client and practitioner in the phone call to set up an appointment, or in the waiting room as the practitioner approaches the client.

The role of the practitioner is to create a climate or treatment framework that will safely contain whatever occurs in the session, be it an emotional release of joy or sorrow by the client, anger that the client expresses to the practitioner because the treatment plan has not eliminated his pain fast enough, and so forth. Emotionally healthy practitioners understand that their role is to facilitate the therapeutic session in a way that will allow the client a safe place to experience whatever may come up. These practitioners are very clear that their role is not to fix, offer advice, or even soothe clients in a way that will interrupt their expression of emotion. It is the client's work to have the experience and see what will unfold because of it.

During a session, a client may feel, as the result of the emotional environment, a sense of safety, concern from the practitioner, cared for, joy, happiness, satisfaction, warmth, appreciation, gratitude, connection to the treatment and the practitioner, dissatisfaction, nervousness, sadness, grief, annoyance, vulnerability, detachment, or indifference. As can be seen, a broad range of emotions can be experienced.

If you have established clear boundaries for yourself, you will be able to manage most clients' expressions of emotion, and work with them to determine if the session should continue or if it should stop. If the session continues, you should still be able to perform an effective treatment.

The other part of this equation is what you are feeling as you are providing the treatment. The emotional environment depends a great deal on your ability to manage personal and emotional issues so that they do not interfere with client-centered treatments. Practitioners who have a lot of **emotional baggage**—latent, unresolved issues; misguided anger; unrealistic expectations—can find that these issues surface as they work on clients. It may be unconscious or conscious, depending on the practitioner's level of self-awareness and self-accountability. Although it is sometimes impossible to completely separate personal and professional issues, we can learn skills to manage whatever is going on in our personal lives while still functioning professionally. In other words, it is our responsibility to be able to set a professional boundary that prevents personal issues from interfering with the client's treatment experience.

Seeking professional counseling is a step practitioners can take if they question their abilities to be honest with themselves about their personal issues, or if they do not feel confident in their abilities to navigate the emotional landscape of the therapeutic environment. A good measure of self-accountability is the willingness of the practitioner to meet with a professional counselor or a respected mentor for supervision. Being open to such self-inquiry will assist the practitioner in developing skills that will prevent burnout, minimize the probability of violating client boundaries, as well as develop an inner core of knowledge that he is making sound choices that will enhance his abilities to have a successful practice.

Transference

Transference means that a client who has unresolved issues in his past is projecting, or transferring, these issues onto the practitioner. These feelings are usually unconscious. In *The Psychology of the Body* by Elliot Greene and Barbara Goodrich-Dunn, transference is defined as the displacement or transfer of feelings, thoughts, and behaviors originally related to a significant person, such as a parent, onto someone else, such as the massage therapist.[6] These transference-related feelings are typically formed in the client's past and transfer to the present moment, making the practitioner the significant person. The practitioner does not have to say or do anything specific to stimulate this reaction nor can he or she stop it from happening.

The client is said to be in a transference relationship when he is projecting thoughts and feelings onto the practitioner. It will also manifest in the behavior of the client believing that the practitioner should behave in the same way as the person the practitioner reminds him or her of. When this does not happen it can be a cause of confusion for both the client and the practitioner because neither is sure why there are feelings of disappointment in the therapeutic relationship.

Positive transference occurs when the client projects positive feelings or good qualities onto the practitioner.[7] In this case, the unconscious memory the practitioner has inspired in the client is a happy one and brings about good feelings such as respect, joy, and calm. Because the practitioner reminds the client of someone significant, the client may reenact the ways in which he tried to make that person happy or feel loved by that person. Clients exhibiting these behaviors may tell the practitioner many times in one session how much they appreciate the practitioner's work or thank them for making time to see them.

Positive transference may occur if the practitioner reminds the client of his ex-girlfriend with whom he is still in love, and so feels attracted to the practitioner. The client is transferring his feelings for the old girlfriend to the practitioner. The client can display this transference by being overly friendly to the practitioner, and talking with her on familiar terms when he comes in for his appointments.

Initially, positive transference could be seen as a win-win situation for both the client and the practitioner. The client is expressing deep appreciation for the bodywork he is receiving; he does all of the self-care homework assignment between sessions, and his friends call to make appointments. All of this can be very flattering and appealing to the practitioner. You need to stay objective and not let your boundaries change for a client who is overly nice and offers lots of compliments or appears to be manipulating you in some way. Remember, these clients *are not aware* of these transference behaviors. It is your responsibility to be able to recognize it when it happens, to maintain clear boundaries, conduct yourself ethically professionally, and not play into the internal drama or suppressed memory of the client.

Transference can also occur if the client takes an immediate dislike to the practitioner, for no apparent reason. This is an example of negative transference, in which the client assigns negative feelings or bad attributes onto the practitioner.[8]

Consider the following: A client is receiving a treatment from a practitioner he has never seen before and suddenly unexplained thoughts and feelings of anger overwhelm him. Because the client is not aware of any unresolved or unconscious feelings he may have, he assumes the practitioner has done something wrong and is incompetent. The client starts to tell the practitioner how to do the treatment, but each time the practitioner does what the client asks it is not good enough and only makes the client angrier. Eventually he demands that the treatment stop immediately. The practitioner expresses regret that the treatment did not meet the client's needs and leaves the room. When the client leaves the room he looks very uncomfortable, almost ashamed. He apologizes over and over again for his behavior, gives the practitioner a generous tip, and leaves the clinic quickly.

In this situation, the client could experience the treatment only through the lens of negative transference. His feelings were very strong, yet unrelated to the present moment. His only coping mechanism was to react with anger and frustration, followed by shame.

Working with clients who experience negative transference can become complex, because you may not be able to get your client to try another treatment as he or she now equates receiving bodywork with feeling bad. As a bodywork practitioner, you are also limited within your scope of practice about how to deal with this kind of client issue. If you have a client who is projecting all his or her anger onto you, you cannot explore the possibilities of what is causing the transference.

It is safest to remain calm and professional. Do not attempt to delve into what is bringing on the negative transference. If you explore too deeply, not only are you going beyond your scope of practice, you also may be setting the client up for experiencing an emotional release that you do not have the training or the skills to handle professionally. Be smart and be safe. If necessary, terminate the session to ensure the safety and well-being of yourself and your client.

Elliot Greene and Barbara Goodrich-Dunn have identified the following as appropriate responses for bodywork practitioners dealing with transference issues:

- Understand and be aware of transference.
- Understand how transference affects the client.
- Understand how your behavior may affect transference.
- Modify that behavior accordingly and appropriately.
- Avoid building or intensifying the transference.[9]

Countertransference

Countertransference is a defense strategy that bodywork practitioners employ when they have unresolved issues from their past, have perceptions about someone from their personal history, or feelings from their past and are transferring these feelings and thoughts onto the client. It is a system of projections by the bodywork practitioner onto the client and includes the practitioner's reaction to the client's transference onto the practitioner. The emotional attitudes that practitioners have toward clients is what forms countertransference.[10] Often, these practitioners are not aware that this dynamic is present.

What they may experience is either feeling good toward the client, or perhaps disliking the client, depending on the past issues. The practitioner may feel drawn to a particular client and look forward to the weekly session. When the client arrives, there is a long conversation before the treatment begins. The treatment generally runs 10 to 15 minutes over each week because the practitioner wants to offer extra time to the client. Conversely, countertransference can manifest as negative feelings, such as unprovoked anger or resentment, toward a client whom a practitioner has just met.

Countertransference results in the loss of objectivity and the practitioner's ability to clearly see the client's role in his or her own therapeutic process. As a result, the practitioner may not choose the correct treatment plan or not hold the client accountable for her part of the therapeutic process.

Warning signs of possible countertransference include the following:

- Unreasonable dislike of a client
- Overemotional reaction or involvement with a client's troubles
- Liking a client excessively
- Dreading a treatment session with a client

- Undue concern about a client between treatment sessions
- Defensiveness on the part of the therapist
- Being argumentative or impatient with a client
- Indifference or inattentiveness to a client
- Being provocative toward a client
- Feeling angrily sympathetic with a client[11]

Managing Transference and Countertransference

Managing transference and countertransference takes sensitivity and self-awareness. It can be a difficult process, however, because often people are not conscious that transference and countertransference are occurring. Self-awareness is essential to bring unconscious thoughts and feelings to your conscious mind as well as to allow you to learn ways to differentiate whether clients have accurate perceptions of you or are experiencing transference, and whether you have accurate perceptions of clients or are experiencing countertransference.

One strategy for dealing with transference issues is to continue to maintain professional boundaries, and not give the client the idea that her feelings will be returned. If it seems that it might be helpful, you can discuss with the client that you are noticing the issue and offer to talk about it. It is important that the client not be made to feel as if he or she did something wrong. You might say, "I'm flattered that you'd like to have a personal relationship with me outside of my office. However, out of respect for you and all of my clients, I don't socialize with clients because I have found that I can't be as focused when working on friends," or, "I've noticed that you've called me 'Margaret' a few times. Do I remind you of someone named Margaret?"

If, however, the interest by the client seems to have grown into an obsession, the best tack you can take is to discontinue seeing the client and refer her to another practitioner, possibly one who does not work in the same office.

One strategy to manage countertransference is for you to be very alert any time you feel other than professional about a particular client. You might ask yourself, "What makes that client special?" "Why do I want to spend more time with her when I don't feel that way with other clients?" or, "Why do I dislike this person so much when I just met him?" These questions will help you reflect on whether there are any similarities between the client and people in your past relationships.

It may be appropriate for you to discuss the issue with the client if it will diffuse the countertransference without harming the therapeutic relationship. For example, you might say, "Your sense of humor reminds me of my favorite teacher in high school." Often, by stating what the past relationship is, the charge is taken out of the present relationship with the client.

If it would be harmful to the therapeutic relationship, it is wiser for you not to discuss it with the client but explore the issue with an objective person, such as a supervisor, trusted colleague, family member, or mentor. That way, you can gain a different perspective. If that is unsuccessful, you may want to consider professional counseling to sort out the emotional threads of your past and deal with the issues that are arising for you.

The worst thing you can do is not address transference or countertransference issues appropriately. By ignoring the feelings, the situation can escalate until you, the client, or both, do something unethical, or possibly dangerous. By acting on the feelings in an inappropriate manner, you or the client may find yourselves in equally unethical or dangerous situations.

Defining Dual Relationships

Dual relationships are defined as those in which a "professional assumes a second role with a client, becoming friend, employer, teacher, business associate, or family member. The dual relationship may begin before, during, or after the professional relationship."[12] As the definition implies, the roles overlap and occur simultaneously, and there can be an exchange of who is in a position of power or expertise.

In a **multiple relationship,** two people have more than two different roles in a relationship with each other. The relationship can also be called multi-layered, because there are multiple ways that two people can connect with each other, most often on professional, social, or acquaintance levels, depending on how intimate the connection is. Examples of such relationships include family members who are business partners, neighbors who are friends and whose daughter babysits for the other family, students who are in the same class and also work together at a restaurant, a supervisor and an employee who hike together on weekends, a woman who is friends with her sister-in-law, and workout buddies who attend the same religious center. People naturally tend to have multiple relationships, and may not even consider their relationships as being defined by roles.

An **overlapping relationship** (Fig. 8.3) is one in which the two people can shift back and forth between roles, depending on the situation and the factors involved. There can be an overlapping of the professional and the personal roles—the practitioner's client is also a friend with whom the practitioner shares intimate details of her life. Another way an overlapping relationship can occur is between professionals—the practitioner's client is also her accountant. Yet another way is a more complex interaction among professional and personal roles—the practitioner's client, whom she has known for years, is also her accountant and has become a good friend.

Role blending occurs when roles and responsibilities are combined. For example, a parent might also be a business mentor to his adult daughter. In this situation, in addition to being a parent, the person is also a teacher, evaluator, and possibly a supervisor. The same is true for people who choose to homeschool their children. This phenomenon exists when social, family, and professional roles meet.

Different from overlapping relationships, **sequential relationships** occur when one set of roles completely ends before a new set of roles begins. For example, a person starts at an entry-level position in a company, then becomes a manager, then works his way into the position of vice president. The relationships he has with the people at each stage of his career are different, and how the person and the people he works with relate to one another changes as he progresses through the sequence.

Food for Thought

Have you ever met someone you instantly liked or disliked? Why do you think that was? Did the person remind you of someone else?

Food for Thought

Think of all the dual and multiple role relationships you have in your life. How do they overlap? What blended roles do you have with others? Does it surprise you to think of these relationships as dual or multiple roles? Why or why not? How well do you and the other people involved function in the different roles you have with one another?

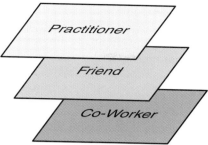

Figure 8.3 An overlapping relationship.

In the bodywork profession, dual or multiple relationships occur when practitioners have two or more roles at the same time or sequentially with a client, relative or friend of the client, other practitioners, other health-care providers, and employers and supervisors. Many bodywork practitioners choose the profession because they enjoy being with people and like the sense of community that can be built with them. For them, the sense of connection extends beyond the treatment room. Because of the intimacy of bodywork, practitioners and clients can also have strong therapeutic relationships, which may naturally carry into the formation of friendships.

Another form of dual relationships is bartering services with others, which practitioners commonly do. For example, a massage therapist may have a client who is a certified public accountant (CPA) and prepares the therapist's taxes each year in exchange for massage. Often practitioners will trade treatments with each other. In this case, the practitioners' multiple roles will be those of colleague, client, practitioner, friend, and possibly mentor to the other.

You always have a choice about dual relationships. You need to carefully consider the consequences of being in a dual relationship, especially one with a client. Therefore, you need to have clarity about your words and actions, and the motivation behind them. You should not just fall into dual relationships with no clear idea of how you got there. The risks of doing so can be enormous. You also need to be aware that there are certain dual relationships you should *never* enter into, such as a sexual relationship with a client.

The very nature of dual relationships raises ethical concerns, including the following:

- Can the boundaries be successfully managed by both the practitioner and the client without damaging the therapeutic relationship?
- What is the motivation behind the practitioner who wants to be in a dual relationship with a client?
- What is the motivation behind the client who wants to be in a dual relationship with the practitioner?
- Can the client be harmed or exploited?
- Would the client expect special care above and beyond what other clients receive because of the dual relationship?

- If the client initiated the possibility of establishing a dual relationship, does the practitioner feel obligated to agree to it out of fear of either losing the client or hurting the client's feelings?
- Would the personal relationship with the client allow the client to think he can dictate the parameters of how the practitioner works with him in terms of time, effort, and compensation?

Because of these ethical concerns, there are differing and conflicting perspectives and viewpoints about the wisdom of entering into a dual relationship with a client. One end of the continuum suggests that it is impossible to avoid dual roles because of the intimate nature of the bodywork profession and the community we live and work in. The opposite end of the continuum states that the intimacy of our profession is exactly the reason dual relationships should be avoided. The intimacy allows for opportunities of exploitation or harm.

Avoiding All Dual Roles

Advocates for avoiding all dual roles state, "Dual relationships tend to impair the therapist's judgment, increasing the potential for conflicts of interest, exploitation of the client, and blurred boundaries that distort the professional nature of the therapeutic relationship."[13] Some people prefer structure and feel safer with hard-and-fast rules that provide clear boundaries and expectations. Therefore, it is very difficult, if not impossible, for them to transition from a professional therapeutic relationship to a dual relationship.

Some feel that because problems are inevitable, it is best not to enter into dual relationships. If a practitioner is not being mindful of her boundaries as well as those of her client, then she can cross them at any time and not notice if an issue arises. Problems will occur for a practitioner who trivializes or disregards his tendency to engage in more than one role with his clients. If it happens on a regular basis in his practice, then he can rationalize that there is no potential for harm and so avoids any responsibility for making a different choice. Consider the following comment: "All my clients are like friends and family to me. Our connection goes beyond the treatment room, which is why I have such intense sessions with my clients. They know I really care about them."

The risk this practitioner is taking is assuming that all clients will want to be considered as friends and family and will be comfortable being in a dual relationship. He is crossing a client's personal boundary by assuming a familiarity that is not necessarily felt by the client. When we do not pick up on our client's cues and assume that he or she wants us to be like friends and family, we are being invasive and potentially harmful to our client's therapeutic process. If a client does not have a solid sense of self, she may go along with the practitioner's agenda. She may offer personal information or engage in intimate conversations that she is not necessarily comfortable with because she does not know how to set a boundary with the practitioner. She is not able to benefit from her bodywork session because she is trying to figure out what the practitioner needs or expects from her and to act accordingly.

Dual or multiple relationships can also occur, and quite often do, between instructors and administrators in bodywork programs and their students because the manner in which bodywork is taught and learned. Because bodywork can be learned only by students actually touching and performing techniques on other people, a certain amount of intimacy is involved. Some bodywork programs require their instructors to receive treatments from students to assess their progress in acquiring skills. Some programs require students to receive treatments from instructors, or even work with a designated instructor, throughout their programs so that the students can feel what professional level skills are like and what they should be striving to achieve.

A blurred boundary could appear in a bodywork program when an instructor socializes with a student outside of school, knowing that it is prohibited but continues to do so. The student is aware that it is prohibited because the student handbook states that it is and, further, the policy has been discussed in class. The student is confused about the reason that the teacher maintains the dual role but does not say anything, both out of respect for the teacher and because it is cool to socialize with a teacher. What is this instructor teaching the student about professionalism and following codes of conduct?

Moderate Viewpoint of Dual Relationships

One cannot deny the intimacy involved in the bodywork profession. It is the human connection with clients that enhances the therapeutic relationship. Dual relationships are complex, but a more moderate viewpoint is that not all dual relationships should be avoided at all times because doing so means that the practitioner is predestined to exploit the client.

There are times when dual roles are unavoidable. Practitioners in small communities may have no other choice but to go to church, bowl, salsa dance, and grocery shop where their clients do. If practitioners are part of an ethnic community in a larger city they may find themselves working, living, shopping, and socializing within a few city blocks. To accommodate these situations and avoid any awkward moments in public, practitioners and their clients may consider having a brief discussion to acknowledge the nature of the dual relationship and perhaps establish some guidelines for behavior. For example, if client and practitioner run into each other at the market, it is fine to say hello, but the practitioner will not ask the client how his psoas is doing in front of his partner. Nor will the client ask to schedule an appointment with the practitioner while standing in line at the movie theater. As simplistic as these examples are, they illustrate the value of clarifying roles and expectations so that both of you will be comfortable when seeing each other in public.

Your job as professionals is to keep the boundaries intact as you thoughtfully engage in a blended relationship. The keys to navigating dual relationships are awareness and motivation. When dual relationships are entered into, you are accountable at all times to manage the professional tone and limits of the therapeutic relationship.

The dual relationship should not be entered into because you think you can get something from a client or a client wants to get something from you. When you are clear and honest about your reasons for being interested in a client beyond the therapeutic relationship, it makes it easier to discern if the dual relationship is appropriate. It also allows for a conversation to take place between you and your client to discuss the ramifications, rather than just falling into the dual relationship and hoping for the best.

The "falling into" the dual role is where problems arise for practitioners. Some can fool themselves into believing that they and a client were meant to be friends, or that somehow this person came to their practice for a reason, and then move right into a dual role without considering the ramifications. Once the glow of the newfound friendship wears off or there is a disagreement, then the therapeutic relationship is affected, usually quite seriously.

Some questions you may ask yourself when contemplating a dual relationship include the following: What is my motivation for engaging in a dual relationship with this client? What will I gain? Lose? What will my client gain? Lose? Is it more appropriate to end the therapeutic relationship and begin a person friendship? Is it possible to do both?

You should be aware of your intellectual, emotional, and mental status as well as that of the client to assess if there is balance in maturity and stability. You will meet fascinating and brilliant people in this profession. However, do you tend to get "starry eyed" by a certain personality type and become charmed, thus making you more susceptible to engaging in a dual role without discernment? The reverse is also true. You will have clients who come to you in great need of being heard and valued. Can you provide that for them without being compelled to be a friend as well?

As stated previously, practitioners and clients always have a choice about whether to pursue a dual relationship. Ideally, the choice begins with the client saying that he or she is interested in pursuing a dual relationship, but sometimes it occurs slowly over time, and suddenly you find yourself in a dual relationship. The moment you recognize that you have a different connection with one client than with others, it is your responsibility to bring that feeling out into the open for discussion and clarification. This does not have to be an intense conversation, but one that simply acknowledges what you have noticed and that you seek clarification.

Consider the following:

Rooney has been seeing Kara for weekly Thai massage treatments for 8 months at her studio. As she was preparing the treatment room today, Kara realizes she is looking forward to seeing Rooney because she has lots of questions about the martial arts class he teaches. During the past 2 months he has been sharing with her the similarities between the work she is doing in his treatments and the classes he teaches. Last week, Rooney and Kara talked for 45 minutes after his session was over about these similarities. At the time, it did not seem out of place to spend so much time talking to him. However, Kara noticed that she does not have the interest or the invitation to talk with any of her other clients at such length. She is concerned about moving into a dual relationship so she decides to bring it up with Rooney. She does not want to give him the impression that she is taking advantage of his time by questioning him about his work. She is acknowledging her awareness of how things are different with Rooney as compared with her other clients.

Risks and Benefits of Dual and Multiple Relationships

In an ideal world, everyone would be able to have any number of relationships. They would always be certain of their intentions; power in the relationship would never be abusive; and there would always be direct communication about the relationships so there would be no misunderstandings, hurt feelings, or even harm. Because this ideal world does not exist, it is necessary that you have the resources and the ability to make intelligent decisions about whether to enter into a certain multilayered relationship, to evaluate the pros and the cons of being in such a relationship, and, sometimes most important, to know when to end a multilayered relationship that is no longer beneficial or useful or that has even become harmful in some manner.

Benefits

One benefit of a dual relationship is that it can enhance the therapeutic or professional relationship. For example, by having a dual relationship with another practitioner, there is the possibility of experiencing a new bodywork modality, receiving support in a project, gaining networking opportunities, receiving technique tips and advice, and having companionship at continuing education events.

In a dual relationship with a client who has become a friend, the therapeutic relationship can be enhanced because you know the client on a more personal level. Perhaps you play sports together so you understand how the client's body moves and where she has restrictions and muscle tightness, and so you can tailor treatments to be more specific to her needs. If you and your client talk about your families, then you will most likely understand the client's style of communication better, know if certain family events are likely to cause stress in her body, and can suggest optimal times for her to receive a treatment.

Benefits should exist for all the people involved in the dual and multiple relationships. In other words, everyone should gain something—for example, a discounted rate for treatments in return for a discounted rate for a haircut, or reduced rates for professional accounting services that are comparable to reduced rates for bodywork treatments. Whatever the benefits are, they should not be at the expense of the other people involved.

Potential benefits, however, can only enrich dual and multiple relationships when all the people involved understand the differing roles in the relationships, and are willing and able to handle the roles with clarity. Dual and multiple relationships work best only when both parties are able and willing to have direct and honest conversations about needs, wants, expectations, and desires. Once these issues are worked out, everyone involved may be open to gaining some incredible experiences.

Risks

Dual and multiple relationships have the potential to impair the practitioner's judgment and increase the chance of conflicts of interest and exploitation of the client. Chapter 6 discusses the concepts of power differences and in this chapter, transference and countertransference. These factors are especially magnified in dual relationships. Because the power differential is increased in dual relationships, there might be a power shift that supports the development of transference and countertransference.

The power differential can be increased in a dual relationship because professionals come into the therapeutic relationship with greater power because of their training, knowledge, expertise, and credentials, as well as the fact that the client is paying for the practitioner's service. Therefore, when there is a shift to a dual relationship, which should be one that has more equality of power, it takes time to find a way to navigate a balance. If the client had come to the practitioner in a lot of pain, and eventually that pain was relieved with the help of the practitioner, then it is possible the client will elevate the practitioner to the status of "miracle worker" or "healer." Therefore, instead of a balance in the dual relationship, the practitioner still has a greater amount of power. In addition, being given a title of "miracle worker" or "healer" makes it hard to shift out of the position of greater power.

Some practitioners like and even cultivate this disproportionate distribution of power. This can manifest in a preference for clients who are passive and willing to give their power to the practitioner. Such clients typically say, "Whatever you think is best. You're the professional," rather than assuming their part of the responsibility for the therapeutic relationship. The more roles a practitioner has with clients, the more power the practitioner may acquire in the therapeutic relationship, which can lead to a client feeling even less powerful.

There is also the unconscious impact of transference and countertransference that both the client and the practitioner must become aware of and discuss. If these issues remain unconscious, it is likely that the power differential will be subtle and have some impact on the relationship. This is the case when a client and a practitioner try to transition to a friendship but there always seems to be something that puts the relationship back in the client and practitioner dynamic.

There is also the possibility that no matter how much discussion takes place, and no matter how aware both client and practitioner are of the transference and countertransference issues, one or both of them cannot make the emotional shift to equalize the power differential. When this is the case, it is best to acknowledge this immediately, end the dual relationship, and resume the initial therapeutic relationship if possible. It may be that one of the parties is too disappointed that it did not work out and choose to terminate all relationships entirely. This may be a wise solution because it allows both parties to learn from the experience and not feel compelled to force a relationship that no longer meets the needs of either one.

Sometimes the practitioner and the client become enmeshed in an unhealthy way. If boundaries are unclear and not maintained with forethought and foresight, the therapeutic relationship can become strained or even disintegrate. The people involved may experience varying levels of frustration, anger, and sadness. Other losses may be financial, educational, social, or personal.

Sometimes the person who has or will have more power in a dual or multiple relationship does not see that there is any harm, even though the person in the more vulnerable position is actually being taken advantage of. For example, in a situation in which there is a difference in age or level of expertise, there is the risk that the person with more experience or expertise, in short, the one who has more power, could take advantage of the other person by manipulating the terms of an agreement, making changes in the terms without regard to the other person, or having unrealistic expectations of the other person while not having the same level of accountability for themselves.

There can be a risk that the people involved did not foresee that one would become dissatisfied with the arrangement and not know how to discuss it with the other person. For example, it may seem that at the beginning the arrangement will be mutually satisfying because both parties involved think they have the same expectations and that they will each meet those expectations in the same way. However, this does not always happen, even if they discuss the parameters of the dual relationship in what they think is the clearest manner possible.

For example, two practitioners who work in the same office decide to trade weekly treatments for 4 months while they are learning craniosacral therapy. As they proceed through their training, one of them is learning at a faster rate than the other, and is becoming more proficient. This practitioner becomes dissatisfied with the other practitioner's treatments. At the end of 4 months the second practitioner asks to continue the trades. The first practitioner says no, without any further explanation. Now, whenever they see each other at work, the second practitioner barely speaks to the first, who is upset and confused by this. He has no idea why the second practitioner is behaving this way.

Resentments or regrets build and interfere with the relationship, and it may be lost entirely. It is important that all people involved be fully aware of what each has to offer in the dual or multiple role, be willing to be accountable, and be willing to hold the others accountable as well, at all times.

In dual relationships that involve practitioners and family members, there is always the risk of creating stress among family members that may get in the way of the professional service that is being shared. For example, family members often have unreasonable expectations of one another based on unspoken family rules. These might include the following:

- Family should never have to pay full price for treatments.
- Family should come before other clients.
- Family should not have to wait for an appointment.
- Practitioners should be available to give treatments anywhere at any time, such as at family functions or while on vacations together.

Many of the unrealistic expectations can be avoided by discussing them ahead of time and making sure there is an agreement on what to expect from you and what is expected from family members. To avoid these issues altogether, some practitioners choose to adopt a policy of not working on family members at all. They have a referral list ready when a family member wants to book an appointment.

It is sometimes hard to change or even end dual and multiple relationships when they are no longer satisfying or useful because of fear of hurting the other person's feelings. Therefore, rather than risk that, some people choose to stay in the relationship and become resentful.

Box 8.1 provides valuable information you can use to determine if your boundaries are at risk in a dual or multiple relationship.

Risk Assessment

Psychologist Michael C. Gottlieb created a decision-making model for assessing the level of risk present when deciding whether or not to engage in a

| Box 8.1 | **FIFTEEN WARNING SIGNS THAT BOUNDARIES ARE AT RISK IN A DUAL OR MULTIPLE RELATIONSHIP** |

1. Feeling overwhelmed by a person
2. Allowing someone to take as much as they can from you
3. Not noticing when someone displays inappropriate boundaries
4. Not noticing when someone invades your boundaries
5. Accepting food, gifts, or touch that you don't want
6. Touching a person without asking
7. Going against personal values or rights to please others
8. Falling in love with anyone who reaches out
9. Letting others direct your life
10. Letting others define you or describe your reality
11. Experiencing feelings of dread at the thought of having to work on a certain person
12. Believing you can anticipate others' needs
13. Believing others can anticipate your needs
14. Falling apart so someone can take care of you
15. Not saying no because you dread the consequences

dual relationship.[14] This model is based on the use of three dimensions that are basic and critical to the ethical decision-making process. These dimensions involve the roles that power differential, duration of the therapeutic relationship, and clarity of termination play on evaluating the level (low, medium, or high) of risk of a dual or multiple relationships. These three components are considered in risk assessment because they are influential factors of the depth of the therapeutic relationship. In fact, these three components are present in varying degrees in all professional relationships.

The power differential takes into account how much separation the two parties perceive between each other. If there is a large power differential, then the risk of causing harm in the relationship is higher because the client places so much power in what the professional says and does that he does not trust his own power. If the power differential were minimal, then the risk would be minimal, because neither party places the other in a superior position.

The duration of the therapeutic relationship provides perspective on how much time has been invested in the therapeutic relationship. If a practitioner has only one or two sessions with a client, then the risk of having problems is minimal as opposed to the client a practitioner sees once a week for several years. The more time you spend with a client, the more information you acquire about him and vice versa. This allows for more opportunities for misunderstandings or getting involved in situations that feel more obligatory chosen. For example, this can happen with a client's appointment time. If than the client has a long-standing appointment on a certain day and time, it may be hard to change it as he may feel proprietary about that appointment time.

You must consider the process in which the client is terminated from services. When it is clear-cut and you know that it is the last time you will see a particular client, you are very clear about where you stand with him. When the client has intermittent appointments with you, you do not know exactly when he will be scheduling them. If you never know when a client may call for an appointment, whenever you see him, in any setting, you must always be mindful not to engage in any behavior or conduct that would reflect poorly on you in the eyes of this client. Until there is a formal termination, there will always be a risk of creating a difficult situation with a client in a dual relationship.

You can use the factors listed in Figure 8.4 when thinking about entering a dual or multiple relationship to determine what investment you have in the therapeutic relationship with the client. Do you have history with this client over a long enough period of time so that you can trust each other? Are you committed to the client on an appropriate level beyond the therapeutic relationship? In other words, have the two of you shared enough history to feel safe in developing another layer in the relationship?

For example, you have performed treatments on a long-term client for more than a year. During that time a level of intimacy and trust has developed because of meeting treatment goals, hearing about the client's personal life, and perhaps sharing in some of the client's life transitions such as the death of a loved one or the joy of getting a new job. The client has also shared in events in your life such as expanding your business, completing a

---

Risk Assessment and Dimensions of the Therapeutic Relationship

Power differential: Assess your level of influence on your client

Low	Does the client see you as a peer? Your client views you as a professional doing the job you are trained to do. The client has no emotional investment in you. The client is simply coming to you to receive a needed service.
Medium	Are you viewed as an expert in your field? Your client is influenced by your expertise and knowledge about the human body as well as your therapeutic skills to help the client's health and well being. The client respects and trusts your professional credentials and will follow your recommendations without hesitation.
High	Do you have an extreme amount of personal influence over the client? Your client has expressed the fact that it is not only your professional expertise that he admires but also your personal perspectives, opinions and thoughts on many topics. Your client may not make decisions for himself, but rather asks what you would do if you were in his situation and follows your advice.

Duration of the therapeutic relationship: Assess your history with the client

Low	Brief — one or a few sessions with the client
Medium	Intermediate — regular sessions over a limited amount of time to accomplish a treatment goal.
High	Long — continuous sessions on a weekly or monthly basis for several years.

Clarity of termination: Assess the likelihood that you and your client will have further professional contact. The client always has the right to renew the professional relationship in the future.

Low	Specific — the therapeutic relationship is set for a specific time and the end of the relationship is clearly stated either by ending the sessions or referring the client to another practitioner
Medium	Uncertain — the treatment plan is completed, but there is still a possibility that the client may return at some point in the future
High	Indefinite — There is no discussion or agreement of when or if termination will take place. It may be a long term client, but the frequency of appointments fluctuates.

Figure 8.4 Risk assessment and dimensions of the therapeutic relationship. *Adapted from Gottlieb, M.C.: Avoiding Exploitive Dual Relationships: A Decision-Making Model, 1993. Retrieved 7 September 2010 from http://kspope.com/dual/gottlieb.php*

second certification program, or having a baby. Sharing milestones such as these increases the level of intimacy because the client and you are both willing to be vulnerable to each other, you have treated each other with respect, and you both have formed a bond of trust.

To assist you in defining what the appropriate parameters for healthy dual and multiple relationships are, you and the other people involved should ask yourselves the following questions:

- What do I have to gain, and what do the other people involved have to gain, by entering into this relationship?
- What do I have to lose, and what do the other people involved have to lose?
- Is there a strong need or emotional component for me or the other people involved attached to entering into the dual or multiple relationship? What are my instincts telling me? If there is a strong need or emotional component tied in, the relationship has a high risk factor, and it may not be the best choice for the people involved.
- Can the dual or multiple relationship cause harm to anyone—myself, to any of the other people involved, to people all of us are associated with?
- Whose needs are being met, mine or the other people's? If there is a lack of awareness or concern about the impact of the relationship on the others involved, then it means you are willing to take advantage of them, which is highly unethical.
- What level of intimacy would be required? Is this level within the bounds of professionalism, or does it go against the profession's code of ethics?
- Who will be responsible for what in the relationship?
- Where does accountability lie? Who is accountable for what in the relationship? If it is unclear or uneven, or if the other people involved are unwilling or unable to discuss this issue, then that is a sign that the dual or multiple role is not a good choice.
- What are the expectations those involved hold?
- How well do we know each another?
- What is the level of trust between us?
- How will the power differences change? Will one person have a disproportionate amount of power?
- Will the therapeutic relationship be enhanced, hampered, or unchanged?
- Will this be a mutually satisfying arrangement?
- Does everyone involved have enough wisdom and self-confidence to handle the shifts in intimacy levels and power differentials while stepping in and out of the various roles, and any other challenges that may come up?
- Is there an exit strategy if the relationship proves to be unworkable? Am I willing to take it?
- What are the consequences of not taking part? What are the possible ways the others could respond if I choose not to participate? It takes skill and sometimes courage to choose not to enter into a dual or multiple relationship, even though that is the right thing to do.
- Can I evaluate the dual or multiple role objectively? This is the most important question. A red flag that you should be on the look out for

is how intense your desire is to have multilayered relationships with clients. Are you not getting social or emotional needs met by friends or family? Are you thinking of using the client base as a place to find friends and dates? Do you feel empowered by the power differential and see the dual or multiple role as a way to maintain that sense of power or respect?

All of these questions are best discussed between and among all of those involved. This can be done as a face-to-face brainstorming session initially, and, if warranted, then certain crucial points can be documented for referral as the relationship progresses. The conversation should take place rather easily. If it does not, perhaps it is not the right time to enter into this relationship, or perhaps the relationship would involve the wrong people.

Accountability is one of the most important factors in participating in dual or multiple relationships. Each person must be committed to and in alignment with what they want to offer and what they want to receive in the relationship. Ideally, all the people involved will have ongoing discussions to monitor how the relationship is working and how everyone is feeling about it. Each person should also periodically spend time in self-reflection to see where they are in the present moment regarding the dual or multiple relationship. These regular times of reflection helps prevent resentments from building up, and can help people identify when something needs to be discussed or changed sooner rather than later.

Defining Appropriate Parameters

If you do decide to enter into a dual relationship, you must be careful to clearly define appropriate boundaries for the relationship. You must not equate dual or multiple relationships with getting something for free or with giving away things for free. Place a high value on your work and contributions to the community. Conversely, you should not ask, "What's in it for me?" for every interaction and connection. If you do, you will place your personal needs above the needs of your clients, choosing to have more than one role with clients to meet your own financial, social, or emotional needs.

Thus you need to carefully assess the risk for conflicts of interest, loss of objectivity, and impact on the therapeutic relationship. All people involved must understand the complexities involved and take equal responsibility for the establishment, continuation, and, if necessary, termination of any part of the dual or multiple relationship. However, keep in mind that you, as the professional practitioner, are ultimately held accountable because you should be aware of the complexities of dual and multiple roles and ethical considerations involved. You need to behave ethically in all aspects of the roles and to trust that the other people involved will behave ethically as well. If this does not happen, then you need to be able to hold yourself and the others accountable.

It is important to have some strategies available when contemplating engaging in a dual relationship. One important strategy is to think through possible stumbling blocks before they occur, then build safeguards into your practice. This preparation will allow both you and the client to be mindful of the fact that you are in a dual role relationship and be proactive about minimizing risks. Some measures to minimize risks inherent in dual relationships include the following:

- Maintaining healthy boundaries from the outset.
- Securing the informed consent of clients and discussing with them the potential risks and benefits.
- Remaining willing to talk with clients about any potential problems or conflicts that may arise.
- Seeking supervision or consulting with other professionals when dual relationships become particularly problematic or when the risk for harm is high.
- Documenting any dual relationships in client files.
- Referring clients to another professional, when necessary.[15]

It is also helpful to consider the following summary of themes surrounding multiple roles in therapeutic relationships, compiled by psychologists Herlihy and Corey, for the mental health field:

- All professional codes of ethics caution practitioners about the potential exploitation in dual relationships, and more recent codes acknowledge the complex nature of these relationships.
- Not all multiple relationships can be avoided, nor are they necessarily always harmful.
- Multiple role relationships challenge us to monitor ourselves and to examine our motivations for our practices.
- Whenever you consider becoming involved in a dual or multiple relationship, seek consultation from trusted colleagues or a supervisor.
- Few absolute answers exist to neatly resolve dual or multiple relationship dilemmas.
- The cautions for entering into dual or multiple relationships should be for the benefit of the clients or others rather than to benefit the practitioner.
- In determining whether to proceed in a dual or multiple relationship, consider whether the potential benefit outweighs the potential harm. To the extent possible, include the client in making this consideration.[16]

Mutual and equal consent to all aspects of the dual or multiple relationship is necessary for all the people involved. Practitioners should be aware that sometimes this can be incredibly difficult to navigate. Thus practitioners need to educate clients about both potential benefits and risks of the relationship, whether it is one initiated by the practitioner or the client. If the primary concern is that the therapeutic relationship not be changed, then a dual or multiple relationship may be too risky and should not be entered into. Practitioners should also be aware that sometimes merely the suggestion of a dual or multiple relationship can change how the people involved relate to each other.

Consider the following:

Vanessa and Diego worked together at the Healing Arts Center for 3 years. During that time they were excellent work companions. They shared a work ethic by showing up early for their shifts to prepare the treatment rooms, turning on the heaters for the heat packs, and making sure the lobby was presentable for the clients. Vanessa told Diego several times it had always been a dream her to own her own business and hire employees.

Eventually she is able to do this. She includes Diego in the planning, invites him to see the progress, and consults him on ideas. However, Diego always defers to Vanessa, saying, "Whatever you think will be fine. I'm just happy you asked me to work for you," to which Vanessa replies, "Diego, you'll work *with* me, not *for* me!"

When the office opens, Diego starts showing up just a couple of minutes before his shifts and leaves soon after. He does not keep up his end of the cleaning schedule, does not cover shifts he has agreed to cover, and continually misses meetings, saying he forgot about them. Vanessa terminates Diego from his position. He leaves without incident, but the two of them never speak again.

When a dual or multiple relationship a practitioner has with a client evolves more into a friendship than just the therapeutic relationship, it may be time to end the therapeutic relationship, refer the client to another practitioner for treatments, and continue developing the friendship.

Practitioners should support clients' freedom of choice in whether they want to enter into dual or multiple relationships. Everyone involved needs to make informed decisions, and have a realistic view. Practitioners should never tell clients that having dual or multiple roles will not affect the therapeutic relationship. In addition, relationships are fluid, and what may have once seemed like a good idea no longer is. Therefore, all people involved need to have the freedom to choose to end the dual or multiple roles at any time.

Dual Roles to Avoid

Certain types of dual relationships are never ethical or appropriate to enter into. The risks are so high and the benefits so low that the relationship is unjustified. For example, a practitioner should never have a sexual relationship with a client. Not only is doing so against the codes of ethics for bodywork practitioners, the intimacy involved in this type of relationship blurs and can even destroy the professional boundaries required for the therapeutic relationship with the client. If the practitioner is being paid by the client for bodywork, this can be construed as prostitution.

Another type of dual relationship that is highly risky and against most codes of ethics is lending money to or borrowing money from clients. Because most people have an emotional attachment to their money, lending or borrowing it can also blur or even destroy the professional boundaries required for the therapeutic relationship with the client. Part of being a professional practitioner is to be self-responsible and self-accountable for finances, and to maintain professional distance from clients' finances.

Box 8.2 lists dual roles that practitioners should avoid at all costs. As you can see, engaging in sexual behavior is first on the list, situations that can be emotionally charged are next, and the rest involve the exchange of money.

Strategies for Managing Dual and Multiple Relationships

Wisdom is the hallmark of successful dual and multiple relationships because it allows all people involved to act with integrity and respect when there are

| **Box 8.2** | **DUAL ROLES THAT PRACTITIONERS SHOULD AVOID AT ALL COSTS** |

- Engaging in sexual behavior, innuendo, and jokes
- Shared emotional venting about family members when they are also clients of yours
- Political discussions
- Lending or borrowing money
- Real estate deals
- Business deals
- Renting office space/home/apartment from clients or to clients
- Providing child care for client's children or client providing for you
- Having a client cater/photograph/organize an important life event such as a wedding, baptism, bar mitzvah, or anniversary party

challenges within the relationship. This means that rather than discontinue all the relationships, the people involved strive to find resolutions that will benefit the primary relationship, make necessary changes in the secondary relationship to preserve the primary relationship, or make changes in the primary relationship to preserve the secondary relationship. Two people meet as client and practitioner but soon discover an attraction to each other and a desire to pursue a romance. Instead of choosing to pursue an unethical dual relationship, the professional relationship is discontinued to allow for a personal relationship to grow.

Ideally, both the practitioner and the client will discuss and create parameters they both agree on. This will provide a sense of safety and clarity of behaviors because both had a voice in what was acceptable and what was not. One of the primary parameters is that the professional therapeutic relationship ends and the practitioner refers the client to another professional so that the romance or the attraction can be pursued.

If the romance ends, or the attraction is fleeting, it is not recommended that the people involved return to a therapeutic relationship. Because of the emotions involved, it is quite difficult to "turn back the clock" to how things were before the intimate relationship started. The most appropriate response is for the practitioner to be professional, maintain boundaries, and not have the former love become a client again.

As has been discussed, making the choice to engage in a dual or multiple relationship should take time and consider the pros and cons of the decision. You should choose actively and not enter into one because a client has invited you and you do not know how to say no or you think saying no will endanger the professional relationship.

For example, there are instances in which practitioners have been known to suffer through endless dinners or social gatherings because they do not trust the professional relationship will stand if the invitation to socialize is turned down. Consider Zorah. She once bought vitamins from one of her clients even though she did not intend to use them because she was afraid the client would stop receiving treatments from her. Zorah went on to justify her choice by saying, "It was the least I could do because the client gets weekly massages from me, and the vitamins lasted for four weeks." This is an example of a practitioner not valuing the therapeutic relationship as it is, and believes that she must reinforce it by accommodating her client's request to buy vitamins. You must be very solid in the belief that your professional expertise is enough to sustain the therapeutic relationship. Taking on a dual role in an effort to please a client undermines the intent of the therapeutic relationship.

The following is an example of how you might respond to a client who invites you to buy products that you are not interested in:

"Thank you so much for telling me about the supplements you're selling and offering them to me at a discount. I'm glad that you're getting positive results from taking them but I'll pass on purchasing any from you, although I'm glad that you are selling a product that you believe in."

This response allows you to express gratitude for the offer of a discount and acknowledge the client's success and passion for the product while declining the offer. You do not need to justify why you will not make a purchase from the client. If the client insists on a yes or on an explanation, then you have another choice to make:

- Can I politely and respectfully decline a client's offer without making a judgment about the product? If the client is persistent, do I want to address the fact that she is not respecting my choice or do I just keep saying no?

Here is another example of a polite refusal to enter into a dual relationship:

- "Kay, it would be great to meet for coffee but I need you to know that I only see my clients at the office during scheduled appointments. I've found that I'm better able to focus on the therapeutic needs of my clients when I don't have a connection with them outside of the office."

This response to an invitation for coffee lets the client know that you do not socialize with any clients outside of the office so that you can maintain your focus on the therapeutic aspects of the relationship. This statement also lets the client know that all clients are given this response so the client will know it is not a personal rejection. If a client is not respectful of this limit and tries to force the issue, then that is more information for you to consider when speaking with this client. Do you want to work with someone who is not respecting your boundaries?

Successful Dual and Multiple Relationships

Successful dual and multiple relationships happen when everyone involved understands the power differentials inherent in the different roles, and do not see them as a means to gain power over others or, conversely, to let go of personal power and be taken care of. In these situations, there are levels of wisdom and self-accountability that ensure a productive structure to the relationships, as well as the means to navigate the terrain of the relationships. Each person involved maintains his or her own sense of self, does not take advantage of the other's, and has the interpersonal skills to communicate directly about the relationship. Each person is able to articulate what he or she is responsible for in the relationship and what the expectations are from himself and the others and has the skills to resolve conflict so that it does not endanger the various layers of relationship.

 Food for Thought
Have you entered into a dual or multiple relationship because you were afraid of what you might lose if you did not? How did you feel in the relationship? Did you communicate your feelings about the situation with the other person or people involved? Why or why not? What would you like to have done differently?

🦉 Words of Wisdom

Once the relationship between massage therapist and client has moved beyond the treatment room, it is forever changed; there is no backing over that threshold. Several areas of potential discomfort exist: as a health professional, you possess medical information about your client/friend that an "ordinary" friend would not. As a businessperson, you charge a fee for time spent with your client/friend. As a receiver of confidences, you walk the knife's edge of appropriateness in your responses, perhaps rendering them inadequate for either client or friend. It can be done, though. My two closest friends now were clients first. It was after only five years had passed, however, and with a snail's pace of progression that we crossed the threshold. My best advice? Move slowly, examine the basis for this relationship very carefully (similar liking for Greek food, scrapbooking, or Chinese films? Having crazy ex-spouses?), and decide before crossing the threshold which relationship, client or friend, matters the most to you. In the time to come, a choice may have to be made.

—Julie Goodwin, ba, Licensed Massage Therapist in private practice since 1987, certified Craniosacral Therapist since 1997, bodywork instructor since 1999

The following is an example of a dual role relationship that embodies these characteristics:

David and Padma have been friends for several years. When Padma completed her shiatsu training, David offered her an office in the building he owns in exchange for four treatments a month, and light housekeeping duties for the other tenants in the building. Before Padma agreed to this offer she and David met to discuss the details of this arrangement. Padma asked David to write down specifically what she was expected to do each week for the light housekeeping duties. She asked David to list each office and what chores were to be done in each, where the cleaning supplies were kept, who was responsible for restocking the cleaning supplies, what schedule the cleaning should follow, and what aspects of the cleaning were negotiable if Padma became busy with her practice. Padma also asked David to make a schedule for his four treatments. She asked David to be specific about the day and time and who would be receiving the treatments. Would it always be David or would it be someone of David's choosing? She also asked what contingency plan David would like to follow if Padma was unable to keep one of the scheduled appointments. David and Padma negotiated a 6-month trial period to see if the arrangement worked. In addition, they agreed to have a phone conversation every other Monday morning to discuss David's satisfaction with Padma's services, and for Padma to give feedback on how she was doing with her cleaning tasks. Finally, they both agreed that there would be 30 days' notice if either one of them decided that this arrangement was no longer viable. All of these agreements were compiled in a written document signed by the both of them.

The reason this dual relationship is likely to be successful is that both David and Padma discussed the arrangement and had input into implementing it. There are also very specific requests made of each of them to delineate exactly what they were each responsible for, and what the timeline was for completion of each component. There was acknowledgment that there might be times that the agreement would need to be adjusted and a plan to do so was arranged. Throughout the entire process both David and Padma were fully engaged and took ownership over what was being created.

Asking for Help

Codes of ethics and codes of conduct can provide some guidelines for you to manage dual and multiple relationships successfully, but there is no substitute for good judgment, being willing to self-reflect about your actions, and being aware of how personal motivations can affect the relationships. Sometimes, however, practitioners may be confused or unsure of themselves and whether entering into a dual or multiple relationship is a good choice or, if they are already in this type of relationship, are having trouble evaluating it. In this case, it may be helpful for you to talk to a trusted friend, colleague, or mentor. The ideal person to ask for help would have experience supervising others, especially in the bodywork profession. Talking with someone outside the relationship may help you gain perspective, and be able to see the whole picture. Asking for help can be especially useful in evaluating dual or multiple relationships if you suspect you have made an error in judgment, and are unsure of what you should do next.

To navigate dual and multiple relationships successfully, refer to Box 8.3.

Ending a Dual Relationship

When is it time to call it quits? How much effort should you put into a dual relationship before the lack of return becomes too much? The answers to these questions, of course, depend on the situation, but the following are some guidelines that may assist you in deciding whether to stay in a dual or multiple relationship:

- What was the original intention of the dual relationship and is that intention still being met? For example, did you originally want to do a monthly trade with a colleague because you could not afford to pay for treatments? Now that you have the income to pay for treatments, do you want to experience other practitioners' work?
- Are you getting out of the dual relationship as much as you are putting in? For example, are you always on time to provide your accountant with his massage treatment, yet he had to file an extension for your taxes because of his lack of organization?
- Do you still have the time to participate in the dual relationship? For example, when you were starting to build your practice, did you have a lot of time on your hands to offer free chair massage at your gym in

---

| **Box 8.3** | **TEN KEY THEMES SURROUNDING MULTIPLE ROLES IN BODYWORK** |

1. Multiple relationship issues affect virtually all bodywork practitioners, regardless of their work setting or clientele.

2. All professional codes of ethics caution practitioners about the potential exploitation in dual relationships, and more recent codes acknowledge the complex nature of these relationships.

3. Not all multiple relationships can be avoided, nor are they necessarily always harmful.

4. Multiple role relationships challenge us to monitor ourselves and to examine our motivations for our practices.

5. Whenever you consider becoming involved in a dual or multiple relationship, seek consultation from trusted colleagues or a supervisor.

6. Few absolute answers exist to neatly resolve dual or multiple relationship dilemmas.

7. The cautions for entering into dual or multiple relationships should be for the benefit of our clients or others served rather than to protect ourselves from censure.

8. In determining whether to proceed with a dual or multiple relationship, consider whether the potential benefit outweighs the potential for harm. To the extent possible, include the client in making this consideration.

9. It is the responsibility of bodywork educational programs to introduce boundary issues and explore multiple relationship questions. It is important to teach students ways of thinking about alternative courses of action.

10. Bodywork educational programs have a responsibility to develop their own guidelines, policies, and procedures for dealing with multiple roles and role conflicts within the program.

Adapted from Corey, G., Corey, M.S., and Callanan, P.: *Issues and Ethics in the Helping Professions*, ed. 7. Stamford, CT, Brooks/Cole Cengage Learning, 2007, pp 269–270.

exchange for advertising and referrals? Now, however, all of your appointments are booked and you could use an afternoon off.

• Are you still invested in the dual relationship or do you want to have just one relationship with this person? For example, ever since you started trading shiatsu treatments with your friend, do you feel disappointed that all you ever talk about is bodywork, and what she wants you to work on the next time you meet? Do you miss going to the movies together and talking about your lives, and now it feels as if you are more colleagues than friends?

Perhaps by asking yourself these questions or noticing how present you are when in the company of the person you are in a dual or multiple relationship with will help you make a determination about whether you want to change the relationship or not. You may discover that the exchange needs to be altered to accommodate the changes that have occurred since the arrangement began, or perhaps the relationship has run its course entirely. Whatever the decision, you have the responsibility to communicate with the other people involved in a timely fashion to ensure a graceful and respectful transition in the relationship.

We cannot predict what will happen as time moves forward and the impact it will have on our feelings toward the other person, the goals we established for the relationship, or the energy we have for the relationship. It is possible that two people can simply outgrow a relationship and no longer have a need or a desire to continue the connection. It is also possible that one of the people in the relationship adopts a different philosophy about an issue that is very important to the other and there is no reconciling the change in opinions. Whatever the reasons may be for growing apart, the right thing to do is recognize the change, discuss the impact it is having on the relationship, and make a determination about where to go from there.

Consider the following:

Justin and Terry have shared a massage therapy office for 4 years. Recently Terry became interested in hypnotherapy and decided to become certified in it. When she puts up a poster in the office advertising hypnotherapy as part of her massage sessions, Justin is not comfortable with it. Even though hypnotherapy is not regulated in their community, he believes it is out of a massage therapist's scope of practice, regardless of Terry's certification. Terry tries to explain to Justin what hypnotherapy is all about, but Justin remains skeptical. Terry decides it is in her best interest to find another office space to work out of. Although she wants to remain friends with Justin, she does not want his attitude about hypnotherapy to have a negative impact on her professional practice.

Clarifying Dual and Multiple Relationships With Family, Friends, and Coworkers

Inevitably one of the first questions that may come up for bodywork practitioners about dual relationships involves family. They may say, "But I don't want to work on my mom. How do I say no and not hurt her feelings?" Coworkers can be a challenge for bodywork practitioners, especially those who are still students. The coworkers may seem to think they should be able to get a treatment from the student anytime they want one. These two examples illustrate the point that it is important for practitioners to set clear boundaries with family and coworkers to let them know when it is appropriate to approach practitioners about receiving bodywork as well as what other appropriate guidelines are.

Often it may be easier for practitioners to tell a stranger that they are not going to engage in a dual relationship because there is no prior relationship, including possible past baggage, with the stranger. With family, friends, and coworkers, however, there are more personal dynamics to manage.

There are a few different perspectives on how to handle the dynamics. Some people believe that it is never a good idea to treat family members, as it allows for the possibility of conflict to arise if there are unresolved family issues. There are also the expectations that some family members have that the bodywork practitioner should always put family first and, of course, offer a discount if not a free treatment. Other family systems see it differently, and would absolutely pay top dollar for the sessions because they see it as supporting their family member's dream. There are some practitioners who refuse to charge family and feel obliged to offer their services for free because that is what their value system tells them to do.

Regardless of where you fall on this continuum, the key is to set clear boundaries around whatever decision you make. If you choose to have the boundary of not charging family and friends a fee, then you need to be clear about when treatments are available so as not to interfere with appointments for your paying clients. If you are not comfortable massaging a family member you do not get along with, you have the right to honor that limit and respectfully decline. Some might argue that that is being rude, and a difficult thing to do with family. However, what is potentially more harmful is for you act against your better judgment. Resentment can then build up, resulting in unprofessional behavior toward that family member or, equally regrettable, you having a sense of powerlessness about the situation.

Although it is impossible to discuss every possible situation practitioners are likely to encounter when interacting with family, friends, and colleagues about their work, there are several that are relatively common. What follows are issues you are likely to encounter, with some suggested methods of handling them.

> *"I've been telling my family members and friends who are practice clients that I'll be graduating from school in 3 months and will be able to charge for my massage therapy treatments. When I said this there was no comment from any of them. Now I am afraid that I have offended them. How do I tactfully bring up the issue of payment for my professional services?"*

When practitioners are getting ready to transition from being students to professionals, it is important to begin thinking several months ahead of time about what they will be charging for treatments. They need to practice what they will say. They need to be direct and sound confident, as if it is the most natural thing for clients to be hearing from practitioners. When presenting the information in such a manner, it lets clients know that you are comfortable with becoming a professional and that you will not shy away from talking about professional issues.

This type of direct communication also works well for family members, as it informs them that you do not intend to give them free treatments. If you want to have a family discounted rate, that could be discussed with your family. However, you should be certain that is what you want to do, not what you think you should do or feel obligated to do. Otherwise, you may become resentful, giving you an additional issue to contend with. You should note that some family members may not expect special consideration, so you should make sure not to assume everyone will be expecting this from you.

The following is a sample script to consider: "I want to let you know that I'll be getting my massage therapy license in 2 months. What this means is that I'll be opening a business and charging $60 for an hour massage treatment. I would really like for you to be one of my first professional clients. Because you're in the family, I'll be offering a family rate of $50 per treatment rather than the full rate of $60."

> *"I have a friend who comes for a weekly shiatsu treatment. During the course of the session there is a lot of conversation back and forth about our lives. I don't feel comfortable with this, and want to change the dynamic to be professional. How can I do this without hurting my friend's feelings?"*

This is an issue that often comes up when two people have a lot in common and enjoy each other's company. This does not have to mean, however, that you cannot set boundaries around the treatment session. In fact, it is a good way to let friends know that you see them as professional clients and not just friends who just happen to pay you for an hour of talking. You can consider talking with the friend before the next session about what you are feeling. You should take responsibility for not having done a sufficient job of setting professional boundaries, and that you want to do so to make sure the friend gets the most out of the treatment. You can assure the client that you do enjoy time spent talking, but it is no longer something that you feel comfortable doing while giving your friend a treatment that he or she is paying for. If the friend balks at your suggestion, kindly let the friend know that it is important to you to set these professional boundaries. Offer to make a plan to get together outside of the scheduled appointment time to catch up.

The following is a sample script to consider: "I've noticed that I talk with you a lot during your shiatsu session and I'm feeling uneasy about my lack of professionalism. What I'd like is for us to find time outside of your appointment to connect so that I'm totally focused on you and the work we are doing in the session."

> *"I am frustrated that my family sees me as their 'personal massage therapist' every time I come over for a visit. As soon as I get in the door they ask where my table is and start directing me to a sore back or a stiff neck. Why don't they get it that I am not working when I come to see them? I don't think they see my work as an actual profession but more of something that can be done anywhere at any time for them."*

Managing perceptions from family and friends about your work can sometimes be challenging. It may seem that either they are so proud that they cannot wait to get an appointment, or they do not understand how you can "rub bodies for a living." An important task, then, is to educate your family on what a professional bodywork practitioner does and the setting in which you work; both of these are part of why the work is so beneficial to and valued by clients. This may seem quite basic, but these situations usually come up because practitioners have not taken the time to inform immediate family about the work that they do, what it entails both professionally and physically, how they have developed their business, how they maintain their business, and how they prefer to be approached about performing bodywork on clients.

What may be the most useful approach is one of excitement and passion, a "Let me tell you what I do and why I love it so much" type of conversation. If you explain to family and friends the structure and boundaries that the bodywork profession demands, then perhaps they will understand, and not be so quick to demand a "rub" from you during, for example, every family get-together.

The following is a sample script to consider: "Dad, I'm so glad that you think I can help you with your sore back, but I'm not able to work on you right now. I just finished a week of seeing 14 clients and I came over to relax and spend some time with the family. If you'd like to schedule some time for me to massage your back, I would be happy to do so in my office. That's where my treatment table is, and I can also use some moist heat packs that may help you feel better, too. What does your schedule look like on Monday?"

> *"How do I maintain my office policies with my family and friends? If clients cancel an appointment at the last minute, I charge them for the missed session. Even if they show up late, I won't alter my schedule to accommodate them. I can't bring myself to do this with my family and friends, so when it happens I get really upset inside and they keep asking me what's wrong."*

Setting and maintaining professional boundaries are hallmarks of the bodywork profession. They are essential to bodywork being recognized and valued as a viable health-care option. Therefore, it is important that you relate this value to all of your clients, especially friends and family. This is so they will understand what your expectations are of them as professional clients.

If there is a pattern of family and friends not respecting office policies, you can ask yourself if they would be so disrespectful of their friends' and family's professions. Would they, for example, simply not show up for an appointment at a friend's hair salon, or would they expect an uncle to rotate the tires on their car even though they arrived 2 hours late at his busy garage? If the answer is yes, then perhaps you need to look at your family system or the culture of your friendships. Does it include an expectation that everyone does not have to follow the rules?

If there is an unspoken rule in your close relationships that it is fine not to be accountable, then you will have a harder time confronting this behavior. Your job will be either to change the expectation or to decide if you want to have these friends and family as professional clients. If you do, then you will have to have a conversation with them explaining your business policies and why you expect them to be followed. You can also invite your friends and family to agree or disagree, and then perhaps create another arrangement that will not be so frustrating for you.

The following is a sample script to consider: "Kyra, before I make another appointment with you I need to clarify a couple of things. You're aware that you were 20 minutes late for your appointment today, and last month you cancelled an hour before your appointment. When my clients do this I don't feel like I'm being respected, and I get a bit angry that my time and my work are not being valued. All of my sessions are important to me and help me maintain my business. When clients who are not friends or family do this I charge them for the session or I give them only a partial treatment because I don't allow their choices to affect my business. However, I haven't been will- ing to apply these policies to my family and friends because it felt like I was being mean. What I need to tell you is if you cancel an appointment with me with less than 24 hours' notice, I will charge you for the session, and if you come late to a session I'm willing to work on you only for the amount of time that is left. I know this may sound harsh to you, but I've discovered I'm not being fair to my business or to you when I don't tell you how it affects me. I don't want our friendship to suffer because I'm feeling resentful about your lateness. Are you willing to abide by my policies or should I make a referral for you to another practitioner?"

There are many layers in the preceding dialogue. However, it is designed to give you an idea of how complicated it can be when you do not hold your friends and families to the same standards as the rest of your clients. As prac- titioners, you must make the choice about what is more important to you— being true to how you want to run your business, or choosing not to combine business with family and friends.

Education Issues and Dual Roles

As discussed previously, bodywork schools and programs provide a context in which students can learn to navigate the complexities surrounding dual and multiple relationships. All of the same dynamics that exist among other people with whom practitioners can possibly enter dual and multiple rela- tionships certainly apply among instructors, administrators, and students.

There are many ways dual and multiple roles present themselves. This is especially true if the school is small and instructors are administrators as well. The following is an example of the different roles that one staff member, Josephine, may assume in a given day:

- As an instructor, the students see Josephine as the one in charge of the material being taught. They have an expectation that she will know the material thoroughly and will teach it to them in a satisfactory way.
- Josephine is also the dean of students at the school and there are times when students from her class need to meet with her to discuss personal issues, such as how they are prevented from being successful in a class because of a conflict with another teacher. In this role Josephine is a supportive listener, allowing students to express their concerns about

the instructor. Josephine will ask questions to assist students in clarifying what they are feeling and what they need to resolve their issues. In this way, while Josephine has an authoritative position, the students see her as being supportive in processing what they are experiencing, looking at their responsibilities in situations, and coming up with some solutions that will help students succeed.

- As a fellow faculty member Josephine has the role of being a supportive colleague and not passing judgment on how other teachers run their classes. Although the director of education is responsible for assisting faculty members when issues arise, Josephine's input is required as an advocate for students.
- Josephine receives treatments in the student clinic on a weekly basis. In this situation, Josephine is a client and students are the practitioners. Granted, Josephine will be giving students feedback at the end of each session and can act as a mentor at that time, but for the 50 to 60 minutes during which they are performing the massage, the students are the ones with the greater power.

As can be seen, the various roles flip back and forth rather quickly. Each role has a value and comes with the responsibility that everyone conduct themselves with integrity.

Inappropriate Dual Roles Instructors Can Have With Students

When boundaries about dual and multiple relationships between students, teachers, and administrators are not clearly stated and enforced, there can be painful consequences. Even a single dual relationship that is not handled appropriately, or a dual relationship that should not have taken place, such as a sexual relationship between a student and faculty member, affects the dynamics of a class, group of students, the entire student body, the faculty, and administration, and may even affect the reputation of the school as a whole.

Consider the following:

Ruth has been a licensed massage practitioner for 22 years and teaches an introductory massage class. She does not agree with the school policy that faculty are not to fraternize with students outside of the classroom. Her belief is that the more one can connect with students on a personal and social level, the more motivated they will be to come to class because it will be fun and meaningful. Ruth goes out every Friday after class for beer and pizza with her students. Often a few of the students end up at her home playing music and talking late into the night. Ruth is considered cool by all of her students because she is relaxed and does not push the students to learn as much as they can.

Other faculty members experience a lot of difficulty in their classrooms with the students because the students resist following the school's code of conduct for the classroom. Behaviors that teachers experience include talking out of turn, arriving late, leaving early, nonparticipation, and general disrespectful attitudes toward the teacher when asked to comply with the classroom behavior agreement. The general attitude of the class is that the only teacher who understands them and has anything to teach them is Ruth. In fact, often the conversations over beer and pizza involve the students complaining about the other teachers and Ruth agreeing with them and not supporting her colleagues.

Ruth is called into the director of education office to discuss her behavior of socializing with her students. She refuses to see that there is a problem. She says, "I've never had an issue with classroom management. My students love me and know that I love them. If the rest of the faculty would get 'real' with the students and stop hiding behind the role of 'teacher' then everything would be fine!"

How would you describe Ruth's attitude toward her colleagues? Toward her students? Toward school policies? How does Ruth's socializing with her students contribute to the lack of cooperation the other teachers experience? If you were the director of education, what would you do?

Megan teaches a continuing education class in chair massage. She has been invited to teach a class in a town 2 hours away. Her regular teaching assistant is not able to attend this workshop so she asks one of her students, Miranda, at the massage school where she teaches. She has noticed Miranda's work in class is advanced and she seemed to have a passion for chair massage. She thinks it would be a good experience for Miranda to help her with this workshop so she could get a sense of what continuing educations classes are like when she graduates in 3 months.

Miranda is very excited and expresses a great deal of gratitude to Megan for this opportunity. Miranda tells all of her classmates about her "teaching gig" and lets everyone know just how crucial her role as teaching assistant in the workshop is.

The Monday after the workshop, Megan and Miranda are talking about the workshop as students are gathering for class. It is quite clear to the other students that the workshop had gone well and that Megan is very pleased with Miranda's participation. After class, Miranda is given a hard time by some of her classmates for being "teacher's pet." They also want to know what she got in return for helping to teach the continuing education class, and tell her she now has an easy A in this class.

What is the level of risk Megan is taking in this dual relationship with Miranda? What is the impact the risk has on Miranda? What responsibilities does Megan have toward Miranda? Toward all of her students? Do you think Miranda's classmates' attitudes and comments are justified? What would you say to Megan? To Miranda?

Instructors Having Students as Private Clients

Some bodywork programs require that students receive professional treatments while they are enrolled so that they can experience firsthand what a professional treatment feels like, as well as experience the professional bodywork setting. Although this can be an invaluable experience for students, faculty needs to follow ethical parameters while engaging in this dual role.

The issue of monetary reimbursement between student and instructor is important to consider if a student has become a client in the instructor's private practice. Is it ethical to have a professional relationship with a client for whom the instructor is also responsible for giving a grade? Is it possible that the student will assume special treatment or for the instructor to be stricter with the student to show there is not favoritism? Does the situation set up a dynamic in the classroom if the other students perceive that their classmate gets special treatment or if it appears that the instructor and the student have become friends? How does money affect dual roles in the classroom?

Some schools develop policies to monitor this situation by saying that instructors may never receive remuneration from a student. Other schools trust that their instructors are professionals and will act ethically at all times. And still other schools have guidelines about when in the student's training they are allowed to receive a professional treatment from an instructor. For example, when the student is enrolled in the instructor's class, the instructor cannot see the student as a professional bodywork client. However, once the student is no longer in the instructor's class, the instructor can see that student as a client.

This issue can be subjective, depending on the perspective of the school administration. It would be helpful to determine the intention behind students receiving treatments from instructors. On the one hand, it is a good way for a student to experience directly what the instructor is expecting in terms of technique competency. On the other hand, it could be seen as an opportunity for an instructor to build a practice by encouraging students to get a treatment from him or her so they will know what the work should feel like. This could be seen as a manipulative tactic on the instructor's part to convince students that if they *really* want to get a good grade in the class, they need to experience the instructor's work.

Another consideration is whether instructors/practitioners can manage their boundaries effectively so as not to let the professional relationship enter into the classroom. For example, an instructor commenting on a student's physical condition in front of the class to illustrate a point could be seen as playing favorites or be seen as a breach in confidentiality. Discretion, wisdom, and a high degree of professionalism are necessary when instructors give students treatments in their private practices.

Dual Roles to Avoid in the School Setting

Certain types of dual relationships are never ethical nor appropriate to enter into in the school setting. The risks are so high and the benefits so low that the relationship is unjustified. One is an intimate, sexual relationship between an instructor or administrator and a student. The damage this type of relationship can do to the student, the instructor, the administration, and the school as a whole is so great, its prohibition is usually delineated very clearly in the school's code of ethics and administrative policies.

Another type of dual role that is usually highly discouraged is an intimate friendship between a student and an instructor, or a student and an administrator. Sometimes, because of the closeness that can develop from learning bodywork, some instructors or administrators develop friendships with students. Certain instructors enjoy being with their students to the point that they socialize with them outside of school.

These dual roles involving intimate friendships and sexual relationships mean that professional boundaries are not maintained. The shifting power differentials can play out in the classroom, no matter how much the people involved think they would not or do not. No matter how discreet the people involved think they are being, those around them pick up on their relationship, especially in the bodywork profession, in which intuition plays a large part. In addition, students who are involved with instructors may not have the ability to separate their friendship or love relationship with the instructor while in the classroom. As a result, they may not think they are subject to the instructor's authority in the classroom and can disregard classroom boundaries and challenge the instructor on a personal level. The chances for the student to learn anything in this situation decrease dramatically.

Those who are aware of the relationship, and even those who are not aware of the relationship but sense that something is going on, will perceive the student as receiving favored treatment, whether this is actually true or not. Human nature being what it is, when one person is thought of as receiving special treatment, the dynamic of the entire group changes. Trust can be lost, resentments can build, and anger or retribution erupt toward the favored person and the associated instructor or administrator. Obviously, the learning environment is compromised.

As happens, relationships end, which can leave one or both parties hurt, confused, and angry. These feelings, too, negatively affect the learning environment. In addition, because it is unethical for the instructor or administrator to have been in the relationship in the first place, the student involved could decide to file a complaint and/or even a lawsuit against the school, which can destroy the reputation of the school and possibly ruin it financially. The instructor or administrator could face censure by the school, be fired, or face legal charges.

Food for Thought

What responsibilities do you think bodywork schools have for teacher training and monitoring? What type of process or protocol should students and faculty follow if a power differential is being mismanaged?

■ CASE PROFILE

Lane is attending massage school. She is in her first semester of a four-semester program. During her first week of school one of her instructors, Ursula, told the class, "Massage school is going to change your lives, and you had better be prepared." Lane was confused about this comment. She had come to school as a fresh start for her young family. She wanted to learn a vocation so she could leave minimum wage jobs behind and work in the wellness field. After class, Lane called Ursula and asked to meet with her to discuss her comment. Ursula says that she would be happy to meet with Lane at a coffee shop near Ursula's home.

Lane arrives at the coffee house at the appointed time, but Ursula arrives 20 minutes late. She apologizes and tells Lane that she's late because she had to drop her 5-year-old off at day care. Lane tells Ursula that she has a 5-year-old also. They have a long conversation about marriage; parenting; and the challenges of balancing school, work, and family. When it is time to go, Ursula suggests that Lane bring her son to Ursula's home on Saturday so the children could play while Ursula and Lane continue their conversation. Lane agrees.

Over the course of the semester, Mary and Ursula met every Saturday morning at Ursula's house so their children can play while Ursula advises Lane on how to make the transition from working full-time to being a full-time student and working part-time. Ursula also gives Lane pointers on how to study for examinations, and on massage techniques and body mechanics. Several times Lane and Ursula share a babysitter so they can go to dinner and the movies with their husbands.

Case Study Continued from page 318

What issues are present in this scenario regarding dual roles?

Describe the power differential between Ursula and Lane.

Describe both Ursula's role and Lane's role in this case profile.

What do you think the impact of Ursula and Lane's interactions are having on the class dynamic?

Chapter Summary

Boundaries create a sense of safety and security, as well as a predictable relationship, for both clients and practitioners. In the bodywork profession, physical, financial, emotional, social, psychological, ethical, and professional boundaries are set by practitioners to determine what appropriate behavior is. Both students and instructors need to identify boundaries, communicate their boundaries to others, recognize when a boundary has been crossed, manage the outcome when the boundary crossing has been acknowledged, and know when to make a boundary more flexible or less permeable, when appropriate.

Successful bodywork practices involve practitioners setting and maintaining healthy boundaries. To develop and maintain professional boundaries, practitioners can self-reflect on what their personal boundaries are first. By setting boundaries for self-care, practitioners can be more available for treatments, and perform better treatments. Self-care plans should include, but are not limited to, specific goals to accomplish an exercise routine and a social plan. If practitioners have signs of needing self-care, then they need to reevaluate their self-care plans and take steps to nourish themselves. Practitioners who work for someone else need to learn how to communicate with their supervisors about what is needed to maintain their self-care.

Through the use of appropriate boundaries, the practitioner sets the emotional environment of the treatment session. This means being able to manage transference and countertransference issues should they come up, and possibly discussing the issues with the client or seeking guidance from a supervisor, trusted colleague, family member, or mentor.

Practitioners may have two or more roles at the same time or sequentially with a client, relative or friend of the client, other practitioners, other health-care providers, and employers and supervisors. To have successful careers, practitioners must be able to navigate these dual and multiple relationships. They need to be aware of the benefits and risks, as well as be able to define appropriate parameters. They also need to know what dual relationships they should *never* enter into with clients and be diligent about avoiding these.

Strategies for managing dual and multiple relationships include knowing how to make appropriate choices, the factors involved in successful relationships, and when and how practitioners should ask for help. Sometimes a dual or multiple relationship becomes no longer manageable or useful and it should be ended effectively and respectfully.

Review Questions

Multiple Choice

1. Which of the following is an example of appropriate boundary setting in the bodywork profession?

a. Offering clients the opportunity to invest in the practitioner's side business selling insurance

b. Making sure to relieve every physical complaint clients have

c. Preventing the client from talking during the treatment session

d. Backing off in a conversation when the practitioner becomes too invested in being "right"

2. Which of the following types of boundaries determine our comfort in connecting with others?

a. Physical

b. Social

c. Ethical

d. Professional

3. The atmosphere or energetic sense of the therapeutic relationship is referred to as:

a. The emotional environment

b. Positive transference

c. Role blending

d. Self-care

4. When one set of roles ends before the beginning of a new set of roles, this is referred to as what type of relationship?

a. Dual

b. Sequential

c. Multiple

d. Overlapping

5. An example of a dual relationship is a client and a practitioner who:

a. Agree that treatments should be paid for with cash

b. Share similar interests

c. Serve on the same volunteer board

d. Have the same political views

6. To navigate a dual or multiple relationship successfully, each person involved needs to:

a. Maintain his own sense of self

b. Communicate directly about needs and expectations

c. Respect the others

d. All of the above

7. When boundaries about dual and multiple relationships between students, teachers, and administrators are unclear and unenforced, what can be affected are the dynamics of the:

a. Faculty

b. Class

c. Entire school

d. All of the above

Fill in the Blank

1. A(n) _____ is a limit set to inform others where one's personal space ends and public space begins.

2. When the practitioner has unresolved issues or feelings from the past and is shifting these feelings onto the client, it is called _____ .

3. Latent unresolved issues, misguided anger, and unrealistic expectations are referred to as _____ .

4. An exercise routine is part of a(n) _____ plan.

5. Shifting back and forth between roles describes a(n) _____ relationship.

6. When considering entering into a dual or multiple relationship with a client, practitioners need to carefully assess the risk for conflicts of interest, loss of objectivity, and impact on the _____ .

7. A type of dual relationship practitioners should never enter into with a client is a(n) _____ one.

Short Answer

1. Explain what boundaries are important for success in the bodywork profession.

2. Give five examples of areas in which practitioners would benefit from setting boundaries with clients.

3. Describe the features of a dual or multiple role relationship and give at least three examples of them.

4. Explain at least three benefits and three risks of dual or multiple relationships.

5. Write three examples of how a practitioner could respond to a client who invites him or her to be in a dual relationship that the practitioner is not interested in.

6. Explain three ways that a practitioner can know when it is time to end a dual or multiple relationship.

7. Give three examples of issues that practitioners are likely to encounter with family, friends, and coworkers. Explain the factors involved and possible solutions to the issues.

Activities

1. In a group setting pass around a ball of string and a pair of scissors. Ask each person to cut off an amount of string that represents of the size of his or her personal boundary, and have each place the string in a circle on the floor around him- or herself. Ask each person to explain how his or her circle of string relates to his or her personal boundary.

2. Design a policies and procedures document based on your professional boundaries.

3. Using whatever means that appeal to you, such as a computer, expressive arts, pen and paper, or collage or other art project, create a self-care plan for yourself that covers a 30-day period. Include the following areas:

- Nutrition
- Exercise
- Spirituality/religion
- Finances
- Creativity
- Sleep
- Hygiene
- Work schedule
- Socializing with friends
- Alone time

4. Make a list of the issues that you believe are or would be potential triggers for you based on transference or countertransference with a client. Reflect on the list, choose two, and develop strategies for managing them.

5. List three dual or multiple role relationships that you are currently in or have been in the past. On a scale of 1 to 5, with 1 being the lowest risk and 5 being the highest risk, rate the risk level for each relationship you are in. Explain why you rated each of them the way you did.

6. One of your clients has invited you to attend a workshop she is conducting called "Money and You: How to Increase Your Income." She has offered to waive your fee for the workshop. Write down the conversation you see yourself having with your client about this situation.

7. Create for yourself a protocol that you will follow when determining whether to enter into a dual or multiple relationship. What questions will you ask yourself? What factors will go into your decision? What do you think will make you ultimately decide whether to enter the relationship?

Guidance for Journaling

Some key areas to think about while journaling for this chapter include the following:

- The importance of boundaries in your life, what personal and professional boundaries you have, and how you maintain them
- How you respond when your boundaries are ignored by others

Guidance for Journaling—cont'd

- The connection between appropriate boundaries and success in the bodywork profession
- How to maintain professional boundaries
- What your self-care boundaries are, and how you feel about them
- Creating a plan for self-care
- What transference and countertransference mean, whether you have experienced these phenomena, and how you felt when they occurred
- What different types of dual and multiple relationships can occur in the bodywork profession
- What dual or multiple relationships you have been in, are in, and could possibly be in, in the future
- Benefits of being in these dual and multiple relationships
- Risks, issues, and challenges in dual and multiple relationships you are facing or may face in the future, and how you would handle them
- What parameters are appropriate for you to be able to manage you dual and multiple relationships
- When you think you might need to ask for help in a dual or multiple relationship, and who you would ask for help
- When and how you have or would end a dual relationship
- The various dual and multiple relationships you have encountered or are likely to encounter as a bodywork student
- What you think about students socializing with faculty

References

1. Adams, J.: *Boundary Issues—Using Boundary Intelligence to Get the Intimacy You Want and the Independence You Need in Life, Love, and Work.* Hoboken, NJ, John Wiley, 2005, pp 2–4.
2. Greene, E., and Goodrich-Dunn, B.: *The Psychology of the Body.* Baltimore, MD, Lippincott Williams & Wilkins, 2004, p 74.
3. Wallace, A.C.: *Setting Psychological Boundaries: A Handbook for Women.* Westport, CT, Bergin & Garvey, 1997, p xi.
4. Adams, *Boundary Issues,* p 29.
5. Greene and Goodrich-Dunn, *The Psychology of the Body,* pp 84–87.
6. Ibid., p 54.
7. Ibid., p 55.
8. Ibid.
9. Ibid., p 57.
10. Ibid., p 58.
11. Ibid., p 62.
12. Purtilo, R., and Haddad, A.: *Health Professional and Patient Interaction,* ed. 7. St. Louis, MO, Saunders Elsevier, 2007, p 218.
13. Corey, G., Corey, M.S., and Callanan, P.: *Issues and Ethics in the Helping Professions,* ed. 7. Stamford, CT, Brooks/Cole Cengage Learning, 2007, p 264.
14. Gottlieb, Michael C. *Avoiding Exploitive Dual Relationships: A Decision-Making Model* (1993). Retrieved 7 September 2010 http://kspope.com/dual/gottlieb.php
15. Corey, Corey, and Callanan, P.: *Issues and Ethics in the Helping Professions,* p 269.
16. Ibid., p 270.

Touch Integrity

LEARNING OBJECTIVES

After studying this chapter, you will be able to:

1. Explain the mechanics of touch and different types of touch.

2. Explain the healing effects of bodywork.

3. Discuss your personal history of touch and explain how it affects your current comfort level of touch.

4. Explain why bodywork students should receive professional bodywork, and why educators need to be mindful in their discussions of desexualized touch.

5. Explain what desexualized touch is and discuss how to create desexualized bodywork.

6. Explain the continuum of sexual manipulation in the bodywork profession.

7. Discuss ways to tell if sexual manipulation is occurring.

8. Explain ways to educate clients about the purpose of bodywork, and outline the steps in the intervention model.

CHAPTER OUTLINE

KEY TERMS

Desexualized touch: touch by the practitioner during treatment that is not in any way erotic or sexual for either the practitioner or the client

Ki: according to traditional Japanese bodywork, the energy or force that gives and maintains life, and also is the connection between organisms and all creation

Neurotransmitters: chemicals released by brain cells (neurons) to communicate with each other

Prana: according to Ayurveda, the energy or force that gives and maintains life, and also is the connection between organisms and all creation

Primary somatosensory area: the area of the brain that receives sensory information from the body and is involved in the perception of the sensation; this area has a "map" of the entire body and so can pinpoint not only what the sensation is, but where in the body it is coming from

Qi: according to traditional Chinese medicine, the energy or force that gives and maintains life, and also is the connection between organisms and all creation

Sensory receptors: specialized nerve endings that respond to various types of stimulation

Sensual: relating to or consisting of the gratification of the senses

Sexual assault: illegal sexual contact that usually involves force on a person without consent or is inflicted on a person who is incapable of giving consent or who places the assailant in a position of trust or authority

Sexual harassment: uninvited and unwelcome verbal or physical behavior of a sexual nature, especially by a person in authority toward a subordinate

Somatosensory association areas: areas of the brain that store memories of past somatic sensory experiences so people can compare current sensations with previous sensations

Tactile: related to touch; tactile sensations include pain, pressure, vibration, itch, and tickle

Therapeutic touch: safe and appropriate placement of parts of the practitioner's body, such as the hands, forearms, elbows, knees, and feet, on a client who has given consent for the purposes of healing or restorative care

Touch overload: a phenomenon that can happen in the bodywork profession in which a practitioner who has been working for a certain period of time no longer wants to touch his clients

Callie is a licensed massage therapist who has been practicing professionally for 6 months. She is employed at a day spa. A new client, Derek, is scheduled with her. Throughout his treatment he lavishes Callie with compliments, calling her an "amazing healer," a "gifted therapist," and that hers is "the best treatment I've ever received." Derek even calls Callie the next day to thank her for the session and to let her know that he feels no pain in his low back for the first time in weeks. Callie is proud of herself and thinks that all her hard work learning massage therapy has paid off in how skillfully she performed Derek's treatment.

Derek schedules another appointment for the following evening. During the second massage, while prone on the massage table, Derek complains that the treatment room is too hot and requests a towel rather than a sheet for the draping. Callie complies, eager to show Derek her continual ability to provide a client-centered treatment. When he turns supine, the towel "accidentally" falls to the floor. As Callie replaces the towel Derek grabs it away and with a large smile tells her it is not needed. Callie is so taken by surprise that she makes a joke about getting fired for not following clinic procedures, to which Derek responds, "I won't tell a soul." Callie does not know what to say so she completes the treatment as quickly as she can, pretending not to notice Derek's erection or the sounds he makes as she massages his adductor muscles. She finishes the treatment, leaves the room as quickly as she can, and does not return until Derek has left the building. When Callie comes back to her room to prepare for her next client she notices a large wet spot on the massage table along with $75.

Callie is caught off guard by Derek's behavior for several reasons. As a new practitioner she is flattered by the compliments he gave her and, based on this, assigns a lot of trust in him that is not necessarily warranted. Derek had an agenda and it is one that he is skilled at executing. He sets the tone for Callie to trust him during the first appointment by being friendly and complimentary. Even his follow-up call the next day was a ploy to further manipulate Callie's perception of him.

During the second treatment he capitalizes on Callie's trust and, perhaps, her naiveté to get his agenda met during the session. Callie is so flattered by his seeming kindness and compliments that she does not recognize that she is being manipulated. And if she did have an idea, it is possible that she ignored it because she could not imagine what Derek really had in mind.

This is why during the second treatment she fails to see the red flags that indicate Derek is sexualizing the massage and putting her at risk. When she finally realizes what is really going on, Callie is so emotionally stunned she freezes and cannot find the words to tell Derek what he is doing is inappropriate, or take other appropriate action such as stopping the treatment immediately and leaving the room. Imagine how further demoralized and insulted Callie feels when she returns to her treatment room to find that her client had ejaculated on the table and left a large sum of money, making the whole situation connect with an act of prostitution.

As illustrated in the scenario above, one of the biggest ethical issues a bodywork practitioner faces is providing safe, nonsexual touch to clients. Given the exaggerated sexualization of our culture in the media and given the historic association of massage with the sex trade, it is essential that practitioners understand how to provide appropriate, therapeutic touch and to avoid sexualizing their work in any way.

In addressing this topic, this chapter first explores definitions of touch, along with the mechanics and different types of touch. Next, we discuss ways to educate clients about the purpose of bodywork and the healing effects of bodywork. Because personal history (both your own and your client's) influences perception of touch, aspects of this history are explained, including family messages or experiences about touch, religious or spiritual beliefs, and other cultural influences such as age and gender. Methods designed to assist practitioners in identifying where they may have challenges in dealing with the amount of touch involved in performing bodywork are presented.

The importance of creating desexualized treatment environments cannot be emphasized enough. How to do this is discussed and includes assisting practitioners in becoming aware of their own sexuality, and ensuring they do not bring it into their bodywork practice. The continuum of sexual manipulation is presented. Because it is sometimes difficult to tell whether sexual manipulation is occurring, we consider some methods to assist you in how to recognize it.

What Exactly Is Touch?

Before we can effectively discuss how to use touch in an appropriate and therapeutic way, we must first understand the importance of touch to humans and define what touch is.

Importance of Touch

Touch is essential for survival. Human beings have an innate need to be touched. Studies have proved that touch is essential for proper growth and development in infants. Dr. Tiffany Field was a pioneer in this research. For more information, see Box 9.1, "Dr. Tiffany Field." However, people at all stages of life need touch for their well-being. For example, touch deprivation has been linked to increased stress, physical violence, sleep disturbances, and suppressed immune responses. It stands to reason, then, that touch serves to soothe and support both the body and mind.

Touch often has profound effects on the client's mind, emotions, and spirit. Through touch, you, the practitioner, can communicate care, compassion, confidence, calmness, focus, skillfulness, anxiety, apprehension, anger,

---

| Box 9.1 | DR. TIFFANY FIELD |

Tiffany Field, PhD, became interested in the problems that premature infants face when her own daughter was born prematurely. As a new mother, she massaged her infant daughter. Later, as a psychology graduate student, she did research on premature infants. Along with her colleagues, she discovered that premature babies who were massaged gained 47% more weight than those who were not massaged.

Field continued research into the beneficial effects of healthy touch, long before massage was even beginning to be accepted by either physicians or the public. In 1992, with a seed grant from Johnson & Johnson, various federal agencies, and private corporations, she established the Touch Research Institutes (TRI) at the University of Miami School of Medicine. Before TRI, no other organization was focused solely on the study of touch.

With more than 100 studies and 350 medical journal articles to her credit, Field is considered a leading expert in touch research, and remains one of its strongest advocates. As she states in her book *Touch*, "Like diet and exercise, people may need a daily dose of touch."

The studies Field and her colleagues at TRI have conducted show that massage therapy enhances growth, decreases pain, decreases issues associated with autoimmune disease, enhances immune function, and increases alertness and mental performance.[1,2]

More information can be found on The Touch Research Institutes Web site: http://www.miami.edu/touch-research.

Source: Field, T.: *Touch*. Cambridge, MA, MIT Press, 2003, pp vii–x.

distraction, disinterest, and lack of confidence. Sometimes practitioners are not even aware of how much their touch affects the client. Therefore, be mindful of your own thoughts and emotions, because these will be communicated through touch to the client, even if not in your words.

Touch can also profoundly affect you, the practitioner. When someone touches another person, the person doing the touching is being touched in return. When you are giving touch, you are also receiving touch. This is one reason giving bodywork can be such a rewarding experience and why bodyworkers like doing it so much.

Defining Touch

Touch is a complex and powerful form of communication involving one person's body coming into contact with an object or another body. The variety of sensations available through touch are numerous and difficult to describe. Touch can be described as light, abrasive, soothing, deep, jabbing, relaxing, sensual, therapeutic, nurturing, inappropriate, cool, painful, and pleasurable, among other things. However, all of these words are subjective, which only adds to the challenge of talking about what touch is. Moreover, practitioners have to not only understand what touch is themselves but also must explain the role of touch in bodywork to clients.

To narrow our focus to what is most relevant to massage practitioners, it is best to define the term **therapeutic touch.** Therapeutic touch is safe and appropriate placement of parts of the practitioner's body, such as the hands, forearms, elbows, knees, and feet, on a client who has given consent for the purposes of healing or restorative care. Therapeutic touch is intended to be physically and emotionally beneficial to the recipient. When therapeutic touch is given, there is a mutual understanding between the client and the practitioner that the touch can cease at any time if one of the participants no longer feels safe or is willing that the touch continue.

More specifically, touch, as it is used in bodywork, often refers to techniques involving either palpation or a stroke:

- Palpation: to handle or feel gently, especially with the hand and usually with the intent to understand or appreciate, such as touching an area of tension on the client's body during a palpation assessment.
- Stroke: to feel, strike, or push lightly, especially with the hand or foot or an implement. This definition certainly applies to techniques and tools used during the performance of bodywork on a client.

In a world where touch has been used as a way to abuse, manipulate, and control others, it is necessary that appropriate touch be recognized as essential for the development of healthy and well-balanced individuals. Bodywork practitioners have a role in this process of reclaiming touch as being positive because each and every time they provide a therapeutic session they are giving one more person the knowledge that touch can be safe and fulfilling.

Physiology of Touch

Essential to understanding touch is to understand the physiological mechanics that underlie this sense. In her book *Touch,* Dr. Tiffany Field states, "Touch is the first sense to develop and it functions even after seeing and hearing begin to fade."[3] As such, it is arguably the most important of the body senses. Through her work, Dr. Field has shown touch to be necessary for babies to thrive and develop. It also reduces aggression in children and increases their ability to learn and to fall asleep. In both children and adults, welcomed touch decreases stress, decreases insomnia, and increases mental clarity.[4]

Touch is a **tactile** sensation. "Tactile" comes from the Latin word *tactilis*, meaning "touch." Tactile sensations include pain, pressure, vibration, itch, and tickle. Tactile sensations arise from external sensory stimulation, primarily of the skin. Internal sensory stimulation comes from deeper structures of the body, such as the muscles, tendons, joints, connective tissues, lungs, heart, and digestive organs. All of these can also project sensations to the skin and are called "referred sensations."

Thus the skin plays a major role in the sensation of touch. It is, in fact, the largest sensory organ of the body. The skin is the organ most directly affected by massage and bodywork, for both the client and you. You receive information about the client's body through touching the skin. For example, areas of muscle tension and adhesions in connective tissue can be felt through the client's skin as it is being contacted by the skin on the practitioner's fingers, hands, forearms, elbows, knees, and feet, depending on the type of bodywork being performed. If the client is fully clothed, as for shiatsu or Thai massage, the practitioner still gathers information by touching the client. The practitioner also imparts touch to the client. The touch is received by client's skin, whether the touch is directly on the skin or through clothing, and transmitted to other systems such as the nervous, endocrine, and muscular systems, causing change in the body.

Specialized nerve endings called **sensory receptors** respond to the various types of tactile stimulation. Receptors located between the epidermis and dermis respond to the lightest forms of stimulation, those located just beneath the skin respond to constant pressure, and those located deep in the

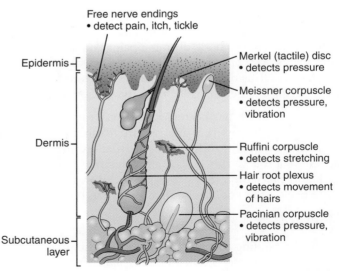

Figure 9.1 Structure and location of receptors in the skin and deep to the skin.

skin can register deeper pressure and temperature changes (Fig. 9.1). Any stimulation that touches the skin is carried into the spinal cord on nerve fibers. If the stimulation is strong enough, the information travels up through the spinal cord to the brain where it is routed to the **primary somatosensory area** and the **somatosensory association areas** in the cerebral cortex (Fig. 9.2). If the stimulation is not strong enough, one of two outcomes could occur. The information may not travel up the spinal cord, so the brain does not become aware of it. The information may travel up to the brain but not reach the primary somatosensory area.

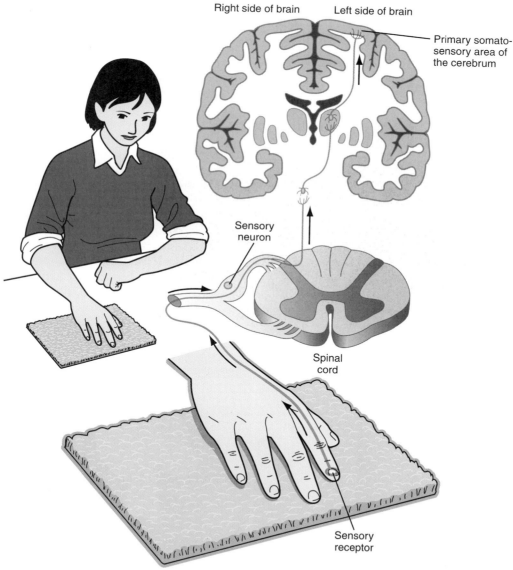

Right side of brain   Left side of brain

Primary somato-sensory area of the cerebrum

Sensory neuron

Spinal cord

Sensory receptor

Figure 9.2 Pathway of information from the skin to the brain.

"Somato" refers to the body. Figure 9.3 shows where in the brain the primary somatosensory and the somatosensory association areas are located in the cerebrum of the brain. The cerebrum is the largest part of the brain. The primary somatosensory area receives the sensation and is involved in the perception of the sensation. This somatosensory area has a "map" of the entire body and so can pinpoint not only what the sensation is but also where in the body it is coming from. This is how, for example, a person can tell he is being bitten by a mosquito and exactly where on his body he is being bitten. Figure 9.4A shows where parts of the body are "mapped" within the primary somatosensory area. Figure 9.4B indicates how much of the somatosensory area is devoted to processing information from receptors in specific areas of the body. For example, more of the primary somatosensory area processes information from the thumb than it does from the elbow.

The role of the somatosensory association areas is to store memories of past somatic sensory experiences so people can compare current sensations with previous sensations. This is how a person knows whether a sensation he is experiencing is a pain or an itch or a tickle. The somatosensory area also allows people to determine the exact shape and texture of an object by feeling it, to determine the orientation of one object to another just by feeling, and to sense the relationship of one body part to another.

Therapeutic touch, as occurs in bodywork, decreases heart rate and the secretion of adrenaline and cortisol, both of which are hormones released during stress. During immediate stresses, such as being nearly sideswiped by a car, the sympathetic division of the nervous system readies the body for action. Adrenaline is released and serves, among other things, to increase heart rate (to pump blood to the tissues faster) and increase muscle tension so that a person is ready to fight or to flee from the threat. During longer-term stresses, such as a difficult semester of school, the sympathetic nervous system does not necessarily keep being activated. Instead, the hormone cortisol is released. It serves to increase blood sugar levels so that tissues can use it for energy to deal with the stress. Even though these

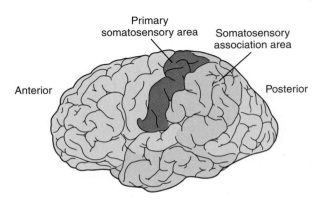

Lateral view of right cerebral hemisphere

Figure 9.3 Location of the primary somatosensory and the somatosensory association areas in the cerebrum of the brain.

Primary somatosensory area

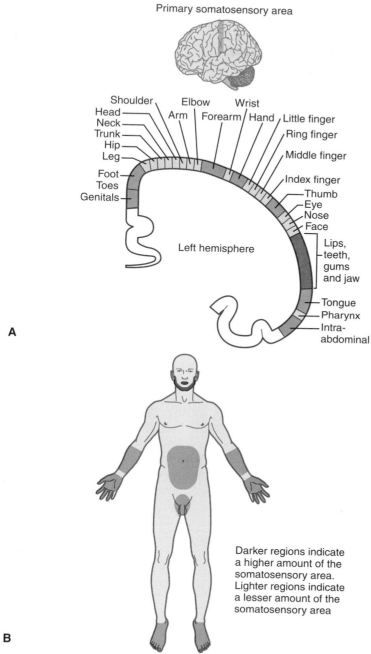

A

B

Darker regions indicate
a higher amount of the
somatosensory area.
Lighter regions indicate
a lesser amount of the
somatosensory area

Figure 9.4 Body map and receptors in the primary somatosensory area. (A) Where parts of the body are "mapped" within the primary somatosensory area. (B) How much of the somatosensory area is devoted to processing information from receptors in specific areas of the body.

are normal, healthy responses to stress, they can take quite a toll on the body over the long term.

The parasympathetic division of the nervous system is responsible for conserving and restoring body energy during times of rest. Ideally, the body is in parasympathetic mode most of the time, with the sympathetic division overriding it only in times of emergency or exercise. Relaxing massage therapy and bodywork treatments stimulate the parasympathetic division, resulting in decreased stress hormone release, muscle relaxation, decreased heart rate, and increased mental clarity. Pain is also relieved because nerve impulses for touch travel to the brain faster than nerve impulses for pain. These changes help to lessen the wear and tear on the body's structures and its immune system.

Inherent in the many types of massage and bodywork is the pleasure of being touched. Dopamine and serotonin are brain chemicals called **neurotransmitters.** Neurotransmitters are the chemicals released by brain cells (neurons) to communicate with each other. Dopamine is released during pleasurable experiences such as an enjoyable bodywork treatment. Serotonin is thought is be involved in, among other things, sensory perception, control of mood, and sleep. These chemicals are part of the creation of pleasurable moods and the feeling of connection during bodywork treatments. These chemical responses to bodywork are one of the main reasons bodywork is therapeutically beneficial. Because touching the client means the practitioner is experiencing touch as well, both can feel centered and relaxed by an enjoyable bodywork treatment.[5]

However, because the perception of pleasure can mean different things to different people, sometimes certain clients will mistake the pleasure they feel in receiving an enjoyable bodywork treatment as sexual stimulation. Perhaps the closest thing to the therapeutic touch they have ever experienced has been sexual experiences. Because the body constantly reacts to new sensations by comparing them to past experiences, it is understandable that a client would interpret these feelings as sexual arousal. This can happen even though you have been diligent in dressing and communicating professionally and have ensured that your touch is therapeutic and not erotic. You then have the responsibility of educating the client on the difference between therapeutic touch and sexual touch. This is discussed in more detail in the section "Desexualized and Safe Touch."

The Energetic Component of Touch

In bodywork, touch is much more than just applying techniques to the client's body. Although there is a physical component, there is also an energetic component, which is equally important in the therapeutic relationship. It, in fact, plays a major role in the connection that can form between you and the client. Although it is not always discussed in Western bodywork, Eastern modalities have a term for the energetic component of the body. In traditional Chinese medicine it is called **Qi;** in the Japanese bodywork modality of shiatsu it is called **Ki;** in Ayurveda, the traditional medicine of India, it is called **Prana.** Qi, Ki, and Prana all refer to the energy or force that gives and maintains life and also is the connection between organisms and all creation.

According to each Eastern modality the energy flows through the body in specifically defined channels, also called meridians. For example, Figure 9.5 shows the channels of Qi flow in traditional Chinese medicine. Along these channels are points where the Qi can be accessed most directly. In acupuncture, needles are inserted at these points; in shiatsu (which is based on traditional Chinese medicine), the practitioner presses on these points using his fingers, thumbs, elbows, and toes.

Optimally, this energy flows within living creatures in a balanced, harmonious way, sustaining health. If it is not flowing properly, disharmony and a lack of balance result, causing illness. In Asian bodywork modalities such as shiatsu, the practitioner uses his own Ki to balance the Ki of the client. The practitioner connects with the client's Ki through touch and receives information about how the client's Ki is flowing. This is the basis for how the practitioner proceeds with the treatment. Energetic connection also occurs in Western modalities, such as massage therapy, even though no name may be given to the phenomenon.

Whether performing Western or Eastern bodywork, however, it is not until you touch the client and feel the client's energy that you have an understanding of what is going on in that person's body. You convey that understanding back to the client through touch. You then work to help clients create change in their bodies through therapeutic touch and the application of techniques, using your own energy to support your clients' energy.

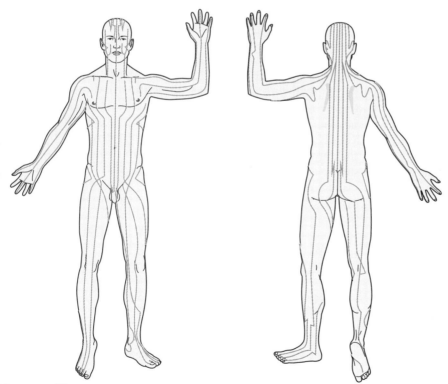

Figure 9.5 The major channels of Qi flow in traditional Chinese medicine.

Benefits of Therapeutic Touch

There is no doubt that humans function best when they have a balance among the physical, emotional, mental, and spiritual planes of existence. This balance takes into account that each factor plays a part in creating a healthy and whole human being. Therapeutic touch can be a tremendous support to those who are struggling to find this balance in their lives.

Therapeutic touch can benefit people on the physical plane because it makes direct contact with their bodies by allowing manual manipulation of the soft muscle tissue to relax tension, bring nutrition to the tissues, and carry wastes away. Structural integration techniques address the skeleton so that bones can be in better alignment, thus creating better movement in the joints. Craniosacral therapy has a healing power for the nervous system and the meninges of the brain to be free of restrictions. Asian bodywork addresses the subtle channels of energy throughout the body, bringing energy to areas that are depleted and dispersing energy from areas that have too much.

Many people use therapeutic touch as a way to regain perspective, and become grounded and centered, and as a means to be positive and stay engaged in all aspects of their lives. The emotional plane is addressed by therapeutic touch within the therapeutic relationship created between the practitioner and the client. By being in a place of safety, the client can let down his or her guard. This allows the client to become vulnerable and release emotions that have been repressed or have been stored as muscle memories or within inefficient postural alignments. Sometimes the emotional healing that takes place has a physical component such as a more aligned posture and muscles that relax in tone. Because it is subjective, emotionally healing may be reported by the client as an enhanced sense of well-being or as better sleep.

Humans exert a lot of brainpower each day navigating this busy and overstimulating world. Many forms of bodywork allow the mind to become still so that meditation or deep breathing techniques can be used to calm the mind. The mental aspect of being human benefits from therapeutic touch because clients have a chance to turn off the mind and not necessarily be so mentally active during the treatment. This can carry over into their everyday lives, and clients can report feeling calmer and having greater mental clarity.

The spiritual aspect of the client can be affected by therapeutic touch in that it allows for the individual to be quiet and still enough to be able to ponder concepts of faith, hope, God, Allah, the Higher Power, and the like. Of course, not everyone is inclined to explore his or her spiritual side, but it is an option if one chooses to take it. Individuals with deep spiritual practices such as meditation, formal religious practice, ceremonial sweats, or yoga as part of a spiritual practice report feeling a greater sense of calm, a greater capacity to face the unexpected, and the ability to stay focused at times of great crisis. Cultivating a healthy spiritual practice is often coupled with receiving regular bodywork sessions. The two complement each other nicely because it seems the more grounded and centered the individual is in his or her body, the more open he or she can be to the spiritual aspects of himself or herself.

Annually, Americans spend quite a bit of money on complementary and alternative medicine. According to the National Institutes of Health,

National Center for Complementary and Alternative Medicine, from 2006 to 2007, 38% of adults used some form of complementary and alternative medicine. They spent $33.9 billion for such things as herbal supplements, meditation, chiropractic care, acupuncture, and massage therapy.[6]

There is a great deal of interest in the unconventional treatments and healing methods. Accordingly, in recent years, research into the health and healing aspects of bodywork for specific conditions or situations has been on the rise. What is being discovered through this research is that therapeutic touch is proving to be quite effective in relieving certain symptoms and conditions.

For example, according to a study conducted by staff at the University of Minnesota in Minneapolis and the United Hospital Department of Integrative Health in St. Paul, Minnesota, "massage therapy and healing touch reduced pain, mood disturbance (anger, anxiety, depression, confusion) and fatigue in cancer patients undergoing chemotherapy."[7]

Another study, conducted by staff at the University of Arkansas for Medical Sciences College of Nursing and the University of Washington Biobehavioral Nursing and Health Systems School of Nursing, shows that "Therapeutic Touch® alleviated agitated behavior, such as mumbling and pacing, in people with Alzheimer's disease, according to a research study."[8]

A study conducted by the University of Colorado Health Sciences Center School of Nursing and the Outpatient Bone Marrow Transplant Unit of the University of Colorado Hospital in Denver found that "massage therapy reduced neurological complications and increased patients' perception of the benefits of therapy following a bone marrow transplant. Both massage therapy and Therapeutic Touch significantly increased patients' comfort after the bone marrow transplant."[9]

Bodywork has been shown to be helpful for survivors of trauma. When working with men and women who have survived physical or emotional abuse it is important that the practitioner clarify before the treatment session what will be happening so that the client can feel safe and have control over what will transpire. Choice was taken away from the survivor when the traumatic experience happened. Bodywork can be a way for the individual to experience making choices about every aspect of the treatment. Examples include whether or not to be clothed (such as for massage therapy); what type of music, if any, to listen to; what type of lubricant will be used (for bodywork that usually uses a lubricant); how long the session will be; and what techniques will be used. The goal is to integrate safe touch into the person's healing process (Box 9.2).

The terminally ill and dying may feel depression, isolation, grief from loss of freedom and friends, fear of abandonment, fear of the disease or aging, or fear of dying. Gentle relaxation bodywork may be able to reduce anxiety, and help the person feel a sense of general well-being. Bodywork may also help the person to release pent-up feelings of frustration, sadness, and anger. Pain that is aggravated by stress may be lessened with relaxing massage.

All of these examples demonstrate that therapeutic touch helps the receiver on many levels. Although sometimes the most obvious effects are physical, the person's mental, emotional, and spiritual aspects also benefit. Bodywork and the therapeutic relationship can help those in every stage of life, from infancy to those near the end of their life, and those who are robust and healthy to those with terminal illnesses.

 Food for Thought

Have you ever received touch that helped you heal in some way? It could be as simple as someone resting his hand on your shoulder when you needed it most to bodywork that helped relieve a specific condition you have had. What was the experience? What did the touch feel like? What were the results? What did you like most about the touch? Was there anything you didn't like? What was it?

| Box 9.2 | **CARSON'S STORY** |

A survivor of trauma, I bring more than biceps and hamstrings to the massage table. I come with a keen sensitivity to the benefits and dangers of allowing oneself to be seen and touched by another person. To lie beneath a sheet and permit someone that I barely know to make physical and visual contact with my belly, thighs, and face is to cruise into the waters of vulnerability. At this stage of my life, having worked through the events that did harm and the wounds that they left, I can tolerate such visibility, but I couldn't always.

To get here I had to navigate the immense need and pain that deprivation and abuse left in their wake, need and pain that became acute when I sought out physical contact. I did not make the voyage alone. I had the help of a skilled psychotherapist. The qualities that made it possible for me to accept her help during that most defenseless of times are the same qualities that I look for when I seek out a massage therapist today. I look for a self-possessed practitioner with a steady demeanor and a measure of emotional intelligence. I look for warmth, compassion, respect, and a willingness to let me determine whether and how much to interact. When I have the pleasure of working with a therapist who integrates these qualities into his or her work, my emotions and thoughts are at liberty to unmoor themselves and sail productively over the seas of my consciousness, while my body lies quietly on the table.

Laying unclothed beneath a sheet, allowing a person that I don't know well to see and touch my body, allowing that same person to witness my retreat into an inwardly focused state . . . I cannot access the benefits of such an encounter if I am not willing to shed the protection that clothing, a guarded posture, and an outward focus generally provide. Dropping these protective covers, however, demands that I trust the practitioner who sees and touches this more vulnerable version of me. For these reasons I seek out therapists who possess the same set of qualities that helped give me safe passage through the harrowing work of learning to tolerate touch and the vulnerability that comes with it. I look for a practitioner whose internal poise and agility enable her to handle whatever I bring to the table, one who possesses a steady demeanor that honors necessary boundaries, one who conveys a sense of warmth and respect for me as a client, and, finally, a quiet presence that allows me to decide whether and how I want to interact.

Intimacy and Touch

To prevent sexualized touch during bodywork, you need to understand more than just the mechanics of touch. You need to have an understanding of how touch is often used to communicate emotional and/or sexual intimacy between people and how you, as the practitioner, need to be careful of the intention behind your touch, as well as how to interpret your client's touch.

"Intimacy" has been defined as physical or emotional closeness to someone else. Note that these two do not necessarily always occur together. Physical intimacy simply means that two people are willing to be physically close to one another, with or without emotional intimacy. For example, you might experience physical intimacy with several strangers on a crowded elevator. Although you are very physically close to these people, you do not necessarily experience emotional intimacy with them.

Emotional intimacy, however, means that someone is willing to be vulnerable with another person and allow her to see a part of himself that he reserves for those with whom he feels safe. There is a high degree of trust for that person based on a history with her. The history can be the length of time the people have known each other or an experience that was very definitive for both parties, such as the death of a loved one or achieving a hard-earned goal together. The ultimate in emotional intimacy is consensual sex between two people as an expression of love. To complicate things, emotional intimacy is often, but not always, communicated by one person to another through physical intimacy.

Physical intimacy is a given in the bodywork profession. As a massage therapist, you will be more physically intimate with your clients than almost any other professional will be. The challenge you face, then, is to maintain an appropriate level of emotional intimacy with your client through your touch, and never allowing this intimacy to cross over into sexual intimacy.

True emotional intimacy occurs when people are choosing to be connected and give equally to the relationship out of trust and respect for one another. This is the type of intimacy that you need to strive for with your clients. The therapeutic relationship is based on sharing common goals, mutual respect for what each brings to the relationship, and the understanding that this is a professional agreement, not a personal friendship. Of course, clients do sometimes become practitioners' friends, but practitioners must not lose sight of the fact that they and their clients have grown close because the clients have chosen them to be their bodywork practitioners. The bodywork session should not become a time to socialize but remain professional in all ways.

Personal History of Touch

History is often a guide that informs individuals what to expect or how to behave in the present based on understanding what issues or circumstances they experienced in the past. When it comes to the concept of touch, everyone's history is rich and diverse, and depends on where they spent their developmental years, what messages or experiences they received in their family of origin about the necessity of touch, and even, perhaps, what religious or spiritual beliefs they hold. All of these factors influence how people view touch, decide on what type of touch they want to experience, and respond to the actual types of touch they receive.

During the 9 months that humans spend in utero they experience constant tactile stimulation. After birth, infants who continue to receive nurturing and consistent touch thrive. Growth will continue as the child matures and achieves other developmental milestones if he or she continues to receive appropriate and healthy touch. These kinds of touch play an active role in these developmental stages because the child feels supported and encouraged to explore, knowing that there is a safe place to return to, such as a parent's arms or a loved one's lap. This helps the child to trust appropriate touch by relying on the knowledge that she or he is protected.

If the child experiences abusive touch, or is neglected, then the child may grow up distrusting any type of touch from anyone. There can be other issues such as fears of being close to or far away from other people, along with having poor physical or emotional boundaries. There is the possibility that the child may grow into a person who only physically contacts others using abusive touch because he or she is unaware that there is any other kind.

Conversely, the child may instead want touch all the time, no matter who it is from or the circumstances in which it is given. This type of child may

Food for Thought
Think of times when you have experienced one or more of the different types of touch. Under what circumstances did you experience these types of touch? What level of intimacy did you feel you had in each of the experiences? How comfortable were you with these levels of intimacy?

grow into a person who, for example, uses sexual intercourse as a means to be touched, but does not make good choices in sexual partners.

Ellen Bass and Laura Davis are the authors of *The Courage to Heal: A Guide for Women Survivors of Child Sexual Abuse,* a guidebook for survivors of child sexual abuse. Although it is written for women, the information applies to both women and men. It is a useful book for bodywork practitioners to consult as it provides extensive information and resources about sexual abuse while neutralizing the anxiety that they may feel when working with a survivor of this type of trauma. The authors' philosophy is that "everyone deserves to heal, and healing is possible for everyone." This philosophy provides a sense of hope and empowerment for everyone involved in the process of healing the past.

The following are key areas of interpersonal development that are negatively affected by abuse:

- **Development of self-esteem.** Children were told directly that they will never succeed, that they are stupid, or that they are only good for sex. They have a difficult time identifying needs, nurturing and taking care of themselves, and recognizing their own interests, talents, or goals.
- **Feelings.** Feelings are not to be trusted, expressed, or even experienced. Depression, despair, anxiety, and panic attacks are common, or feelings alternate between overwhelming anxiety, fear, or rage and being numb and shut down.
- **Body.** The body is a place where frightening and painful things happen; therefore, they think the world and their bodies are not safe. They learn to ignore the body and live mostly in their heads. Often they are unable to relax or feel physically safe, they mistrust and blame their bodies, and they feel numb or disconnected from physical sensations.
- **Intimacy.** They lack the capacity for intimacy because they have experienced deep betrayal and a violation of trust by adults who were supposed to protect and provide safety. They feel alienated or isolated, do not know whom to trust or trust too readily, or feel taken advantage of.
- **Sexuality.** Natural sexual development is stolen; therefore, sexual arousal becomes linked to feelings of shame, disgust, pain, and humiliation. Pleasure is tainted and desire is dangerous.
- **Parenting skills.** Because they did not witness healthy modeling by their own parents, they may repeat the same damaging patterns they grew up with by abusing, neglecting, or failing to protect their own children. They may choose not to have children at all.
- **Family relationships.** Essential trust, sharing, and safety are missing, and in their place there is secrecy, isolation, and fear. They may feel crazy, invalidated, and/or depressed when visiting family. Sometimes they are alienated or completely estranged from family members.[10]

In his book *Compassionate Touch: The Body's Role in Emotional Healing and Recovery,* Dr. Clyde Ford draws a parallel between abuse survivors and emotional dysfunction. Ford states that the persistent emotional and psychological scars of abuse have a strong somatic component that results in lowered self-esteem, lowered self-worth, and a sense of helplessness and powerlessness. The resulting feelings of guilt and shame experienced by the survivor are centered on the body, manifesting into behaviors such as obsessive-compulsive behavior, self-mutilation, and perpetration of abuse.[11]

States Ford, "With the body so directly involved in the long-term consequences of sexual abuse, I've sought ways to directly involve the body in the treatment of abuse . . . ultimately therapeutic gains are consolidated and the survivor emerges with greater empowerment to continue living, healing, and recovering."[12] Bodywork provides a safe place for the survivor to consciously reunite with her body and integrate her past with the present. Touch is no longer the enemy.

Being informed about these issues allows you to be present with your client should she confide in you or if you sense the possibility that she is a trauma survivor. If you are a survivor of trauma, this information will assist you in maintaining professional boundaries and manage any transference or countertransference you may experience without bringing harm to your client.

Other life events can influence the perception of touch. For example, people who have undergone painful and extensive medical interventions or had serious accidents, especially at a young age, may have quite a different view of touch than does someone who did not experience these. Men and women who have children may view touch differently from those who do not have children. People who have much contact with animals may also give and receive touch differently from those who have not.

Other Factors Affecting Personal Perception of Touch

Once individuals achieve autonomy and move beyond their family of origin or outside their cultural surroundings they may adopt different behaviors or perceptions about the role touch will play in their lives. For example, a woman who grew up in a very close household may have felt stifled by all the togetherness. She may choose to seek space in her life away from home, and so is hesitant in her contact with others. Conversely, a young man who experienced a lot of pressure to be tough and strong for the first 20 years of his life may not have experienced soothing touch from loved ones. That may have been considered "sissy" in his household. As an adult he may seek a community that allows for him to balance his masculine and his feminine qualities, such as bodywork. The type of experience one has and the people who made that experience happen have the biggest influence on how the individual will embrace touch for the rest of his or her life.

Each person defines an area around himself as personal space, and the distance encompassed by this personal space differs from person to person and culture to culture. Bodywork enters this personal space. Because of this, practitioners must be aware of and sensitive to the various factors that influence people's responses when their personal space is entered. More than one practitioner has been caught off guard by an unexpected response from a client in response to the touch given. The receiver of bodywork may interpret the practitioner's touch in a way that was not intended. He or she may project his or her own issues regarding touch onto the practitioner. The touch may even be perceived as abusive or sexual when the practitioner had no such intention.

Words of Wisdom

As a cancer survivor, I have an understanding of health and wellness from the perspective of being seriously ill. Along with traditional cancer treatments, I received massage therapy, which really helped me through this difficult experience. It made me want to give to others what I have been given, and the best way I can do this is through being a massage therapist. I enjoy being around people, and it feels good to help people reduce their stress and feel better in their bodies.

—JANNA HARVEY,
Licensed Massage Therapist
since 2009, cancer survivor

Food for Thought

Think of a time when your personal space was entered without invitation. How did you feel? How did you react?

Cultural backgrounds also influence the perception of touch. While not everyone in a certain culture can react a certain way, sometimes there are certain tendencies within a culture. For example, in her book *Touch,* Dr. Tiffany Field states, "In African cultures . . . people live skin-to-skin with virtually everyone. . . . Some cultures do more touching than others. For example, the French touch people more than the Americans or the British."

You might want to examine your own cultural views of touch to see how well these views enhance how you give bodywork, as well as what challenges they present for you. In addition, you are likely to have clients from a wide variety of cultural backgrounds. It is virtually impossible to know how every possible different culture views types of touch. You should also not make assumptions about a person's perception of touch based on the person's culture. Instead, be sensitive to the fact that different people have different views of touch. You should also remain professional at all times, and talk about the touch used in bodywork in terms that are designed to leave no doubt in the client's mind that it is therapeutic. You can observe how clients act and model from them, following the client's lead. Ask questions and let the clients be the educators about themselves and their culture.

Women and men sometimes have different concepts of the appropriateness of touch. In general, women tend to have somewhat smaller and more approachable personal space. Men tend to have larger, more structured personal spaces that they are most comfortable having others enter only by invitation. Of course, these patterns are also influenced by cultural customs and family history.

Male practitioners working with women clients should also be mindful that most cases of sexual harassment and abuse are committed toward women. It is likely that some of their clients will have such a history. It is also possible that the women may not recognize these past experiences as affecting them in the present. What this means is that these clients may have a sudden, unexpected response to touch that neither they, nor the practitioner, were aware would happen.

Age is another factor in the perception of touch. Some may consider touching very young people appropriate but may be more cautious about touching older people. Or perhaps older people may be more hesitant about being touched than a younger person might. In addition, the touch of a young practitioner may be interpreted differently from the touch of an older practitioner, even if the skill and expertise levels are the same. For example, the older practitioner may be seen as more experienced, wiser, and calmer than the younger practitioner. Clients may think, then, that the older practitioner's touch is more therapeutic, whereas the younger practitioner's is less experienced.

There is no other way to be a bodywork practitioner than to have intimate contact with another through touch. The practitioner's comfort level must be genuine and authentic or else clients will be able to pick up on the hesitancy and discomfort and not be satisfied with the work. Conversely, a practitioner could be so at ease with the power of touch that she has poor boundaries around providing touch. She may be the type of practitioner who touches everyone who comes within 3 feet of her, usually without asking permission first.

Assessing Touch Comfort Levels

A person who has made the decision to become a bodywork practitioner would benefit greatly from reflecting on his personal "touch timeline." This can give the person information about how well suited he is for this intimate profession. Figure 9.6 shows an example of a touch timeline. Practitioners are encouraged to fill one out for themselves. Make sure it includes family history of touch, as well as cultural influences.

People may realize they have challenges in giving and receiving touch that they were completely unaware of. They then have the choice of working on the challenges if they want to become a bodyworker, or choosing another, less touch-intensive profession. Conversely, people may discover just how completely in tune with therapeutic touch they are, and are completely comfortable with becoming a bodyworker.

Rebecca Martinson

Family only shows physical affection (in the form of hugs) throughout lifetime.

1960 **Birth.** Youngest of four children. Held a lot by siblings and aunts (as reported by her sister). Kissed parents goodnight regularly.

1965 **Started school.** While boarding the bus to school, was pushed down on the steps by someone from behind her. Began standing in the back of the line to get on, and sitting alone on the bus, if possible, or with sisters.

1968 **Dance lessons.** Learned paired dancing; didn't like it at all.

1970 **Held hands** for the first time with a boy at school, during a movie.

1974 **First date and first kiss.** Slow danced with a boy (in a hugging position)

1978 **Graduated high school.** Dated on and off throughout high school but had minimal physical contact during the dates (hand holding, a few kisses).

1978– **College years.** Involved with church group; had a great deal of camaraderie. Group members hugged each
1982 other, held hands and massaged each others' shoulders in a platonic fashion.

1979 **First sexual experience.** Enjoyed it but the relationship did not last long.
1981 **Date raped.** Was told by her date that "she made him do it." Felt a great deal of shame and responsibility. Was told by her family and friends to keep it quiet.

1983– **Started career as an accountant.** Went out on a few dates but nothing serious. Formed a large network of
1988 friends that demonstrated affection through platonic touch.

1990 **Received first massage.** From a female practitioner. Enjoyed it.

1991 **Becomes frustrated with job.** Having received massage on a regular basis for two years, starts to explore it as a career option.

1992 **Started massage school.** During the program, instructors bring to her attention that she never pairs up with male students to practice during class. She also stiffens up every time a male instructor or teaching assistant touches her when showing her practice partner how to perform techniques properly. In her student clinic, her female clients have positive feedback about the treatments they receive from her but her male clients dislike the treatments they receive. Rebecca states she had no idea this was happening. She agrees to meet with her massage instructors on a regular basis to work on these issues. She also decides to see a professional counselor on her own.

1993– **Owns a successful massage therapy business.** Has many satisfied male and female clients. Has been
present in a happy, long-term, committed relationship since 1998.

Figure 9.6 Example of a touch time line.

It would be beneficial for the new bodywork student to interview practitioners who have been in the profession for 4 or more years to gain insight about how they manage the issue of being comfortable with the level of intimacy and what measures they may have taken to reach their current level of comfort if it did not come naturally. Discussing these findings, as well as the practitioner's own touch timeline, with a trusted mentor or supervisor will help the student gain perspective on the situation as well as develop strategies, if necessary, to fully embrace the role of bodywork practitioner.

Other resources also exist for those who have a history in which touch was used against them, and now tend to have a more difficult time receiving appropriate and therapeutic touch. Seeking help is sometimes not easy to do, but professional counseling services could be crucial for healing the past and integrating it into the future. Professional counseling may bring awareness to many issues, such as transference and countertransference, that could prevent the bodywork student from being successful. It can help the person determine what it is they want to achieve by using therapeutic touch, rather than denying themselves the experience of safe, therapeutic touch.

It is essential that bodywork practitioners make an effort to understand how their past experiences with touch are influencing them now. This self-reflection as well as the knowledge gained gives practitioners opportunities to create a life that is rich and fulfilling instead of one perhaps filled with anger or fear. Not only will this help practitioners to become more comfortable with themselves, it will help them better relate to clients who have a similar history. This gives bodywork practitioners the ability to educate clients on the healing powers of touch by being present and focused in the therapeutic relationship.

Touch Overload

In the bodywork profession, a practitioner who has been working for a certain period of time may no longer want to touch his clients. This could be seen as burnout or **touch overload.** It can happen if a practitioner has not been practicing self-care, and has performed many treatments without a break or has not taken any time off to recharge. It can also happen if a practitioner uncovers some emotional information that was previously hidden from his consciousness. Sometimes practitioners may feel emotionally vulnerable and just not have the energy to work on clients. Whether the practitioner is aware of what is happening, or just has a gut feeling that something is amiss, the result is that the practitioner wants to stop touching others.

Practitioners who practice healthy boundaries and maintain a balanced work and relaxation schedule will have greater success at not experiencing touch burnout. This is not to say that the occasionally "off day" or bad mood will not happen. The key to a successful practice, though, is how the practitioner manages his response, and manages his resources.

Touch in Bodywork Programs

Students attending school to learn bodywork have, of course, a personal history around the role touch has played in their lives. This history is important for the student to explore as it will have an impact on the student's ability to embrace the intimacy of bodywork as well as the level of success the student will have in gaining skill and competency. The more self-aware and comfortable the student is with touching and being touched, the more ease the student will experience while learning as opposed to the student who has little self-awareness and is fearful or indifferent to the experience of touch.

Bodywork students who have challenges around touch can choose to grow into a zone of comfort and ease with it. If they do not, they will not be successful practitioners. However, they must be honest with themselves, and be willing and able to make adjustments. This process should be assisted by meeting with a mentor or a trusted faculty member. These students benefit from having an objective person listen and bear witness to their experiences with touch as well as their concerns, challenges, and successes. A starting point for such a discussion is to share candidly about what it feels like to have such intimate contact with others, and what self-care measures are in place or are lacking.

New Students

A recent interesting phenomenon some massage and bodywork schools have been experiencing is the rising number of new students who have never received a professional bodywork treatment. This brings up some good questions. How do these students know they want a job performing bodywork if they have never received a treatment? How do they know they will like to be touched in the ways required to learn bodywork if they have never received a professional treatment? Are they fully aware of the level of intimacy, both emotional and physical, it requires to be a successful bodyworker?

When asked why they have chosen to become bodyworkers, the answers may vary from, "I want a job where I can help people feel better" to "I want a job where I am my own boss" to "It sounds like a fun job." All of these are valid reasons for wanting to become a bodyworker. However, this brings up the question of whether the connection has been made in the new student's mind that he or she is entering a profession that is not like most 9-to-5 jobs.

Some practitioners refer to their work as a calling or as a vocation. They feel compelled to learn the craft because they themselves have benefited so much and they want to be a part of helping others to have the experiences they have had. Some individuals who choose to attend bodywork schools describe it as a personal development program where anatomy and physiology and bodywork techniques happened to be taught, too. In other words, attending school to become a bodywork practitioner can change lives. If students are willing, school has the potential to open their eyes and hearts to the human experience as no other school can.

Why can this happen? Perhaps it is because, as a student, the individual was willing to open herself up to the unknown. The student was willing to be vulnerable to be touched in a way that was safe and therapeutic on a physical level as well as an emotional level. The student was willing to look deeper into his or her own life experience and explore how touch and intimacy contributed to her personal growth and development.

To be vulnerable in this way can open the person to all sorts of discoveries such as the following:

- How she formed ideas and opinions about the world, or even discover that she has few ideas or opinions
- Who has influenced her the most prior to this point in life
- What the level of trust she has in order to be honest with others . . . especially people she does not know well

All of the work is essential because it mirrors what you expect your clients to do each and every time they come in for a session—be vulnerable and willing to trust that you will provide a safe environment in which to experience therapeutic touch. If practitioners are unwilling to do this, how can they expect this of their clients?

Consider again the new student who has never had a bodywork treatment before enrolling in school; that student needs to be reassured that she has indeed chosen a great profession. But the student should receive a professional treatment as soon as possible so that she can begin to map her own journey of discovering how bodywork will affect her life.

Some of the waypoints you can use on your journey include considering the following:

- What does it feel like to have a stranger touch me?
- Do I find therapeutic touch comfortable or does it feel awkward?
- Has anyone ever really touched me in this way before?
- Are there functional limitations in my muscles or joints that I did not know about before receiving the treatment?
- How did my body become the way it is now?
- How can bodywork help increase my health, strength, and movement?
- What is it like to be quiet for the entire time that the practitioner is giving the treatment?
- Am I comfortable with the silence or do I need to talk a bit during the treatment? If so, why do I need to talk? Is it to decrease the anxiety I feel?

The point of all these questions is to create an understanding of the role touch has played in the past for you as well as the role it will play in the future. Sometimes new students believe that they are entering a trade school and there is nothing else involved except performing the manual techniques on the clients and scheduling them for their next appointment. This belief system does not take into account that therapeutic touch is central to this vocation, and it is not just a series of well-performed massage strokes or other bodywork techniques.

Educators

Bodywork educators have a responsibility to prepare future practitioners for what is waiting for them in the real world in terms of understanding the impact that one's sexuality has on his or her ability to be an ethically sound bodywork practitioner. Sexuality is part of being human. It is shaped by the following:

- Family history of how issues of sexuality were discussed or not discussed
- Early experiences of touch and sexual experimentation

Food for Thought

Why did you decide to become a bodywork practitioner? What in your life brought you to the point where you wanted to learn your particular modality? What role did your experiences with touch play in your decision?

- How comfortable practitioners are with their own sexuality and sexual identity
- How aware they are of what arouses them or what makes them uncomfortable in terms of sexuality
- How they define "intimacy," "sexuality," "sex," and "eroticism"
- How they acknowledge a very human part of themselves while remaining ethical bodywork professionals

Encouraging this kind of exploration and reflection can be a daunting task for educators and students alike. However, it is necessary so that practitioners will become conscious about what role sexuality and intimacy plays in their ability or inability to connect with clients on a therapeutic level.

In addition to raising the awareness of these issues, educators must also be mindful of their presentation styles.

Consider the following: Sheila is a new student at massage therapy school. She almost leaves the program after the first week because she is uncomfortable with the emphasis that the instructors put on making sure that the students understand that they are learning "nonsexual, therapeutic" massage. It is also continually emphasized that it is the obligation of all practitioners to make clients understand that nothing torrid is going to happen during a session. At one point, she tells her husband, "I feel like I'm being primed to be a pioneer for making sure the profession would never be maligned." Some of the instructors use humor when describing the various uncomfortable situations practitioners may find themselves in. In addition, her classmates giggle and make inappropriate jokes about the topic to one another. All of this annoys Sheila and makes her question the intentions of her educators and classmates.

Sheila decides to stay in the program. Eventually she comes to realize that although she is uneasy with the topic, she is also projecting some of her unresolved feelings around experiencing inappropriate touch herself. She decides to seek professional counseling to make sense of her reactions because she does not want to let go of her desire to become a bodywork practitioner. Once she gets some perspective, and develops skills to communicate to others about being respectful of the bodywork profession she no longer has the desire to leave school.

As this scenario illustrates, educators must be conscious about the many levels students can be affected by this topic. Sometimes appropriate humor may be used by educators to ease the tension that this subject can create or that may be found offensive by students. Educators must also be mindful that they do not present this material in such a manner that it instills fear in the students. They can never know what history students bring with them; it is likely some will be incest or sexual assault survivors.It is the job of educators to be as professional and direct as possible when discussing sexuality, and they need to be sensitive and respectful as well.

Desexualized Touch

Touch is one of the five senses, which makes it, by definition, **sensual**, relating to or consisting of the gratification of the senses. Being sensual usually implies a connection to the physical body. Sometimes people in our society have mistaken and continue to mistake the sensual nature of bodywork as being sexual, thus associating bodywork with sexual gratification. Sensual touch does not have to imply foreplay to sexual activity, however. It can imply nonsexual pleasure, enjoyment, satisfaction, or relief. These states are all appropriate outcomes for a therapeutic bodywork session.

With advertisers in our culture sexualizing any and every product to get our attention, how do we as bodywork practitioners navigate our way through this maze to promote our businesses? We need to do so with care, with knowledge, sound intention, and carefully scripted dialogues to diffuse uncomfortable situations.

Defining Desexualized Touch

What exactly is desexualized touch? And why do bodywork practitioners have to desexualize touch if they are not the ones making it sexual? The reality is, however, that it *is* the responsibility of practitioners to desexualize bodywork, because many times the public does not. As has been discussed, current culture is saturated with images of sex appeal as a means to get attention. Because this is a given, it cannot be ignored but instead needs to be faced and the public educated.

To sexualize experiences means to make the event, procedure, or conversation something that is sexual or could be interpreted as sexual. **Desexualized touch,** then, means the practitioner ensures that the way he or she touches the client during the treatment is not in any way turned into an erotic or sexual experience for either the practitioner or the client. In addition to desexualized touch, practitioners need to make sure their verbal and nonverbal communication is desexualized as well. This includes being diligent about the words they use and how they say them, as well as their body language.

Ethically appropriate touch does not just happen. Practitioners must have awareness of their own sexuality and be willing and able to keep it separate from all aspects of their professional bodywork career. They must be absolutely professional at all times. In addition, they need to be prepared to deal with the physiological, mental, and emotional reactions of arousal if and when they occur, either in themselves or in their clients.

Creating Desexualized Bodywork

As has been discussed previously, there is no doubt that much of modern American culture is sexualized. Bodywork, especially massage therapy, has long been erroneously linked to sexual acts and sexual services. There is no doubt that current views on sexuality, and the fact that it is rampant throughout all forms of entertainment and advertising, tend to perpetuate the association of sex and bodywork in the minds of some consumers, no matter how hard members of the bodywork profession work to promote the fact that the touch used in bodywork is therapeutic, and that this type of touch has healing benefits. Even though bodywork has made great strides in gaining respect and acceptance in recent years, the words "bodywork" and "massage" still conjure erotic thoughts in the minds of many.

Sometimes practitioners think that a desexualized treatment environment means only that the practitioner does not flirt with, attempt to date, or have sex with clients. In fact, when bodywork students and some professional practitioners are asked what it means to be ethical, the almost universal answer is usually, "Don't sleep with your clients." Although this is certainly true, the reality is much more complex than that.

Issues are not always clear. For example, certain practitioners may not realize the image they are projecting is a sexual one and do not understand why clients flirt with them or ask them out on dates. Other practitioners do realize they are projecting a sexual image but think that is normal and acceptable because current culture is highly sexualized—provocative clothing and sexual language are the norm in entertainment and advertising. Some of these practitioners may be blindsided one day by a client who assumes they will provide sexual services during bodywork and will not take no for an answer. Yet other practitioners may be diligent about dressing and speaking professionally, but think that they need to tolerate flirty and sexualized behavior from clients, no matter how uncomfortable it makes them, because they feel that the client is always right.

Practitioners have the right to be treated with dignity and respect. They also have the obligation of ensuring that the bodywork profession is treated with dignity and respect. Although it is certainly true that practitioners cannot control the behavior of others, they do have control over their own behavior. Also, although practitioners are sexual beings, they do have control over when and how they express it. This is the difference between sexuality and sexual activity. Practitioners cannot divorce themselves from their sexual nature, but they can control their sexual activity by being responsible and appropriate.

The first step for you to create desexualized bodywork is awareness of your own sexuality. You can start by asking yourself the following questions:

- When you find someone attractive, does your behavior become flirty, no matter what the setting? If so, why do you think that is? If not, why not?
- Does your conversation usually include sexual language of some sort? If so, what are some of the terms you use?
- How do you think your sexuality affects the therapeutic relationship?
- Have you observed sexuality in your bodywork program experience and in your practice sessions or conversations about bodywork so far? If so, how did that make you feel? Why do you think you felt that way?
- Do you think you have ever made unconscious judgments or comments about a client regarding his or her sexuality?
- How would you feel if a client, practitioner, colleague, family member, or friend made a sexual comment about bodywork? Why do you think you would feel this way?
- How would you respond to someone who makes a sexual comment about bodywork? Why would you respond this way?

Answering these questions provides an opportunity for you to examine your motivations and commitment to your bodywork career as well as a chance for you to develop self-awareness and self-accountability, which are the foundations of ethical behavior and professionalism.

If you are unsure whether you display sexual behavior, intended or not, you can ask a trusted colleague or mentor for an honest evaluation, and you should be willing to listen without comment and be open to feedback.

When a practitioner is trying to change a pattern of behavior, he must first be aware that the pattern exists, and then he must be committed to breaking the pattern.

It would be wise for practitioners to take a look at how they dress, how they carry themselves (there is a difference between a confident bearing and a sexual one), and whether they seek attention for their physiques. The evaluation can include the volume of the practitioner's voice, the expressions on the face, and body gestures and hand movements when speaking, both in person and on the phone. Is any of it flirtatious or could it be misconstrued by someone else as an invitation to ask for a date or sexual favors? Does the practitioner seem more polite and accommodating to clients whom the practitioner finds attractive, and less so to those the practitioner is not attracted to?

The evaluation can be extended to the practitioner's treatment space. Are there any sights, sounds, or smells that can be considered erotic? In the case of bodywork that requires clients to remove clothing, such as for massage therapy, does the practitioner always use proper draping techniques? Is a robe provided in case the client needs to make a quick trip to the bathroom? When giving a treatment, is the practitioner mindful of body contact during the session? Is the contact appropriate for the treatment, or are there times when inappropriate contact seems to happen? Does the practitioner maintain professional boundaries at all times, or does she seem to lapse somewhat around people she finds attractive?

Nonsexualized interactions begin with practitioners making the conscious choice that they are not going to engage in such behavior. In addition, they ask their peers, friends, and colleagues to point out if they do engage in telling off-color jokes, acting flirtatiously, or dressing for work in a provocative manner.

Once practitioners are aware of their own sexuality and how it can possibly manifest in bodywork, they will be more able to recognize inappropriate language and behavior from others. There is, in fact, an entire continuum of sexual manipulation that can occur in the bodywork profession. In fact, every profession has to deal with these issues on some level. Most of these issues are also struggled with in some form in every culture as well.

Continuum of Sexual Manipulation in the Bodywork Profession

The most effective tool that a practitioner has to combat sexual manipulators or predators is awareness. The more aware and vigilant a practitioner is about the games and tactics used for illicit sexual gratification at another's expense the less likely the practitioner will be at risk for being violated. Practitioners should understand, however, that even if they do and say everything in an appropriate manner, certain people may still behave in inappropriate and threatening ways. Practitioners are not responsible for the behavior of these people; they are only responsible for their own.

Predatory behavior is defined as "greedily destructive; greedily eager to steal from or destroy others for gain; extremely aggressive; determined or persistent." How is it possible that someone with these goals would see bodywork as a means to achieve them? It is because this behavior is about people exerting power over others as well as getting needs met in a way that generates excitement for themselves at the expense of another. This happens in every profession and every walk of life.

Defining the Continuum

In all relationships, each person carries 50% of the responsibility for what goes well and what goes poorly. In a professional relationship, however, the practitioner is held to a higher standard than the client because the practitioner is the one with the expertise as well as the obligation to do no harm, either by neglect or abusive behavior, to the client.

The continuum of sexual manipulation begins as "harmless" flirting and can escalate to sexual activity between the client and the practitioner (Fig. 9.7). Flirtatious behavior, behaving in a playfully alluring manner, is not appropriate behavior for a professional practitioner to engage in. Sometimes certain practitioners will use this behavior in an effort to gain more clients or to receive higher gratuities. However, it sends a mixed message to the client—on the one hand the practitioner is presenting himself or herself as a professional bodyworker, and on the other hand is hinting that he or she is receptive to a more personal relationship with the client. Whether that is the actual intention, it demeans the profession. Practitioners who do this are also putting themselves at risk. Flirting can be easily interpreted as an actual invitation. More than one practitioner has been caught by surprise, to say the least, when a client took the flirting seriously. These practitioners might have thought that the client understood that it was all in fun. Some practitioners have actually been assaulted by clients when the clients assumed the flirting meant something more. Granted, the client chose to commit the assault, but the initial flirting on the part of the practitioner may have set the whole unfortunate situation in motion. If practitioners do not see the harm in some "innocent flirtation," then they should seek counsel from a respected supervisor or mentor.

The use of vulgar language, sharing off-color jokes, or telling explicit stories about one's sexual encounters are all examples of sexualized behavior

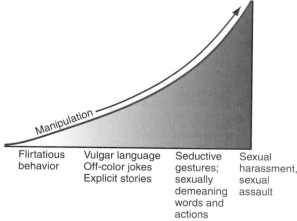

Figure 9.7 Continuum of sexual manipulation.

further along the continuum. It is being used to seek attention and to get a reaction out of another person. An individual with healthy boundaries, self-respect, and respect for others does not take part in this type of conversation. Practitioners who engage in public conversations such as this demean the profession by placing it right back in the realm of sexual services and prostitution. As peers and colleagues, practitioners should challenge one another about such behaviors and their impact on the profession.

If a conversation of this type occurs, the listener can ask the speaker why he or she is sharing this. The listener can then tell the speaker that he is not interested in what the speaker is saying, and ask the speaker to refrain from sharing. If the speaker continues, then the listener can make a choice about whether he wants a client, friend, or colleague who does not respect the boundary he has set. Practitioners always have the option of terminating the conversation and terminating the relationship.

Further along the continuum are gestures or expressions that are seductive or sexually demeaning. These can include sexual comments about either the practitioner's or client's body or clothing; strong interest in or disapproval of the client's or practitioner's sexual orientation; comments made during a treatment or pre- or post-treatment interview about sexual performance; conversations about sexual problems; the practitioner's or client's preferences or fantasies; failure to ensure a client's privacy by using improper draping; not providing a gown; opening the treatment room door while the client is dressing or undressing; unnecessary physical assessment of the breast and/or genital areas; inappropriate touching of the client or the practitioner; and unwelcome touching, hugging, and kissing.

Verbal sexual harassment includes inappropriate ways of addressing a person, such as calling another practitioner or a client "honey," "babe," or "sweetheart"; use of sexually explicit language; or using words that refer to the breasts or genitalia. It can also involve displaying visually explicit material, regardless of whether that material is intended to offend.

All of these activities can, in fact, be considered **sexual harassment** or even **sexual assault,** both of which are criminal acts. Sexual harassment is defined as "uninvited and unwelcome verbal or physical behavior of a sexual nature especially by a person in authority toward a subordinate (such as an employee or student)." Sexual assault is defined as "illegal sexual contact that usually involves force upon a person without consent or is inflicted upon a person who is incapable of giving consent (because of age or physical or mental incapacity) or who places the assailant (such as a doctor) in a position of trust or authority." Practitioners must not only be aware of sexual misconduct in the treatment setting, they must also be aware of sexual harassment in the work environment as well, such as between coworkers or from supervisors. Practitioners should also keep in mind that sexual harassment can be perpetrated by members of the same sex as well as the opposite sex.

Both sexual harassment and sexual assault are serious crimes. Should a practitioner who is an employee experience sexual harassment the practitioner needs to document the incident(s) and inform his or her supervisor unless, of course, the supervisor is the one performing the sexual harassment. In that case, the supervisor's superiors need to be notified, as well as law enforcement. If the practitioner is self-employed, the practitioner needs to notify law enforcement. If a practitioner is sexually assaulted, law enforcement needs to be contacted immediately. In any of these situations, the practitioner may also need to seek counseling from trusted mentors and colleagues, or from a professional counselor.

Sometimes it is difficult to tell if sexual manipulation is occurring. Unless it is blatant, some people may not be aware they are being manipulated by others. Usually during manipulation one person is acting in a devious and disingenuous manner. Their words and actions are not straightforward. One measure to determine if behavior is sexualized is for you to assess how you feel while it is happening, and when the encounter is over. Do you feel let down? Are you titillated? Did the encounter feel creepy? Are you confused, angry, or feeling nauseous? A yes to any of these responses is your body and intuition telling you that something was not above board or safe in this encounter. To assist you in recognizing when clients are not being appropriate, Box 9.3 lists sexually manipulative behaviors and Box 9.4 lists sexually inappropriate behaviors they may exhibit.

Another way you can recognize sexual manipulation is by honestly assessing your feelings if you regret some action, a comment, or an opinion you shared against your better judgment. Did you end up saying something you had not intended to? In that case, the other person may have been using manipulation. Or did you say it with the intention of gaining something from

---

Box 9.3 | **CLIENT SEXUALLY MANIPULATIVE BEHAVIORS**

- Excessive compliments about your physical attributes, e.g., your eyes, hair, and legs
- Questions about your personal life such as, "Where do you like to go out?" "Do you like to dance?" and "Are you seeing anyone?"
- Excessive comments about how lucky your wife, husband, partner, girlfriend, or boyfriend is to come home to you every night
- Flirting with you and either hinting at or asking outright about going out with you after the session, or that you and the client should get to know each other better
- Telling jokes or stories with sexual innuendo

Box 9.4 | **CLIENT SEXUALLY INAPPROPRIATE BEHAVIORS**

- Continued flirting with you when you have told the client to stop
- Grabbing or caressing your hands, legs, buttocks, breasts, or genitalia
- Asking sexually explicit questions about your personal life
- Asking your opinion of sexually explicit topics
- Telling sexually explicit jokes and stories
- Receiving massage with the intent of sexual arousal and/or release
- Masturbation during the massage
- Excessive moaning that resembles orgasm
- Male clients who grind their penis into the table when prone
- Male clients who continually readjust their genitalia during the session
- Asking for sexual favors, e.g., oral sex, manual stimulation, or intercourse

Have you ever come into contact with someone who sexually manipulated you? What was the experience like? What did you feel? What did you say and do? Knowing what you know now, what would you do differently?

Have you sexually manipulated someone else? If so, what did you say and do? Why did you do it? What were you hoping to gain? What was the experience like? What did you feel? Knowing what you know now, what would you do differently?

the other person? In that case, you yourself may be the person doing the manipulating.

For clients who have a pattern or tendency to sexualize or be manipulative, it is your role as the practitioner to inform them of their behavior and tell them to stop. If they do not take you seriously, then this is critical information you need to consider when determining if you will continue seeing the client.

Educating Clients About the Purpose of Bodywork

Bodywork practitioners have a tremendous ability to be influential in educating people who are unaware of the benefits of bodywork. Some new clients may be skeptical about the efficacy of bodywork because they have heard some misinformation about it, or they have a hard time trusting that someone would touch them without expecting something in return. They may even be touch deprived, and therefore are fearful about what may happen to them during the treatment.

The best place to start in the education process is to explain to clients how the touch is administered during the treatment, what the benefits of therapeutic touch are, what the client can expect to experience in a bodywork session, what the client can expect from the practitioner, informing the client of the best way to receive a bodywork session, and, most important, informing the client that he or she can stop the session at any time.

Giving the client permission to give feedback if something is not feeling right is another important aspect of educating potential clients. It is also helpful to schedule extra time for the first session to allow for the client to ask questions. While explaining the process of receiving a session it is also appropriate to explain what the equipment is and how it works and what choices the client has about disrobing. It is also wise to go over the treatment plan step by step so that the client can give informed consent and so that there will be no surprises for the client, or the practitioner.

Educating clients about the purpose of bodywork begins from the first contact with the client, whether it is by phone or in person, and may continue throughout the entire therapeutic relationship. The screening process, pretreatment interview, the treatment itself, and the post-treatment interview are all opportunities for practitioners to make clear verbally, physically, and environmentally that the session involves therapeutic, not illicit, touch.

In an initial phone conversation with a potential new client, you can make the purpose of bodywork clear by stating, "I provide nonsexual, therapeutic bodywork for the sole purpose of reducing stress and facilitating health and healing in the client." If the client has called looking for a sexual experience, this brief yet direct description ideally should clarify for the caller the intention of your work. You should note, however, that some clients will still persist in requesting sexual services or may even ask you for a referral to an establishment that performs them. At this point, your best response is to hang up on the client.

When meeting with the client in person, you should be dressed professionally in clothing that does not draw attention to your body. You should use verbal and body language that is professional, and related specifically to the therapeutic nature of the treatment. There should be little confusion about what type of treatment is being offered. Informed consent should be presented in such a verbal and written manner that there is no doubt that the treatments given are therapeutic and nonsexual.

The physical environment of the treatment space is also a precise way to demonstrate that the session is health-care related and not intended for sexual gratification. For example, the room can be decorated with items such as muscle and bone charts, chakra diagrams, or figures with shiatsu channels (meridians) located on them. Tasteful, nonerotic artwork is also a good choice. The lighting in the room should be appropriate for the interview. It should not be too dim because certain clients may perceive that as seductive. The lighting can be changed to a lower, more soothing level during the session. The music chosen should be appropriate and not have any sexual lyrics or moaning sounds.

Once a client experiences the professional tone of the interview, gives informed consent for the treatment plan discussed, and notices the professional environment of the office, optimally he or she knows that the bodywork treatment is about healing and rejuvenation. However, certain clients will still hope, or even think, that you will provide more than a therapeutic treatment if asked or offered more money. This may be done before the treatment starts, or during the treatment itself. In either case, you need to make it absolutely clear that the client will be receiving no sexual favors.

To assist you in how to handle these situations, an intervention model is presented.

Intervention Model

Some practitioners may think that they will never have to experience an interaction with a client who is being inappropriate. Perhaps it never occurs to them because they regard bodywork as part of health care, and they are always diligent in their professionalism. Others may think that they simply will not emanate an aura that would draw clients to them who have questionable motives. Yet others may think it happens to someone else, and will not happen to them.

However, it is usually not a matter of *if* it will happen, but *when* it will happen. There always have been, and always will be, people who think they are entitled to receive what they want when they want it. This includes sexual experiences within a bodywork treatment. Although it may be uncomfortable to think about, it is better to plan for the unexpected than to be confronted with a situation for which you are completely unprepared.

The following are some examples of scripts that you can use when a client requests a sexual encounter or alludes to the fact that he or she is interested in one.

Scenario One

Client: Are there any techniques you can use to release the tension in my groin?

Practitioner: Are asking if I will perform a technique that is sexual in nature?

Client: Ah, well maybe, if you can.

Practitioner: No. The techniques that I use are therapeutic and nonsexual. If that is not your intention for making an appointment with me, then I must ask you to leave.

Client:	Um, no. That's okay. I was just joking around. It's all good.
Therapist:	Actually, I don't think it's all good. I take my work very seriously and I do not appreciate your joke. Not only will I not give you a treatment today, I will not schedule another appointment with you.

You might also say the following: "You say that you are 'just joking around' but I have to be honest with you and let you know I do not appreciate it. In fact, I find it offensive and disrespectful. I expect my clients to respect me and my work and not make lewd suggestions. If you are capable of abiding by my standards, then I would be happy to continue working with you. If not, then I will end this session and not schedule another one with you. What would you like to do?"

When a client acts like a predator it is useful for you to say back to the client exactly what you are hearing the client request. When the client hears it said out loud it often takes the thrill out of the request, and requires the person to answer for his or her behavior.

In the last response, the practitioner is actually giving the client a chance to redeem himself or herself. The practitioner might also say, "I know you said that you were joking but I am not that kind of practitioner. Let's just focus on this session and get to work. " In this case the practitioner has put the comment aside and is willing to do the treatment. However, once the treatment is over, the practitioner is under no obligation to reschedule with that client.

Sometimes, however, it is wise to take a nonconfrontational approach to the get the client out of the office as soon as possible for your safety.

Scenario Two

Client:	I got a treatment here a while ago and the one who worked on me was really nice. He told me it was okay if I didn't want to be draped. I hope you're okay with that.
Practitioner:	Actually, I'm not okay with that. I'll use the draping technique that is required of all practitioners in this clinic, as well as what is required by law.
Client:	Oh come on! I won't tell anyone. No one will know.
Practitioner:	No. I won't perform this treatment if you're not willing to follow the draping protocol. The draping is required by law, but I also require it as I don't appreciate being exposed to your genitalia and gluteal cleft. I understand that you have a preference for how you want to receive this treatment. However, I have standards for how I provide treatments and I'm unwilling to compromise that standard.
Client:	Okay, have it your way.
Therapist:	Thank you for respecting my standards.

Some may think that the practitioner was not being tough enough to the client by saying thank you at the end or by even agreeing to continue with the session. The point of resolving conflict with clients is for the practitioner to state what the appropriate choice is for her while not shaming the client. For example, it could be that the client in the scenario feels very comfortable being nude and has no other agenda than feeling a cool breeze on the whole body during the session. However, the client is not honoring the clear boundary that the practitioner put forth. As always, it is up to you to decide whether you feel safe continuing with the session. If not, you have every right to refuse to work with the client.

If this occurs in a clinical or spa setting, you will likely have formal policies and procedures to follow when choosing to refuse working with a guest, such as documenting the incident. It is in everyone's best interest if the spa is supportive and trusts your decision to not work on the client. It is also possible that refusing to work on a guest, no matter what incident transpires, is not an option for practitioners. It is important that practitioners who are employees know the policies and procedures of their work settings, and be willing and able to abide by them. However, if your safety is at risk and your workplace environment does not ensure your safety, then it would be wise to find another place to work that does.

During the treatment, if a client touches you inappropriately, appears to be sexually aroused, makes sexual comments, or otherwise appears to be sexualizing the experience, the following are steps you can take to address the situation:

1. Stop the session and redrape the client (if performing bodywork in which the client is unclothed, such as massage therapy).
2. Describe the behavior you are observing.
3. Ask the client to clarify the intent behind his or her behavior.
4. Restate the intent of your bodywork and your professional boundaries.
5. Listen to the client's response.
6. Continue or discontinue the session as you find appropriate.
7. Document the situation.

After the client leaves, some practitioners may choose to make a follow-up phone call to the client about his or her behavior. Other practitioners may be reluctant to contact clients who have behaved in this manner. However, making a follow-up call can bring some closure to the incident. Even if practitioners do not talk to the client directly but leave a voice mail message, it is still beneficial to say, in a professional manner, what the practitioner needs to say to let go of the incident and move forward.

In addition, the practitioner should seek out the support of a supervisor or a trusted mentor to discuss what happened. Having a trusted colleague listen to what transpired will help practitioners work through the emotions these types of incidents generate. Often practitioners come out of such a situation feeling "dirty," disturbed, angry, and violated. It is essential to talk about these feelings so they do not linger and so practitioners do not bring them into the next treatment.

■ CASE PROFILE

Marquette decided to go to massage school after working 3 years as a server in a popular sports bar. She grew tired of having a job that did not allow her any room for advancement. During Marquette's student clinic rotation, her clientele tends to be male, and most of them request

Case Study Continued to page 358

Case Study Continued from page 357

her every time they come in for a treatment. As a result, Marquette feels very confident in her massage skills and often brags to the other students that she will be able to build her private clientele easily from her clinic clients.

However, Marquette's clinic supervisor, Han, has noticed a certain pattern of behavior from Marquette's clients that concerns him. He has observed that Marquette's clients do not hesitate to tell her how beautiful her eyes are, or ask personal questions about her life outside of school, and some have even asked her out. Each time Marquette's response is to laugh it off and say, "Maybe next time." Han has also observed that Marquette lets the other students know about what great tips she gets. She says, "It feels just like my old job. I was the top server and always made the most tips!"

Han requests a meeting with Marquette and asks that the other clinic supervisor, Bonnie, attend the meeting. The intention of the meeting is to bring to Marquette's attention the concerns Han has about what he has witnessed. He wants to discuss the fact that Marquette is not behaving professionally by setting limits with her male clients, and that she does not seem to make the distinction between her role and responsibilities as a massage therapist and her previous role as a server in a bar.

What history does Marquette bring with her to a new career as a bodywork practitioner?

How would you address these issues with Marquette?

What insights would you want Marquette to take away from this meeting?

What do you think is the purpose of having Bonnie in attendance during the meeting?

If you were Marquette, how would you respond to Han's concerns?

What steps would you recommend to Marquette to address the concerns that are raised in this scenario?

What to Do If a Client Has an Erection

A male client with an erection does not automatically mean that he is sexually aroused or has the intention of sexualizing the bodywork treatment. It could be that the erection is the body's natural response to relaxation, as discussed previously in this chapter, or it could mean that the man has to urinate. Making a determination about what to do when this occurs will depend on what your perception is of the client's intent for receiving the massage, your level of comfort with the fact that an erection occurred, and your willingness or need to address it with the client. Therefore, there is a range of options for how to proceed:

Say nothing and disguise the erection. If there has been no sign of inappropriate behavior that would indicate that the client wanted a sexual experience (e.g., verbal comments with sexual innuendo, movement of the pelvic region into the table, inappropriate moaning and gasping) then it is appropriate to continue the treatment without commenting. Some practitioners provide a draping technique on the anterior body that provides some slack in the sheet over the groin area. These folds of sheet allow extra room should the client experience an erection. Other therapists choose to place a blanket or towel over the client's midsection to achieve the same goal. The placement of the blanket or towels allows the practitioner to continue the treatment without seeing the erection. Again, these methods should be used only if you do not feel threatened by the client and you are confident that there is no sexual intent.

Say nothing but change location, rhythm, and pace of strokes. If you have determined there is no sexual intent from the client, you may choose to change the location of your strokes as well as the pace, rhythm, or pressure in an effort to interrupt the sensory flow near the groin area, for example, moving from the inner leg to the feet. Another example, in massage therapy, is to move from giving long and slow gliding strokes on the quadriceps muscles to faster kneading strokes. If you are working on the abdomen when the erection occurs, you can complete the area and move to the head or the feet, depending on which direction your treatment is going.

Talk to the client. There are two reasons you may choose to talk to the client. The first is if, even though you know there is no sexual intent, you are unable to continue the treatment because it makes you uncomfortable not saying anything. This is a tricky situation because you are putting your needs before the client's. However, if you know that your work will be compromised and decrease in quality unless you discuss the situation, then you should do so. The key to this option is to be very clear that even though you understand that the client is having a natural relaxation response and is not sexually aroused, you have a need to mention it so that you can focus on your work. This may result in an awkward conversation that could ultimately embarrass your client more than your inability to continue the treatment. If you choose this option, be direct and brief when explaining that you do not expect him to change anything but you just needed to state the obvious so that you would no longer be distracted.

The second reason you might talk to your client about his erection is if you believe there is sexual intent. In this case, you need to follow the seven steps in the protocol presented in the previous section, "Intervention Model." This option should be used if you feel unsafe, or if you have observed or experienced inappropriate behavior and language from him. In some cases, it may be that the client needs to be educated on how to receive a professional bodywork treatment as well as informed that any sexual overtones will not be tolerated. If the client is clearly inappropriate and suggestive with his behavior, then you must stop the treatment immediately and tell the client to leave.

Chapter Summary

Touch often has profound effects on the mind, emotions, and spirit of the client. Because current culture society tends to sexualize many arenas to attract people's attention, bodywork practitioners need to ensure that they provide desexualized treatments and be diligent in their professionalism.

Relaxing massage therapy and bodywork treatments stimulate the parasympathetic division, resulting in decreased stress hormone release, muscle relaxation, decreased heart rate, increased mental clarity, and pain relief. Therapeutic touch can also be a tremendous support to those who are struggling to find balance in their lives. Research shows that therapeutic touch is proving to be quite effective in relieving certain symptoms and conditions.

All types of touch land on a continuum of intimacy based on personal comfort and willingness to be touched by another. Personal history influences perception of touch. Personal history of touch may cause bodywork students and bodyworkers to experience challenges in giving and receiving touch that they were completely unaware of. They then have the choice of working on those challenges if they want to become a bodyworker, or choosing another, less touch-intensive profession. New bodywork students are encouraged to receive professional bodywork treatments so that they have an understanding of the amount of touch involved in performing bodywork. To create desexualized treatment environments, practitioners need to have an awareness of their own sexuality, and ensure that they do not bring it into their bodywork treatments.

Educating clients about the purpose of bodywork begins from the first contact with the client and may continue throughout the entire therapeutic relationship. During the treatment, if a client touches the practitioner inappropriately, appears to be sexually aroused, makes sexual comments, or otherwise appears to be sexualizing the experience, the intervention model has steps practitioners can take to address the situation.

Review Questions

Multiple Choice

1. "Tactile" means:
   a. Sensual
   b. Touch
   c. Sexual
   d. Restoration

2. The largest sensory organ of the body is the:
   a. Brain
   b. Nose
   c. Eye
   d. Skin

3. Which of the following is an example of what the somatosensory association area does?
   a. Respond to tactile stimulation
   b. Pinpoint exactly where in the body a sensation is coming from
   c. Allow the comparison of current sensations with previous sensations
   d. Transport nerve impulses up to the brain

4. Dopamine and serotonin are examples of:

a. Neurotransmitters

b. Tactile sensations

c. Sensory receptors

d. Areas of the brain

5. In a professional relationship, the practitioner is held to a higher standard than the client because the practitioner is the one with the:

a. Most power

b. Obligation to do no harm

c. Most education

d. Expertise in techniques

6. Which of the following is considered sexual manipulation?

a. A practitioner flirting with clients to get larger tips

b. Unwelcome erotic advances of a supervisor toward a practitioner

c. Erotic jokes told by a client to a practitioner

d. All of the above

7. If the client behaves sexually during a bodywork treatment, which of the following is the practitioner's most appropriate response?

a. Make a joke out of it

b. Ask the client to clarify the intent behind the behavior

c. Ignore the observed behavior

d. Finish the session as quickly as possible

Fill in the Blank

1. In Eastern modalities the term for the energetic component of the body is __Qi__.

2. Specialized nerve endings called __receptors__ respond to the various types of tactile stimulation.

3. The part of the brain that has a "map" of the entire body and so can pinpoint not only what a sensation is, but where in the body it is coming from, is the __primary somatosensory area__

4. Touch can help people create a __balance__ in their physical, emotional, mental, and spiritual planes of existence.

5. Gentle relaxation bodywork may be able to reduce __anxiety__ in terminally ill and dying clients.

6. Touch overload occurs when a practitioner no longer wants to __touch his or her clients__

7. The uninvited and unwelcome verbal or physical behavior of a sexual nature, especially by a person in authority toward a subordinate is the definition of __sexual harassment__

Short Answer

1. Briefly explain five physiological responses of the body to welcomed touch.

2. Briefly explain the energetic component of touch.

3. Describe three benefits of therapeutic touch.

4. Explain how a person's history of touch influences his or her present perceptions of touch. Give at least three examples.

5. List five questions a bodywork student can ask him- or herself when discovering how bodywork will affect his or her life.

6. Describe five ways that a practitioner can ensure the treatments he or she performs are desexualized.

7. Explain three ways a practitioner can educate a client that bodywork is not sexual.

Activities

1. List all the adjectives you can think of to describe different types of touch. Which of these would you use in connection with bodywork? Why would you use these instead of other words when talking about bodywork and touch?

2. Do an Internet search for an article, other than the ones discussed in this chapter, on the healing benefits of touch. It might be one on how touch is beneficial in general, or one on a specific disease, condition, or situation. Write two or three paragraphs on what you discover by reading the article.

3. Create your own continuum for your experience of intimacy. Place a low level of intimacy on the left of your continuum, and a high level of intimacy on the right. Be specific about naming the behaviors that fall along the continuum. For example, hugging an acquaintance for a couple of seconds might be on the low end of the continuum, whereas hugging a close friend whom you have not seen for several months might be higher on the continuum, and hugging a significant other could be on the highest end of the continuum.

4. Write a script of what you would say to a friend or family member who continually makes disparaging remarks about you attending bodywork school. Be mindful of the role practitioners have in educating the public about therapeutic nonsexual bodywork. Be sure to consider preserving a positive relationship with your friend or family member.

5. Write a self-reflection essay discussing your current comfort level with working in a profession that requires intimate physical contact with clients. Include in your discussion answers to the following questions:

- Has your level of comfort changed from the time you began training in the bodywork profession? If so, how and why? If not, why not?
- What specific client behaviors have you experienced that have influenced your degree of comfort in the bodywork profession?

6. You are responsible for developing a workshop for new bodywork practitioners to discuss the role sexuality plays in the profession. What topics would you want to be sure to cover? Create two role-play scenarios that could be acted out in the workshop.

7. Describe how you will evaluate whether a client's behavior is sexually motivated. Write a script of how you would handle the situation if you determined the behavior is inappropriate.

8. Describe how you would respond to a client who is "playfully" suggestive during a treatment and makes vague sexual comments. What limits would you set for clients regarding this behavior?

Guidance for Journaling

 Some key areas to think about while journaling for this chapter include the following:

- The healing effects of bodywork
- What the different types of touch mean to you
- The levels of intimacy associated with each type of touch
- What your personal history of touch includes
- How various cultural influences have had an effect on your perception of touch
- What your comfort levels with touch are
- Any challenges you might have with being touched, and how these challenges can interfere with your success as a bodyworker
- How touch is or was presented in your bodywork program
- What desexualized touch means to you
- How you create desexualized bodywork
- Awareness of the continuum of sexual manipulation
- How you can tell if sexual manipulation is occurring
- Ways you would educate clients about the purpose of bodywork
- How you would address sexual behavior from clients before and during a treatment

References

1. Field, T.: *Touch*. Cambridge, MA, MIT Press, 2003, pp vii–x.
2. Menehan, K.: (2006) Tiffany Field on massage research. *Massage Magazine*, 2006. Retrieved 13 October 2010 from http://www.massagemag.com/News/2006/January/125/Tiffany.php
3. Field, *Touch*, p 8.
4. Ibid., pp 41–43, 52–53, 99, 133–134, 146–147.
5. Tortora, G.J., and Derrickson, B.: *Principles of Anatomy and Physiology*, ed. 12. Hoboken, NJ, John Wiley & Sons, 2009, p 448.

6. National Institutes of Health, National Center for Complementary and Alternative Medicine. Americans spent $33.9 billion out-of-pocket on complementary and alternative medicine. National Institutes of Health, National Center for Complementary and Alternative Medicine website, 2009. Retrieved 14 October 2010 from http://nccam.nih.gov/news/2009/073009.htm

7. Massage and health touch ease cancer symptoms. *Massage Magazine,* 2009. Retrieved 14 October 2010 from http://www.massagemag.com/News/massage-news.php?id=5444&catid=233&title=massage-and-healing-touch-ease-cancer-symptoms)

8. Therapeutic touch eases agitation in people with Alzheimer's. *Massage Magazine,* 2009. Retrieved 14 October 2010 from http://www.massagemag.com/News/massage-news.php?id=5440&catid=233&title=therapeutic-touch-eases-agitation-in-people-with-alzheimers)

9. Touch therapies reduce complications, increase comfort after bone marrow transplant. *Massage Magazine,* 2009. Retrieved 14 October 2010 from http://www.massagemag.com/News/massage-news.php?id=5387&catid=232&title=touch-therapies-reduce-complications-increase-comfort-after-bone-marrow-transplant

10. Bass, E., and Davis, L.: *The Courage to Heal: A Guide for Women Survivors of Child Sexual Abuse,* ed. 4. New York, HarperCollins, 2008, pp 3–12.

11. Ford, C.W.: *Compassionate Touch: The Body's Role in Emotional Healing and Recovery.* Berkeley, CA, North Atlantic Books, 1999, p 137.

12. Ibid., p 138.

Support for Ethical Practice

LEARNING OBJECTIVES

After studying this chapter, you will be able to:

1. Explain types of support available for bodywork practitioners.
2. Define "mentoring," and discuss how to find and choose a mentor.
3. Describe the factors involved in being a mentor.
4. Explain how to terminate a mentoring relationship.
5. Define "peer support."
6. Explain ways to identify appropriate peers.
7. Explain how to know when support is needed, how to get the most out of support, and how to choose the best type of support.
8. Describe how to build and use support networks appropriately.

CHAPTER OUTLINE

Identity: the essential characteristics that the practitioner recognizes and names as belonging uniquely to him- or herself

Mentoring: a professional relationship in which a person with greater experience and skill provides support, encouragement, and career expertise to one with less experience and skill in the profession

Peer: one who is of equal standing with another

Peer support: the interaction among practitioners who have similar levels of skill and experience to encourage and maintain appropriate professional and ethical practice

Supervision: periodic review of the bodywork practitioner's professional actions by an authority in the work setting

Support network: an interconnected group or association of people who can provide the practitioner with encouragement, assistance, and resources as needed

---

Lucia works at a resort as a massage therapist. She asks her mentor, who is not employed at the spa, for support regarding a business idea that she has implemented. It involves giving in-room massages after 10:00 p.m. because the spa closes at 9:00 p.m. She provides these massages without the knowledge of the management because she knows they would not be supportive of this after-hours work. She explains to the resort guests that these treatments are part of her private practice and not a service provided by the spa. She also stresses to the guests that these treatments are not to be mentioned to any of the resort staff or management.

Lucia's decision to work with a mentor is prompted by the fact the she is feeling overwhelmed by the late hours she is working. She often shows up for her scheduled shifts at the spa exhausted. She also wants some direction on how to manage inappropriate behaviors from male clients that she is encountering during her after-hours treatments. She is confused about why this has never been an issue in the spa. Finally, she is hoping that a mentor can support her creativity and ingenuity in her new business venture because she is not being supported by her peers who do not work for the resort. In fact, when she offered to include one of her colleagues in her plan, she was flatly refused and told she was running an unethical practice.

Lucia's mentor points out that Lucia is, indeed, running an unethical practice. Offering these treatments after hours is in direct competition with the spa, Lucia's employer. Therefore, if resort management does find out about her side business, it is likely that Lucia will be fired. In addition, because Lucia is choosing to work late hours, it is no wonder she is exhausted before her day begins for her regular shifts. This means she is unable to give the high-quality treatments the spa expects from her, and for which the spa is paying her. Finally, Lucia's mentor points out the risks Lucia is taking with her safety. The male clients who are behaving inappropriately when she provides massages after hours in their guest rooms are probably thinking that she is available for sexual services.

Although Lucia's mentor does applaud Lucia's creativity and ingenuity, she is able to help Lucia see that her plan is not really working. Granted, she has an increase in income, but she has placed herself in jeopardy. She may lose her main source of income as a spa employee, she can possibly be harmed by a guest who has other ideas of what she should be providing after hours in the guest's room, and she is in danger of losing the respect of her peers and colleagues for running an unethical business. Lucia decides to stop providing the after-hours treatments immediately. Shortly thereafter she is once again able to arrive for her regular shifts at the spa full of energy and ready to go. With the help of her mentor, she has developed a new, long-term plan for her career in which she works hard to become a spa manager.

As this scenario demonstrates, having someone to support your ethical practice as a bodywork practitioner can be a lifesaver. As a student, you likely have had (or have) the opportunity to study, discuss, role-play, and dialogue with others about ethical situations that may occur with clients, other students, family members, and friends. However, it is when practicing as a professional that you will come face-to-face with your true self. Human interactions are often complex, especially in the bodywork setting, and you may realize you are not as equipped to deal with some real-life challenges and conflicts as you had thought. Most practitioners need advice and support from others to navigate all of these challenges and conflicts successfully.

Support can take many different forms. Close family members and friends you trust can be incredible resources. Depending on your situation, family and friends may provide a shoulder to lean on, an ear to listen, advice, financial support, and even hope and inspiration.

Not every practitioner, however, has family and friends on whom they can rely or who understand the unique challenges that can arise in the bodywork profession. They may not know how to approach circumstances involving ethics or not understand why the practitioner is struggling. They may think that bodywork is like any other work and not realize the physical, emotional, and mental preparation it takes to perform treatments. Boundaries surrounding the client–practitioner relationship may be completely uncharted territory for them, and they may have no idea of the factors involved in creating therapeutic relationships.

Fortunately, there are other types of support available to you, including supervision, mentoring, and peer support, which are the focus of this chapter. All of these are meant to provide needed sounding boards for practitioners by practitioners, although mentors can also come from other professions. The purpose is to gain insight with the help of others who have been in similar situations or who at least understand what it is like to be in the bodywork profession. The chapter also considers how to recognize when you need support and how to choose the best type of support. Finally, the chapter covers how to build a support network and use it appropriately.

✳ Supervision

The first type of support we will consider is supervision. **Supervision** involves periodic review of a bodywork practitioner's professional actions by an authority in the work setting. The supervision can be direct, as when a supervisor observes you at work, or it can be indirect, as when a supervisor discusses professional practices with you.

Ideally, supervision is a helping relationship. Supervision assists practitioners in maintaining ethical practices and reduces burnout. One practitioner, the supervisor, has more experience and insight into the profession and can assist less-experienced practitioners in developing a deeper understanding of their professional work, leading to better fulfillment. Supervisors are in a position of authority; most are found in practitioners' places of employment. However, you may also choose to be supervised by someone outside of your work setting.

Supervisors are generally involved in areas such as the development and approval of treatment plans, scheduling, disciplinary matters, and instruction. Optimally, they suggest—in a manner that is affirming and not shaming—ways you can improve your performance. Supervisors should encourage the awareness that mistakes are an important part of the learning process. They should also have the ability to truly listen to you and allow you to discover for yourself appropriate choices and responses to your experiences.

An effective supervisor will help you explore what you are experiencing mentally and emotionally. A supervisor can also help you define appropriate boundaries between yourself and clients and determine what actions may help in given situations. The focus should be on you developing problem-solving skills, leading to increased confidence in your abilities. If the supervisor tells you what to do and say all the time, it can diminish your belief in yourself as well as your ability to take initiative and be creative. Ultimately, supervision is about you, as a practitioner, facing reality. The supervisor's job is not to "fix" or soothe you but to point out areas of challenges and strength that will enhance your therapeutic work with your clients.

You, as the practitioner being supervised, need to enter this relationship with the desire to receive support and feedback on how to be successful. This mutual purpose allows for effective communication and a productive outcome.

Effective supervision has a lasting impact after the session is over. Ideally, ideas, comments, or "Aha!" moments will occur that will motivate you to embrace and embody the values and principles of ethical bodywork practices. These insights will also assist you in having a fresh perspective about your practice. It is important that you be self-accountable. Therefore, ultimately supervision means being held accountable by a more experienced practitioner.

Supervision can be conducted one-on-one or in a group setting. Each has its own merits. Individual supervision can be more personalized. Time is not shared with other practitioners, and you do not have to listen to issues concerning other practitioners. In addition, the supervisor's attention is solely focused on you and is not fragmented.

Conversely, group supervision allows many practitioners to share in the supervisor's time and experience at once. This can be an effective process because practitioners may gain insight into issues they may not have considered until others brought them to light. It also provides for a richer experience, as a variety of ideas may be generated. If group supervision is successful, and the practitioners like and respect one another, they then have a broader support system to call on in between meetings if something comes up that they need to discuss.

The specifics of the supervision process, such as how the supervision is conducted and how often you will meet with the supervisor, will likely be discussed with you before or at the start of your employment. If you can, ask for this information during the interview process. Doing so will show that you are proactive in the development of professional skills, knowledge, and experience. It also shows commitment to the place of employment.

Mentoring

Another option you may consider is finding someone who is not necessarily in a position of authority over you but can advise you. Such people are called mentors. **Mentoring** involves a professional relationship in which a person with greater experience and skill provides support, encouragement, and career expertise to those with less experience and skill in the profession.

Practitioners often choose this option as part of their commitment to becoming a better professional. Perhaps they are in sole practice and have no one else to bounce ideas off. They may be new to the profession and want to ensure that they are on the right track or may be finding themselves in situations for which they feel completely unprepared. They may be dissatisfied with the supervision they are receiving as an employee and want other ideas and opinions.

Because mentors do not have the capacity to hire, fire, or discipline you, there tends to be more freedom in the relationship. With mentors, you may feel more able to discuss issues without feeling inadequate or fearing reprisal. The relationship with a mentor is not as formal as with a supervisor because it does not involve a direct working relationship.

Some mentors are willing to donate their time and expertise. Others choose to charge a fee, which may vary, for their services. If a fee is charged, an amount comparable to what is charged for one bodywork session may be discussed.

Although it is true that a mentor is someone you can turn to in times of struggle and confusion, do not look to the mentor to be the "fix-it person" when perplexing situations arise. The role of the mentor is to help you become aware of who you are as a practitioner and how you can learn to manage the problems you encounter yourself. The mentor helps you discover how you are being challenged in difficult situations, with difficult clients, or during personal issues. You can use the mentor's experience and expertise as a guide to seeing actions and behaviors that are getting in the way of being successful in your work.

Core mentoring skills that are involved in effective mentoring include the following:

- Listening actively. The mentor pays close attention to what the mentee is saying and reflects back the mentee's words and ideas so that both are in alignment.
- Building trust. The mentor projects an attitude and presence of believing in the inherent worth of the mentee.
- Encouraging the mentee. The mentor provides supportive and motivational comments that will inspire the mentee.
- Identifying goals and current reality. The mentor provides an honest reflection of the reality of the situation that the mentee is facing, and sets specific goals that will meet the needs of the supervision sessions.
- Providing corrective feedback. The mentor is direct in pointing out behaviors and attitudes that are limiting the mentee's success.[1]

 Food for Thought

What qualities in a supervisor would benefit you the most? What would you do to get the most out of being supervised? How would you like supervision to help increase your professional skills?

Benefits of Mentoring

A mentor helps you discover your **identity.** In this context, the term "identity" is used to describe the essential characteristics that you recognize and name as belonging uniquely to yourself. In Parker J. Palmer's book *The Courage to Teach,* he states, "Good teaching cannot be reduced to technique; good teaching comes from the identity and integrity of the teacher....my ability to connect with my students, and to connect them with the subject, depends less on the methods I use than on the degree to which I know and trust my selfhood—and am I willing to make it available and vulnerable in the service of learning."[2] Although Palmer is discussing teachers and students, it can also be applied to mentors and bodywork practitioners. Practitioners who know and trust themselves to be authentic with clients will have a deeper experience in the therapeutic relationship as well as a deeper connection to his or her work. As a result, the client may experience a deeper connection, as well.

Identity is akin to one's personality. Yet when it comes to the professional self, sometimes practitioners think their identities should be hidden or that they should have a professional identity that is completely different from their personal identity. The difference, they assume, is that as a professional their true personality should not be brought into the treatment room. In addition, they think they should always look good on the outside when they are engaged in a professional relationship with their clients, peers, or colleagues, regardless of how they are feeling on the inside.

It is certainly true that professionalism involves ensuring your personal thoughts, feelings, and beliefs do not intrude on the therapeutic relationship. It is also true that professionalism means working on clients even when you do not feel particularly motivated to do so or when doing something else, such as taking the day off, is more appealing than working.

However, if you completely conceal your true identity behind a veil of professionalism, you may have difficulty having an authentic and genuine therapeutic relationship with clients. Helping you identify and address this issue of "split personality" is precisely the role and responsibility of a mentor. In so doing, the mentor educates you on the importance of trusting your true self and allowing it to come forward in your work with clients.

Your mentor should be able to point out the disconnect between how you *think* you should act or feel regarding a particular issue and how you *actually* act or feel. It can take a lot of energy and emotional stress to keep up such a façade, or pretense. This energy is better spent on learning to accept the parts of yourself that you know are worthwhile and seeking support for the parts of yourself that you know need transforming.

Mentoring is about finding alignment between personal and professional identities. Mentoring can assist you with this process so that you do not have to pretend to be someone you are not. At the same time, wise mentors will guide you in how to behave professionally while remaining true to yourself.

David Stoddard states in his book *The Heart of Mentoring: Ten Proven Principles for Developing People to Their Fullest,* "Mentors never settle for mediocrity. People perform at the level of their internalized standards. . . . People are more capable than they think and they need a change in their expectations. Therefore, mentors should expect more of the mentee than the mentee expects of herself."[3] Therefore, a mentor should be skilled at encouraging and inspiring professional growth by not allowing the mentee to settle for behaviors that have not proved successful.

Consider the following: Jaye is naturally very outgoing, warm, and welcoming to anyone she meets. Because of the training she received in setting and maintaining boundaries, Jaye thinks she should have only sterile and clinical relationships with her clients. She politely sidesteps personal questions and redirects the client back to the treatment. Even when she feels inclined to offer a client a word of encouragement or disclose a personal fact that may help the client, she stays silent and merely smiles, nods, or says something noncommittal. Jaye feels like a phony, but she believes that she is behaving according to the profession's standards.

Jaye seeks mentoring when she realizes just how unhappy she is in her work. Jaye speaks with Romero, her mentor, about how she just cannot seem to connect with her clients in a way that works for her. Romero and Jaye begin exploring why Jaye is denying her true nature as well as her instincts about connecting with others. Romero is able to help Jaye look at the fact that she has been hiding her identity as a warm and giving person in an attempt to follow what she thought were mandatory rules of the profession regarding boundaries. Through mentoring she learns that boundaries can be maintained without being cold and distant to clients. Romero helps Jaye understand that one of her tasks as a professional is to find an appropriate balance between her innate qualities and the behaviors necessary for an ethical professional. Once Jaye understands that healthy professional boundaries may involve her personal identity and traits she is able to recommit to her work and her clients. As a result, her practice begins to thrive.

Receiving mentoring on a regular basis is a sign of a conscientious bodywork practitioner. You do not necessarily have to see a mentor every week. The mentor and you will mutually determine the frequency of the meetings. The frequency of meetings can also be determined by the severity of the issues that you are experiencing.

How to Find a Mentor

A mentor is typically someone with whom practitioners have a history of familiarity and connection. Many practitioners choose mentors based on how they have seen them work and interact with others. They like his or her style. Often, mentors are teachers in practitioners' bodywork programs or professionals from whom they have received bodywork in the past or on a regular basis, and practitioners feel a connection to them. A mentor might also be one who provides quality continuing education classes, or simply an individual whom the practitioner has heard good things about and believes could guide him or her in problem solving, recognition for work well done, and analysis of behavior and choices when necessary.

However, those mentoring bodywork practitioners do not necessarily need to be practitioners themselves. Various health-care professionals, such as nurses, counselors, and psychologists, struggle with issues similar to those in the bodywork profession. Some practitioners may in fact feel comfortable seeking a mentor outside the bodywork profession because they may get a more objective viewpoint.

The personality of the mentor is important. Ideally, it would match the comfort level of the practitioner without being too similar. A good mentor is one who is at ease in the role, is comfortable with him- or herself, has good communication skills, and can break a situation down into relevant issues for the practitioner to understand and work with. As discussed previously, active listening skills are the primary skills of a good supervisor. A mentor is concerned with the successful career growth of those they mentor.

Mentors to consider would be experienced bodywork practitioners who have successful practices, are well respected, have volunteered their time for bodywork organizations and learned skills beyond the treatment room, and are also instructors.

For mentors outside of the bodywork profession you can get recommendations from trusted colleagues, friends, and family members; and contact professional organizations, such as nursing or mental health associations.

Choosing a Mentor

When choosing a mentor it is important to select a person who is similar to you personally and professionally. For example, you will want to choose someone who shares your core belief systems: work ethic, honest representation of self, and respect for others regardless of differences. When you match these fundamental qualities, you can move more quickly toward setting goals rather than spending time (and perhaps money) getting to know each other.

Consider choosing your mentor from a group of professionals that you have been in contact with through taking continuing education classes, reading articles they have published, or being in the same network group. Witnessing their interactions with others and noticing how you respond to their behavior will give you insight into whether a particular person will be a comfortable fit for you. It is also helpful to ask for a consultation interview to get to know him or her before making a decision. Questions you may consider asking may include the following:

- What inspires you about your work? About your life?
- What are your strengths?
- What challenges you?

You must be clear about who you want to work with and why. It is useful for you to know what type of support you are looking for, how that support would look, and what the person you are thinking of asking has to offer along those lines. Do not choose a mentor simply because you like a person or think he or she is charming. Nor should you choose a mentor because you have the impression that the person can do no wrong.

Consider the following: Gail received her acupuncture training at a private school that had a core group of teachers who taught most of the classes. One instructor, Miguel, impressed Gail with his extensive knowledge of traditional Chinese medicine, skillful technique with the needles, and down-to-earth lecture style. Gail had found the clinical aspect of the training to be quite challenging. She did not feel comfortable talking to people she had just met, and she had a hard time piecing all the information together to form a treatment plan. Each week she would watch Miguel respectfully and compassionately ease into conversation after conversation with all of the clients. She had never met anyone like him, and decided that she would ask Miguel to be her mentor when she started her clinical rotation at the local wellness center.

During their first mentoring session, Gail discusses a client who had many complaints and was difficult to treat. To Gail's surprise, Miguel says the client would never benefit from the treatments because she is such a negative woman. Miguel advises Gail to conduct a general session that does not address the issues the woman has. He says, "She'll never know. Get her settled in the room and get on to your other clients who are more interesting." When Gail brings up her next client for discussion, Miguel's cell phone goes off and he takes the call, leaving the room for 20 minutes. When he returns he asks if there is anything else Gail needs. Gail says no and leaves the office. She is disappointed that Miguel did not behave in the way she expected. He was nothing like the person she saw when she was in the student clinic. Gail decides to stop the mentoring sessions with Miguel.

This scenario depicts what happens when practitioners discover that their heroes have human failings. It is human nature to want to place those whose skills and personalities one admires on a pedestal. However, this is risky if you do not know anything about them other than what you see during a few hours in a controlled environment, such as the classroom. When choosing a mentor you must be willing to see the person with your eyes wide open. You must also be willing to change your mind if you discover you have misjudged the person's ability to be a helpful mentor. Deciding not to work with someone does not have to be a personal indictment of character. It simply means the person does not meet your mentoring needs.

Approaching a mentor could be an anxiety-provoking prospect because you are asking someone of higher status and experience if he or she would be willing to help you. If the power differential is so great that butterflies in your stomach become unmanageable, perhaps this is an indicator that there might never be a comfortable exchange between you and the prospective mentor, and that you would be better off looking elsewhere.

Box 10.1 presents a model for a mentoring session.

How to Be a Mentor

As practitioners gain experience and skill, and as their practices become successful, some may consider becoming a mentor to less experienced professionals. Practitioners who are considering doing so need to be clear about their motives for becoming a mentor. Being a mentor means making a commitment to the practitioner being mentored. If that is not a comfortable position to be in, then the practitioner should decline the request and suggest someone else if possible.

If you are considering becoming a mentor you should ask yourself the following questions:

- Is it ego?
- Do you think you have something genuine to give others?
- Do you want others to learn from your mistakes?

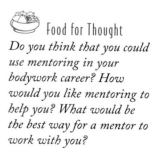 Food for Thought
Do you think that you could use mentoring in your bodywork career? How would you like mentoring to help you? What would be the best way for a mentor to work with you?

| Box 10.1 | A MODEL FOR A MENTORING SESSION |

In his book, *A Hidden Wholeness: The Journey Toward an Undivided Life*, Parker J. Palmer discusses the value that supervision and mentoring provide for people who want to fully engage with the people in their life, whether they are students, clients, or loved ones. He uses the phrase "a circle of trust" to describe this gathering. Palmer defines a circle of trust as a "community of solitudes where people come together in a way that gives every participant a chance to attend to the inner teacher and learn from one."[4]

The group has a facilitator to keep participants on task and to ensure the safety of the group. His or her role is also to be fully engaged in the group process so that there is no sense of division or hierarchy. Once a member has finished speaking, the other members ask questions to help clarify what has been said. There is an agreement that no one is responsible for offering advice or ways to "fix" a situation except the person sharing. This allows each member take responsibility for the resolution of an issue; the questions being asked by the group members help guide the speaker to a workable solution.

An effective mentoring group meets at least once a month in a setting that offers privacy and confidentiality. Members are asked to make a commitment to attend a designated number of sessions with a limited number of absences. This will ensure continuity of group members and help establish rapport. If someone is not able or interested in continuing with the group he or she is not obligated to stay.

The following is a sample schedule of a mentoring session group of four people, including the facilitator:

7:00 p.m. Group members gather and share intentions for the session.

• Each participant states his or her intentions for the meeting.

7:10 p.m. The facilitator reviews the guidelines of the session.

• Timeframes for length of sharing are established (maximum of 30 minutes each).
• Group members are reminded that there are no interruptions while the person is sharing.
• The person sharing will indicate when he or she is ready for questions.
• The group is reminded that there is no "fixing."

7:15–8:50 p.m. Each group member has time to share and receive feedback.

• Feedback is offered in the form of questions.

8:50–9:00 p.m. Closing comments and announcements are made.

• Any group member can make comments.
• Announcements pertaining to anyone who may not be attending the next session are made.

• Are you willing to be honest about your failures as well as your successes?
• Did someone mentor you and you would like others to benefit from the experience the way you did?

By answering these questions honestly, you will have a better idea of what kind of mentor you would be. If you are doing it out of ego, the chances of having a successful mentoring relationship with a less experienced practitioner are small. If, however, you are willing to be honest about your experiences, and not control the outcome of the mentoring sessions, there is a much greater chance of a successful mentoring relationship.

According to the Web site The Mentoring Group (http://www.mentoring-group.com), the following are key components of a mentor:

1. To be a mentor you must be very clear on what your purpose is. Do you want to be a sounding board for your mentee, or do you want to teach and guide your mentee toward new behaviors and attitudes? Do you want to provide a combination of both?

2. Both you and your mentee need to be committed to the relationship; it must be a high priority for both of you. Be trustworthy and consistent in your policies, procedures, and behaviors. Do not cancel appointments without a good reason, talk negatively about others, or make excuses about why you cannot follow through on your commitment to the relationship. Keep confidential the information your mentee shares with you. All of this will inspire confidence and trust.

3. Make sure you and your mentee are clear about why you are working together. You need to discuss and agree about what you will work on. Also decide how the two of you will measure progress. Throughout the relationship you should check in to see if you should change your purpose or focus in some way. When the mentee has accomplished his or her goals, you should be willing to see the partnership shift focus or even end.

4. How you communicate is important. Inspire confidence and trust through your choice of words, tone, and nonverbal language. Be willing to be direct when what you say may not be comfortable for the mentee. Also, be an active listener and remember what your mentee tells you. Ask appropriate questions and share appropriate, relevant information about yourself. However, make sure the mentoring sessions are not all about you. Ask your mentee to give you suggestions about how the two of you can communicate better, and be willing and able to implement his or her ideas.

5. Have a system for giving feedback. Although it is important that you be willing and able to give corrective or difficult feedback, you must also focus on the positive things that your mentee is accomplishing. Discuss in the first meeting how the mentee best receives feedback and how you best provide it.[5]

Terminating the Mentoring Relationship

Knowing when to stop seeing a mentor or seek a new mentor is an important consideration. Some practitioners seek a mentor when dealing with a difficult situation. If this is the case, then the relationship ends when the situation is adequately resolved. A relationship may also be terminated if the practitioner no longer thinks that the mentor is meeting his or her needs.

If the mentoring sessions become more focused on what the mentor believes to be important than on what the practitioner wants to discuss; if the mentor talks about him- or herself rather than about the practitioner's experiences; or if the mentor appears to be uninterested, then these are all signs that a practitioner is no longer being helpful. These behaviors could signal that the practitioner has outgrown the relationship and is no longer benefiting from it. It could also mean that the practitioner's goals and plans have changed and he or she needs to make adjustments concerning who will now meet those needs.

Another reason for terminating the mentor/mentee relationship is if you feel confident in your practice and no longer have the need for a coach or sounding board. It is always possible to leave the door open for future sessions should you need or desire to meet again.

Finally, if it feels as if the mentoring sessions have become a social gathering rather than a work-oriented session, then it is time for you to move on. Although spending time relating socially enhances the mentoring relationship, if it becomes the core of the meetings then it is time to reevaluate goals and the purpose of the mentoring.

Terminating the mentoring relationship does not have to be a somber occasion. In fact, it can be a reason to celebrate the practitioner's ability to grow professionally or move through a difficult time. It can also be an acknowledgment that the practitioner feels capable of moving forward with the skills and insights gained from the mentor.

As you wind down and end the formal aspect of your mentoring relationship, consider the following:

- Discuss what you have learned through mentoring.
- Show your appreciation for the mentor's help.
- Give respectful feedback to your mentor about how he or she could mentor better.
- Discuss future options for the relationship.
- Decide what, if any, contact with each other will be made in the future.[6]

Peer Support

Peer means one who is of equal standing with another. In the bodywork profession, **peer support** is the interaction among practitioners who have similar levels of skill and experience to encourage and maintain appropriate professional and ethical practice. It is an opportunity for colleagues to support one another as well as challenge one another to adopt fresh perspectives on issues and situations they encounter in their practice.

In *Issues and Ethics in the Helping Professions*, Gerald Corey, Marianne Schneider Corey, and Patrick Callanan state that "Sidney Jourard (1968) made a comment many years ago that still seems timely. Jourard warns about the delusion that one has nothing new to learn. He maintains that exciting workshops or contact with challenging colleagues can keep therapists growing. He urges professionals to find colleagues whom they can trust so that they can avoid becoming "smug, pompous, fat bottomed and convinced that they have the word. [Such colleagues can] prod one out of such smug pomposity and invite one back to the task."[7]

For the bodywork profession, this holds true as well. Practitioners should never feel that they have nothing new to learn. Finding other practitioners they can trust and interacting with them with an open mind will help keep them from becoming, to reword Jourard's phrase, "smug, stagnant know-it-alls who are convinced they are the universe's gift to the bodywork profession." No matter how skilled and experienced a practitioner is, it is always good to remember that one of the hallmarks of a professional is genuine humility and a desire to improve.

Peer groups can help decrease the isolation that practitioners who are in sole practice, or who are the only bodywork practitioner in a work setting with other professionals, may feel. They are also ways in which new practitioners can support one another, as well as benefit from wisdom gained by practitioners who have been in the profession longer.

These groups can also provide support and networking prospects. Practitioners can blow off steam and relieve the stresses and strains of being in the bodywork profession. In a well-functioning peer group, there is the safety of speaking freely about experiences (while maintaining client confidentiality, of course) with other practitioners who understand how they feel.

The role of the group is to listen and offer questions that may inspire group members to find solutions for their dilemmas. The understanding is that members are not to shame, belittle, or try to fix the other members' problems for them. Support comes through active listening and asking mindful, open-ended questions.

In some peer groups, there is no one person who facilitates the meetings. The role of facilitator is shared and rotates among the member for each meeting. Some practitioners are more comfortable with this setup because they do not feel as on the spot as they might with a more formal facilitator who calls on them. Rotating the task of group facilitator allows each member the opportunity to be a leader in the group. However, some groups choose to have a professional facilitator for the sessions. This choice is made by practitioners who want the group experience while having the expertise of the facilitator. In this case, the practitioners should share the fee for the facilitator.

The members of a peer group should all be willing to receive support as well as provide support. The members should also be grounded in a shared sense of purpose for the group as well as the bodywork profession. It is not beneficial to be in a peer group with individuals who do not respect one another or are judgmental. Receiving and offering feedback is a very intimate exchange. You must be willing to share the experience with whoever is in the group. It is counterproductive to change how you are just to accommodate the group's expectations or to impress an individual group member. You have to be yourself; by not doing so, not only will the group not meet your needs, it could also make the issues that caused you to seek support worse.

It is essential that guidelines and parameters be established for the group to ensure safety, accountability, and confidentiality. A confidentiality agreement, preferably a written one, is essential if the members are going to share what is deeply personal to them. Establishing parameters in terms of how often the group will meet, the timeframe of the meetings, the location of the gathering, and how the group will be facilitated are factors that provide structure and security for all involved.

It is useful to have a policy about how often a group member can miss a meeting so that each person can decide if he or she is willing and able to make a commitment to the group. Continuity in a group is important so that healthy group dynamics can be established and built on in each meeting. Some practitioners feel comfortable sharing information about themselves only after they have known others for some time. Not knowing who will be attending the meeting each time can be disconcerting to them.

Asking group members to be accountable for their participation in the group is a teaching tool that will help the members to become invested and have ownership of the group process. The bottom line is that peer supervision groups are most successful when there is mutual respect and an agreement among all members about how the group will function.

Practitioners must be mindful of who they consider to be appropriate peers for offering and receiving support. As stated previously, being a peer means that both people are of equal standing with each other. Although it is helpful to share ideas and strategies with someone else of equal status, it is important that practitioners be selective in exactly which peers it would be the most beneficial to do this with.

Consider the following examples:

Ana is a great person to party with during school. She is easygoing and very approachable, and she seems to quickly pick up the bodywork techniques taught. However, she often arrives late to class, and is always talking about how she stays out until 4 a.m. Sometimes she looks as though she has not showered. Ana may be a fun person to be with, and she may have a high level of skill, but is she the best choice for peer support? What if issues of professionalism arise?

Caleb has been a practitioner for 4 years and he has built a steady clientele. His treatments are relaxing as well as educational because he incorporates new techniques as soon as he learns them. However, he constantly talks about how much his clients love his work, and he calls all the women in the office "babe." How good a listener would Caleb be? How respectful would he be to other practitioners?

Julia has been a practitioner for 20 years, and has a flourishing practice. She learned her particular modality by apprenticing with a more experienced practitioner. Because she lives outside the city limits, for most of her career she has not needed a license to practice. However, state licensure was recently passed, requiring all practitioners, no matter where they live in the state, to become licensed. Julia thinks this is nonsense. She says that a license does not guarantee that a practitioner is competent; it is used only as a means to generate money for the state. She refuses to become licensed and thinks that anyone who attends a bodywork school and becomes licensed has been brainwashed by politicians. Even though Julia is a successful businessperson, how ethical is she? How open minded would she be about the issues and dilemmas other practitioners face?

It might be tempting to ask a group of friends you already know to come together on a regular basis to share work experiences and get support for managing successful practices. Friends are an essential ingredient to a well-rounded life. Yet when it comes to wanting someone to hold you accountable for your actions, sometimes a friend may not be the right choice. Everyone is different, of course, but sometimes friends are reluctant to speak frankly about challenges you need to work on because they are afraid of harming your friendship.

Conversely, having a history together that dates back to attending bodywork school together means that you are likely to have the same pool of knowledge and experience. You may be less inhibited with them than you are with other friends and will share more honestly about your doubts and fears. But you should also keep in mind that it can also be useful to choose practitioners who have a background that is different from yours. These practitioners can give fresh, differing perspectives on what it is like for them in their practices.

It is also important that practitioners respect their peers' choices, behaviors, and attitudes when it comes to professionalism. It can be divisive to a community of professionals if there are one or more practitioners that hold themselves above others rather than seeking to find common ground. This does not mean lowering standards or trying to change the ways of others. Instead, an awareness that there are many ways to embody professionalism without violating boundaries or codes of ethics is a much healthier way to interact. The diversity of the bodywork profession is one of the reasons people are attracted to it. It is also a fact that people who enter the bodywork profession come from a variety of educational backgrounds and professional and personal experiences. Figure 10.1 shows the relationships of practitioners and peers, mentors, and supervisors.

Knowing When You Need Support

Sometimes it is quite apparent when you need support. Perhaps you are blindsided by a client's inappropriate behavior, or maybe it is difficult to get along with coworkers. Other times there may be no defining moment when it is obvious that support is needed, but you just have a feeling that it would be nice to talk with others who understand the bodywork profession.

For self-employed practitioners, it may appear easy because no one is telling the practitioner what to do. However, working in isolation can cause some practitioners to feel disconnected from their support networks, and perhaps suffer burnout. Some sole practitioners become complacent about bodywork if it starts to feel repetitive and boring. Working in isolation can also cause some practitioners to not hold themselves accountable to certain standards of care because "no one will know the difference." This lack of self-accountability

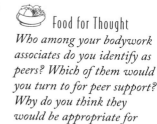

Food for Thought
Who among your bodywork associates do you identify as peers? Which of them would you turn to for peer support? Why do you think they would be appropriate for peer support?

Supervisor

High professional relationship
Low personal relationship
In workplace settings; paid for duties
Follows strict guidelines

Mentor

Mod-high professional relationship
Some personal relationship
Not part of workplace settings
May or may not be paid
Much freedom in the interaction

Peer

Mod-low professional relationship
Highly personal relationship
May or may not be part of workplace settings
Not paid
Much freedom in the interaction

Figure 10.1 The relationships of practitioners and peers, mentors and supervisors.

is dangerous when it comes to making ethical decisions and choosing appropriate behavior. Although self-accountability is an individual responsibility, it is helpful to have a trusted support system to help stay in alignment with core beliefs and principles.

It may be time to seek support if you:

- Feel ineffective in your work.
- Have lost clientele.
- Are lonely.
- Are disheartened about your work.
- Are overwhelmed by clients.
- Feel emotionally spent.
- Find yourself slacking off in your treatment skills.
- Have considered behaving, or actually have behaved, unethically.
- Are bored.
- Have your social needs met by your clients.
- Cannot keep a job.
- Have a crisis with a client.
- Have a pattern of blaming the clients when sessions do not go well.

The common thread in each of the above examples is that they all indicate being disconnected with yourself and your purpose in doing bodywork. This disconnect is typically the signal of deeper issues at play. It could mean that you are no longer interested in doing bodywork but do not know how to acknowledge that fact. Perhaps you have stopped growing professionally and have become stagnant in your work.

Note that these feelings do not necessarily mean it is time to end your bodywork career. Too often good practitioners get tired of what they are doing and misread that as a sign that they should leave the profession. However, being aware of the feelings is the start of discovering what is truly going on for you. Getting support to work through the feelings is the next, quite important, step. With some guidance and assistance to sort out the complicated layers of life and work, it is possible for you to have more clarity about how to proceed with your career.

Getting the Most Out of Support

The issues discussed in support sessions, whether they involve supervision, mentoring or peer support, vary. However, the most common are issues surrounding transference and countertransference, preventing or acknowledging burnout, wanting to fix clients, overextending one's self, problem solving around difficult clients, forming business strategies, and sharing personal reflections. Patterns in behavior can be pointed out by your supervisor, mentor, or peers if you are unaware that they exist, and are confused about why certain issues keep resurfacing. Effective support people do not take care of your issues for you. Instead, they hold a mirror up to you so you can see more clearly what is going on.

If you are seeking support, you will get more out of the process if you are able to:

- Be open to feedback.
- Discern what support and feedback are necessary and true for you.

- Implement useful feedback in a timely fashion.
- Not back down if the feedback given does not feel accurate.
- Be honest about what you are lacking or what may be causing you fear.
- Have an authentic desire to grow emotionally and professionally.

Being open to feedback requires that you listen before deciding on a response. It is not useful to ask someone for help and then argue or disagree with him or her at every turn. If need be, you should also be willing to acknowledge how painful it is to learn something about yourself that you were not aware of. Pretending that everything is always fine is not being authentic. This is not to say that everyone experiences traumas on a daily basis, but real life is complicated.

Along with the openness to feedback, you must also be able to judge or measure how much of what is being shared is applicable to you, and how much is not. As in any helping relationship, you must be careful to not make the other person or people more powerful or more knowledgeable to the point that you do not listen to your instincts. It is possible to respect someone's input without agreeing with it. Your job as the person receiving feedback is to make a decision about whether the feedback is suitable for you.

Making an action plan as a result of supervision is an example of implementing feedback. Although it is important to talk about what is wrong and what needs to be done to change it, it is just as important to take action to make necessary changes. You should be willing and able to create manageable and effective steps to make the changes you want to see in your personal and professional life.

Choosing the Best Type of Support for You

What should you look for when choosing the best type of support for yourself? This varies depending on your personality and what goals you want to achieve. If you are quiet and have a hard time finding your voice in a group, you might find a group setting intimidating and perhaps not be willing to speak. The opposite may be true as well. If there is an overpowering practitioner who really wants to be the leader, he or she may use the group setting as an opportunity to take control and demonstrate to others how much knowledge he or she has. If you are a practitioner with this type of personality you may benefit more from one-on-one mentoring. In this case, there would not be other practitioners in the mentoring session to try and impress, and your mentor may point out your need for control and perhaps explore how this behavior surfaces when you interact with your clients.

The following are questions you can ask yourself to determine what type of support you would feel the most comfortable with. Do you:

- Like discussing things in groups of people?
- Prefer discussing issues one-on-one with another person?
- Prefer to work alone and occasionally discuss issues with others on an as-needed basis?
- Need to talk regularly with other practitioners?
- Want to discuss issues only with practitioners in the field?
- Want viewpoints and experiences from those in other professions?

Building Support Networks

One of the most successful ways for bodywork practitioners to get support and feel connected to others is to build networks. A network is a usually informally interconnected group or association of people such as friends or professional colleagues. Therefore, a **support network** is an interconnected group or association of people who can provide you with encouragement, assistance, and resources when you need them. Everyone chooses their support systems for different reasons as well as from different circles of friends, family, colleagues, and peers. The general reasons for needing a support network are:

- Emotional issues.
- Business advice/coaching.
- Health and fitness.
- Spiritual matters.

The typical sources to provide support are:

- Trusted friends and family.
- Professional counselors and therapists.
- Financial advisers or planners.
- Business coaches.
- Life coaches.
- Fitness trainers and nutritionists.
- Spiritual leaders.

Emotional issues typically center on matters of the heart and spirit such as self-worth, relationships, and validation. When the emotional state is being challenged because of anxiety, fear, anger, confusion, or time constraints, practitioners need to talk about these feelings without feeling judged, dismissed, or belittled or fear that it will be used against them at some point in the future. Everyone undergoes times of struggle. It is part of being a fully alive human being.

This is especially true for people who have chosen a career that focuses on helping people. Sometimes caregivers think that it is not reasonable for them to have a difficult time because they must be there for others first. The result may be stuffing feelings down and hoping they go away, or that these feelings will become routine. These choices do not help. Instead, they keep practitioners from believing they can feel better.

Sometimes bodywork practitioners are unable to recognize when they need help and support. Many have trained themselves to think, or have the inherent belief, that they should put everyone else's needs before theirs. However, it is an important part of self-care to reach out to others for help when necessary. Sometimes the struggle cannot be avoided but that does not mean practitioners should go through it alone if help is available.

Types of Support Networks

Sometimes asking for help with finances or with business start-up can be a source of shame and anxiety. Some practitioners may feel shame because they are not successful at managing their money or their business. Practitioners may feel anxiety because the issues seem so big that they cannot imagine finding a new way of running their business. Finding someone who will work with them to explain what they need to know and give them some sound strategies on how to improve or enhance their financial situation can be enormously helpful. Allowing someone with expertise in an area that they are being challenged in takes pressure off so practitioners can concentrate on finding workable solutions.

Spiritual or religious support is sought when one is feeling an emptiness or a loss and no longer seems to be leading a life of purpose. Spirituality can have many interpretations. However, it does speak to the fact that humans tend to seek a place to belong and feel accepted. When that sense of belonging is absent, people tend to feel alone and detached from others.

Spiritual or religious matters are best supported by working with someone who has training in this area. They can help practitioners to determine what these issues mean to them. It is important that practitioners work with someone who does not have an agenda other than helping them. When feeling vulnerable, some people are easy to take advantage of and easily persuaded that certain beliefs will fix every problem. Practitioners certainly can find comfort in those beliefs, but they still have to apply their own hearts and minds to find a solution that matches their belief systems.

Networking groups are a specialized gathering of people in similar professions that can assist one another in meeting business contacts. The local chamber of commerce often has social gatherings for small business owners to meet one another and learn how they may help each other professionally and personally. Sometimes these groups provide members with discounts as an incentive to participate. Because many bodywork practitioners go into private practice, these networking groups help to bring a sense of belonging to the owners.

Some network groups are very fluid and allow members to come and go from the group. Others are very specific and require mandatory attendance unless otherwise noted. Some networking groups are committed to community service projects as a way of getting to know other people in the same field. Other networking groups may focus solely on business.

There are a variety of reasons why you might seek support as well as a variety of resources for you to seek out support. You need to be consciously aware of the specialized roles each of your supporting networks have. This will give you the best information when you are determining who will be the best resource for a particular problem you may be having. This determination is based on being able to accurately identify for yourself what the core issue is and who would be best suited to assist you.

Consider this scenario: Ariel works at a local country club giving Watsu and craniosacral treatments. She is very open with her clients about her personal life, particularly her rocky relationship with her mother. One of Ariel's clients, Corinne, is an elderly woman who has several children and grandchildren. Corinne often shares stories with Ariel about the family gatherings she has and the weekend trips she takes with her daughters. One Saturday, Ariel has a major falling out with her mother. She is so upset that she calls Corinne Sunday night.

She is crying, and tells Corinne what happened at great length. Corinne listens but does not have much to say. Eventually, Ariel feels better and thanks Corinne for being such a good friend, and for showing her how a "real" mother acts. Corinne does not show up for her next Watsu treatment on Wednesday. Ariel leaves several messages for Corinne but none are returned. On Thursday, Ariel receives a disciplinary notice, and is put on probation by the manager of the country club. Corinne filed a complaint about Ariel's behavior.

Ariel did not make a wise choice about whom to talk to about her fight with her mother. Not only was it a boundary violation to call her client to discuss a personal issue, Ariel also projected her desire for a "real" mother onto her client. This projection, along with sharing such a personal issue, made her client so uncomfortable that she chose to discontinue the therapeutic relationship as well as any personal contact.

The backlash of Ariel's poor professional judgment resulted in several losses—the loss of a client, the loss of integrity when Ariel realized how her behavior had negatively affected her client, the possible loss of her reputation among other country club members, and finally the loss in confidence by her employer.

Practitioners should not burden clients with stories of strife and struggle; nor should the practitioner expect the client to be the sole provider of support and comfort. Practitioners who continually talk about the hardships they are having in their life are at risk of alienating, offending, and losing clientele.

In addition, you should not rely on one person or network for every issue you encounter in your life. This can place a great deal of stress on that one person or network, and dual roles can overlap in such a way that it can be hard to navigate them. Also, each person and each network has unique viewpoints, skill sets, and ways of assisting. It is unfair to ask a person or network for aid that the person or network is unable or unwilling to give.

Food for Thought

Whom do you turn to for help with emotional issues? Business advice? Health and fitness? Spiritual matters? Why do you go to these particular people or networks? How are each of them uniquely qualified to help you?

■ CASE PROFILE

Randy is in his last semester of training at the Tucson School of Massage Therapy (TSMT).

One day, just before his clinic class starts, Jason, the clinic instructor, observes Randy switching client file folders with another student. When Jason asks what is going on, Randy replies, "I can't work on this client because she is too big and it grosses me out. I worked with her 2 weeks ago and it was terrible. I know that I didn't help her so it's better to let another student work on her."

Jason reminds Randy that he is not allowed to trade his client for another one without discussing it with Jason. Jason says he would assist Randy throughout the session so that he could work on his attitude and work through his resistance for massaging clients with a larger body size. Randy refuses and walks out of the clinic. Another student therapist is assigned to Randy's client immediately, and Randy receives an absence for class.

Case Study Continued from page 384

When the clinic is over, Jason calls Randy to set up an appointment to talk about what happened in clinic. When Randy arrives for this appointment, he is upset about losing his attendance points in class. He says, "The issue was not that big a deal. We have been told throughout this program that if we feel our boundaries are being violated, then we should take action. Plus, I was not going to be able to give my client a good treatment and that would have been unprofessional. I was just trying to help her and now I'm the bad guy. It's not fair."

1. What type of support should Jason give Randy as they discuss his behavior?
2. How could Randy benefit from this type of support?
3. Do you think Randy will be open to the feedback Jason gives him? Why or why not?
4. What type of support would you give Randy for him to have an ethical practice?

Chapter Summary

Support can take many different forms for practitioners. Supervision involves periodic review of the bodywork practitioner's professional actions by an authority in the work setting. An effective supervisor helps practitioners develop problem-solving skills, leading to increased confidence in abilities. Mentoring involves a professional relationship in which a person with greater experience and skill provides support, encouragement, and career expertise to those with less experience and skill in the profession. Practitioners can use the mentor's experience and expertise as a guide to seeing actions and behaviors that are getting in the way of being successful in their work. Peer support is the interaction among practitioners who have similar levels of skill and experience for the purpose of encouraging and maintaining appropriate professional and ethical practices. Practitioners must be mindful of who they consider to be appropriate peers for offering and receiving support.

One of the most successful ways for bodywork practitioners to get support and feel connected to others is to build networks. Practitioners need to be consciously aware of the roles of each of their supporting networks, and use each supporting network appropriately. In addition, practitioners should not rely on one single person or network for every issue they encounter in their lives.

Review Questions

Multiple Choice

1. Periodic review of the bodywork practitioner professional actions by an authority in the work setting is called:

   a. Peer support

   b. Supervision

   c. Mentoring

   d. Identifying

2. Mentors differ from supervisors in that mentors usually:

   a. Have more experience than the practitioner

   b. Offer the practitioner encouragement

   c. Cannot discipline the practitioner

   d. Help the practitioner find solutions to problems

3. Which of the following is a way that practitioners can find a mentor?

   a. Asking trusted colleagues for recommendations

   b. Identifying successful bodywork professionals

   c. Recognizing exceptional bodywork instructors

   d. All of the above

4. The primary role of a mentor is to:

   a. Solve problems for the practitioner

   b. Point out all the things the practitioner is doing wrong

   c. Give the practitioner praise no matter what

   d. Guide the practitioner's actions and behavior for career success

5. Which of the following is a sign that a mentoring relationship needs to be terminated?

   a. The mentor talks solely about the issues the mentee is experiencing

   b. A difficult situation the mentee is dealing with is unresolved

   c. The mentor is meeting the mentee's needs

   d. It seems as though the mentor is uninterested

6. A practitioner is most likely needing to seek support if he:

   a. Has a successful practice

   b. Blames clients when for unsuccessful sessions

   c. Feels satisfied in his work

   d. Has behaved ethically throughout his career

7. A practitioner who would enjoy a peer support group is one who:

   a. Wants many different viewpoints at the same time

   b. Dislikes discussing things with many people at once

   c. Prefers discussing issues one-on-one

   d. Prefers to work alone

Fill in the Blank

1. Supervisors are generally involved in such areas as the development and approval of treatment plans, scheduling, _____ matters, and instruction.

2. The practitioners being supervised need to have the desire to receive support and _____ on how to be successful.

3. The term _____ is used to describe the essential characteristics that the practitioner recognizes and names as belonging uniquely to him- or herself.

4. When practitioners think there is a complete separation between professionalism and their true identity, they may have difficulty having a(n) _____ therapeutic relationship with clients.

5. If the practitioner feels capable of moving forward with the skills and insights gained from a mentor, then it is time to _____ the mentoring relationship.

6. A _____ is one that is of equal standing with another.

7. When one is feeling an emptiness or a loss in leading a life of purpose, _____ support may be needed.

Short Answer

1. Explain at least three ways an effective supervisor helps a practitioner.

2. Explain at least three reasons a practitioner would choose to be mentored.

3. Briefly describe five key components of being a mentor.

4. Explain at least five benefits of peer support.

5. Describe at least three characteristics of appropriate peers.

6. Briefly describe each of the types of supporting networks practitioners can build for themselves.

7. Explain how to appropriately use supporting networks; give examples.

Activities

1. Other than the issue presented in the Case Profile in this chapter, name at least four other issues that could cause a student or a professional practitioner to seek supervision/mentoring. Choose one of the issues and make a list of what may be contributing factors. Write down possible questions you would ask this practitioner to help him or her explore the issue and the impact it is having on him or her and the practice.

2. Using the Internet or local Yellow Pages, create a referral list of resources that you could contact for support or networking purposes. For each resource, identify the area of expertise.

3. Spend some time reflecting on your life, both professionally and personally, and identify any issues with which you believe you could use some mentoring or support. Journal your reflections along with some ideas on whom you would choose to help you and why. Are any of the issues you thought about too difficult to share with another person? If so, why?

4. Write down the qualities and characteristics you would want in a mentor.

5. Choose one of the following statements. Make an argument for the reason it is incorrect, and then rewrite it.

    - Asking for help is a sign of weakness. I can handle my problems myself.
    - I won't ask for help because I don't want to burden anyone. Besides, it's my fault I'm in this predicament.
    - It's my fault I am in this situation. I don't deserve to get any support because I should have known better.

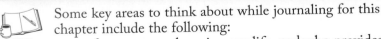

Guidance for Journaling

Some key areas to think about while journaling for this chapter include the following:

- What types of support you have in your life, and who provides that support
- What types of support you do not have and wish you did
- How you plan to get the support you need
- How you have been supervised in other work settings, and how successful that supervision was
- How you would like to be supervised as a professional bodywork practitioner
- How you think mentoring would or would not help you as a practitioner
- Who you would choose as a mentor
- Whether you would like to be a mentor
- How you would terminate a mentoring relationship
- Who you see as your peers
- How you would choose appropriate peers to give you support
- How you would use peers for support
- How you would identify when you need support

References

1. Jones-Phillips, L.: Mentoring is in the details. The Mentoring Group Web site, 2003. Retrieved 24 November 2010 from http://www.mentoringgroup.com/html/articles/mentor_5.html
2. Palmer, P.J.: *The Courage to Teach.* San Francisco, CA, Jossey-Bass, 1998, p 10.
3. Stoddard, D.: *The Heart of Mentoring: Ten Proven Principles for Developing People to Their Fullest.* Colorado Springs, CO, NavPress, 2009, p 7.
4. Palmer, P.J.: *A Hidden Wholeness: The Journey Toward an Undivided Life.* San Francisco, CA, Jossey-Bass, 2004, p 212.
5. Jones-Phillips, L.: 2004. Effective mentoring relationships: The mentor's role (part 1 of 2). The Mentoring Group Web site, 2004. Retrieved 24 November 2010 from http://www.mentoringgroup.com/html/articles/mentor_43.htm
6. Jones-Phillips, Mentoring is in the details.
7. Corey, G., Corey, M.S., and Callanan, P.: *Issues and Ethics in the Helping Professions,* ed. 7. Stamford, CT, Brooks/Cole Cengage Learning, 2007, p 344.

Answers to Chapter Review Questions

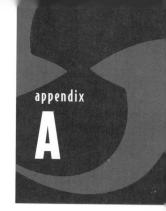

Chapter 1

Multiple Choice

1. a
2. c
3. b
4. d
5. a
6. d
7. c

Fill in the Blank

1. therapeutic relationship
2. misunderstanding, creative interaction
3. body language
4. authentic communication
5. peacemaker (turtle)
6. verbal
7. actions, words

Chapter 2

Multiple Choice

1. c
2. d
3. c
4. b
5. a
6. b
7. d

Fill in the Blank

1. auditory
2. Any three of the following: clothes that fit; clothes that match; clothes that are appropriate for the work setting; clean clothes; neat clothes; no strong scents; clothing that is free of advertising, words, and logos; clothes that are thick enough that underwear is not seen through them; clean footwear and socks
3. Image
4. Empathy, genuine interest
5. Mission statements
6. Any three of the following: business cards; brochures and pamphlets; cover letters; résumés; business letters to other professionals; intake forms; documentation forms; calendar of appointments
7. Double-booking clients

Chapter 3

Multiple Choice

1. c
2. b
3. a
4. d
5. a
6. c
7. d

Fill in the Blank

1. client retention
2. client base
3. feedback
4. breathe, pause, separate
5. closed, open
6. behavior
7. receiving

Chapter 4

Multiple Choice

1. d
2. a

3. a
4. c
5. c
6. d
7. d

Fill in the Blank

1. communication gaps
2. understanding, respect
3. teach or preach
4. meta communication
5. collaboration
6. timeline
7. solutions

Chapter 5

Multiple Choice

1. b
2. b
3. d
4. c
5. a
6. b
7. a

Fill in the Blank

1. consciences
2. "Am I doing the right thing?"
3. code of ethics
4. codes of conduct
5. Ethical congruency
6. Ethical dilemmas
7. cultural relativism

Chapter 6

Multiple Choice

1. b
2. c
3. d
4. b
5. a
6. a
7. d

Fill in the Blank

1. perceive
2. Empower

3. Expertise
4. crisis intervention services
5. Accountability
6. polling
7. relational

Chapter 7

Multiple Choice

1. b
2. d
3. c
4. d
5. a
6. d
7. c

Fill in the Blank

1. Scope of practice
2. assessment, diagnosis
3. certification
4. confidentiality
5. Documentation
6. The Health Insurance Portability and Accountability Act, or HIPAA
7. Business privilege

Chapter 8

Multiple Choice

1. d
2. b
3. a
4. b
5. c
6. d
7. d

Fill in the Blank

1. boundary
2. countertransference
3. emotional baggage
4. self-care
5. overlapping
6. therapeutic relationship
7. sexual

Chapter 9

Multiple Choice

1. b
2. d
3. c
4. a
5. b
6. d
7. b

Fill in the Blank

1. Qi
2. receptors
3. primary somatosensory area
4. balance
5. anxiety
6. touch his (her) clients
7. sexual harassment

Chapter 10

Multiple Choice

1. b
2. c
3. d
4. d
5. d
6. b
7. a

Fill in the Blank

1. disciplinary
2. feedback
3. identity
4. authentic
5. terminate
6. peer
7. spiritual or religious

Glossary

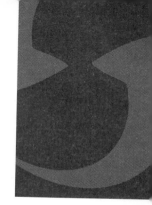

A

Assessment Evaluation

Auditory A component of communication that involves hearing

Auditory processors People who process information most effectively when they hear it spoken. They are very attentive to the tone and rhythm of speech and will often hum, talk to themselves, and listen with their eyes closed or when gazing off into the distance.

Authentic communication Communication characterized by an honest presentation of oneself and a lack of pretension

B

Boundary A limit set to inform others where one's personal space ends and public space begins

Business privilege license Required by municipalities for individuals or businesses that sell products

C

Certification A process in which a person has completed a formalized program of study, and has passed one or more tests demonstrating competency in the area of study

Chronological résumé Lists employment history in order of dates of employment

Client base A core group of people who come to see the practitioner on a regular basis

Client retention Keeping a person as a client over a period of time and for repeated treatments as a result of providing satisfactory services

Closed questions Questions that most often result in a yes or no answer

Code of ethics A set of guidelines that delineates the standards of behavior for the members of a group or profession

Codes of conduct Sets of rules listing the proper practices and responsibilities of an individual, organization, or profession

Communication gaps A difference in understanding between two people that causes problems in communication

Competency The ability to perform a specific task, action, or function successfully

Confidentiality The safekeeping of clients' personal knowledge. It is considered nondisclosure of privileged information; it may not be divulged to a third party.

Conscious communication Communication in which a person thoughtfully considers how what he or she says will affect the other people involved, both in the short term and the long term

Consensus General agreement, or the judgment arrived at by most of those concerned

Countertransference A defense strategy that bodywork practitioners employ when they have unresolved issues from their past, have perceptions about someone from their personal history, or have feelings from their past and are transferring these feelings and thoughts onto a client

Critical thinking The process of conscious thought based on weighing all the facts that are known to form an opinion about something

D

Desexualized touch Touch by the practitioner during treatment that is not in any way erotic or sexual for either the practitioner or the client

Diagnosis To assign a name or label (such as disease, disorder, or condition) to a certain group of signs or symptoms. Diagnosing falls only within the scope of practice of medical physicians.

Disclosure Revealing information

Dual relationship A relationship in which a professional assumes a second role with a client, becoming friend, employer, teacher, business associate, or family member

E

Emotional baggage Latent, unresolved issues; misguided anger; unrealistic expectations

Emotional environment The atmosphere or energetic sense of the therapeutic relationship

Empathy Having an understanding of the feelings or the difficulties another is facing

Empower The process of helping people who do not have power gain it so they can improve their personal or professional circumstances

Ethical awareness Self-awareness and willingness to continually ask, "Am I doing the right thing?"

Ethical congruency Being authentic in both words and actions and having behavior that matches with declared personal ethical standards

Ethical dilemmas Situations that require considering information that requires an opinion, a response, or an action in a situation that challenges a person's ethics

Ethics A system or set of principles that are used as a framework for choosing between right and wrong behavior and for determining what is good and what is bad

F

Feedback A process in which information is relayed to a person about how his words and actions affect other people

Functional résumé Organizes experience by category

G

Group ethics The behaviors and attitudes that a culture, community, organization, or profession determines best reflects its goals and desires

H

Healthy insulation barrier A boundary structure that is permeable enough to allow experience to penetrate the inner self but solid enough to protect it from being overcome by internal impulses and external demands

HIPAA The Health Insurance Portability and Accountability Act; a law enacted in 1996 to protect the privacy of people's health-care records

Homogeneous A term meaning "the same"

I

Identity The essential characteristics that the practitioner recognizes and names as belonging uniquely to him- or herself

Informed consent The process by which clients have been fully informed about what to expect during the bodywork treatment

Innuendo Hinting at something, but not quite coming out and saying it

Integrity The quality of transparency and accountability in words and actions

Intimacy Something of a personal or private nature; the quality or state of being familiar; acts of a sexual nature; the degree of closeness in a relationship

K

Kanji The term for Chinese language symbols

Ki According to traditional Japanese bodywork, the energy or force that gives and maintains life, and also is the connection between organisms and all creation

Kinesthetic processors People who communicate most effectively when using touch and body language. When speaking, they tend to use "feel" words (such as "that hit me really hard" and "the story was really touching").

L

Language A system of communicating ideas, thoughts, and feelings by the use of words, their pronunciations, and the methods of combining them as has been agreed upon by a community; communication using sounds, gestures, or symbols

Lingo Vocabulary that is specific to a particular field

M

Mentoring A professional relationship in which a person with greater experience and skill provides support, encouragement, and career expertise to one with less experience and skill in the profession

Meta communication Used to describe the hidden or underlying meaning behind spoken words

Mission statements Brief statements of the purpose of a company, an organization, a group, or an individual

Morals Standards of judgment about behavior and character

Multiple relationship A relationship in which people have more than two different roles with each other

N

Neurotransmitters Chemicals released by brain cells (neurons) to communicate with each other

Nonverbal communication Communication without using words, such as facial expressions or body gestures

O

Occupational license A license needed by people who provide services, such as attorneys, chiropractors, and bodywork practitioners

Open questions Questions that invite an expanded response

Oral language Communication in which the lips and tongue form words

Overlapping relationship A relationship in which two people can shift back and forth between dual or multiple roles, depending on the situation and the factors involved

P

Peer One who is of equal standing with another

Peer support The interaction among practitioners who have similar levels of skill and experience to encourage and maintain appropriate professional and ethical practice

Personal bias The tendency to interpret a word, an action, or a person in terms of some personal significance assigned to it

Positive transference A situation in which the client projects positive feelings or good qualities onto the practitioner

Power The capacity to influence the behavior of others and to resist their influence on oneself

Power difference Occurs when, in a relationship, one party has greater control, or power, over the other

Prana According to Ayurveda, the energy or force that gives and maintains life, and also is the connection between organisms and all creation

Presence The quality of staying focused and centered, specifically during client interactions and treatments (as in being present), but applicable to any interchange

Primary somatosensory area The area of the brain that receives sensory information from the body and is involved in the perception of the sensation; this area has a "map" of the entire body and so can pinpoint not only what the sensation is, but where in the body it is coming from

Principles Behavioral guidelines based on a person's morals, which can vary widely from person to person

Q

Qi According to traditional Chinese medicine, the energy or force that gives and maintains life, and also is the connection between organisms and all creation

R

Revolving door syndrome A situation in which a bodywork business does not have a stable clientele and instead continually relies on new clients for income

Role blending A situation in which roles and responsibilities in dual or multiple relationships are combined

S

Self-care The ability of practitioners to ensure a healthy emotional state, a sound physical state, and the awareness of how self-care affects the practitioners' work

Self-disclosure The process of deliberately revealing information about oneself that is significant and that would not normally be known by others

Self-empowered Having the means within ourselves to overcome doubts and insecurities rather than relying on an external support system

Sensory receptors Specialized nerve endings that respond to various types of stimulation

Sensual Relating to or consisting of the gratification of the senses

Sequential relationship A relationship in which one set of roles completely ends before the beginning of a new set of roles

Sexual assault Illegal sexual contact that usually involves force upon a person without consent or is inflicted upon a person who is incapable of giving consent or who places the assailant in a position of trust or authority

Sexual harassment Uninvited and unwelcome verbal or physical behavior of a sexual nature especially by a person in authority toward a subordinate

Somatosensory association areas Areas of the brain that store memories of past somatic sensory experiences so people can compare current sensations with previous sensations

Status The position of an individual in relation to another or others; a socially valued quality that a person carries with her or him into different situations, where power and dominance are likely to be seen as a personality trait

Stay solid To know oneself and so not be swayed to deny personal feelings or change them because someone disagrees with them

Supervision Periodic review of the bodywork practitioner's professional actions by an authority in the work setting

Support network An interconnected group or association of people who can provide the practitioner with encouragement, assistance, and resources as needed

T

Tactile Related to touch; tactile sensations include pain, pressure, vibration, itch, and tickle

Therapeutic relationship The bond formed between the practitioner and the client that is necessary for a positive treatment outcome for both the practitioner and the client

Therapeutic touch Safe and appropriate placement of parts of the practitioner's body, such as the hands, forearms, elbows, knees, and feet, on a client who has given consent for the purposes of healing or restorative care

Touch overload A phenomenon that can happen in the bodywork profession in which a practitioner who has been working for a certain period of time no longer wants to touch his clients

Transference A situation in which a client who has unresolved issues in his past is projecting, or transferring, these issues onto the practitioner

V

Values What a person finds desirable

Verbal communication Communication using words, either written or spoken

Visual processors People who communicate most effectively when creating pictures in their minds and using many descriptive words as they "paint" word pictures during conversation. They tend to use "see" words (such as, "Let's take a look at this," and "If we view it from this angle . . .") and want to make eye contact when conversing.

W

Work ethic A drive within a person that motivates him or her to arrive at work on time every day, do the best work at all times, work until the work is done, not take excessive amounts of time off, and cooperate with colleagues and supervisors

Index

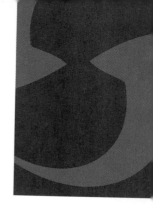

Note: Page numbers followed by "b," "f," and "t" indicate boxes, figures, and tables, respectively.